ARTICULATION

A PHYSIOLOGICAL APPROACH

ARTICULATION
A PHYSIOLOGICAL APPROACH

SAMUEL G. FLETCHER, PH.D.

President, The Talk Foundation
Birmingham, Alabama
and
Professor Emeritus
The University of Alabama at Birmingham
Birmingham, Alabama

SINGULAR PUBLISHING GROUP, INC.
SAN DIEGO, CALIFORNIA

Singular Publishing Group, Inc.
4284 41st Street
San Diego, California 92105-1197

© 1992 by Singular Publishing Group, Inc.

Typeset in 10/12 Times by CFW Graphics
Printed in the United States of America by McNaughton & Gunn

Library of Congress Cataloging-in-Publication Data

Fletcher, Samuel G. (Samuel Glen)
    Articulation : a physiological approach / Samuel G. Fletcher.
      p. cm.
    Includes bibliographical references and index.
    ISBN 1-879105-89-6
    1. Speech — Physiological aspects. 2. Articulation disorders.
  3. Motor learning. I. Title.
    [DNLM: 1. Articulation Disorders — physiopathology
  2. Articulation disorders — therapy. 3. Motor skills. 4. Speech
Therapy — methods. WL 340 F815a]
  QP399.F54   1992
  816.85'5 — dc 20
  DNLM/DLC
for Library of Congress   91-41499
                                              CIP

CONTENTS

PREFACE

Since the days of Aristotle, science has wrestled with the physical concepts of matter and motion and their more recent biological structure and function parallels. In this book, we address many of those same issues as we confront the problems of how to describe, quantify, and change patterns of articulation.

Giving effective assistance to those with speech disorders demands accurate descriptions of articulatory gestures in terms of postures, movements, and interarticulator relationships. Our current physiologic concepts of speech production stem from traditional beliefs about articulatory place and manner. The information on which these beliefs are built has been derived primarily from acoustic impressions and introspection. The logic of these beliefs has been justified by observations such as when the lips, jaws, and tongue are placed in certain positions and a flow of air is channeled through the vocal tract, the acoustic characteristics of the output are accurately predicated.

Modern technology enables us to control and manipulate many different speaking conditions as we seek to discover the basic building blocks of speech production. On the basis of findings to date, we can predict that when the physical bases of speech are fully identified, the elements will consist of a limited set of articulatory postures that, when combined in different ways, form the structure of sound production. Current trends in basic physiological theory also predict that the system, as it emerges, will be hierarchically organized and molecular in its nature. The evidence summarized in this book suggests that specific postures may exist which function as the predicted elements of speech production. Dynamic, rhythmical action sequences of these postures are found in exquisitely controlled combinations that appear to serve as the basic molecules of speech production. Speech is thus conceived to be a hierarchically organized set of postures, gestures, and action sequences organized under central motor command to generate meaningful messages. Procedures are outlined to use this conceptualization in assessing articulatory postures, gestures, and movement sequences in the process of examining, defining, and delineating speech articulation functions and deviations.

The terms *normal* and *natural* are used to define articulatory deviations. Articulation assessment and training also makes use of these terms in describing dynamic feedback to guide talkers toward specified speech patterns. Speech production is defined as *normal* when the articulatory postures, gestures, and movement patterns of a talker are similar to those of most other talkers of the same age speaking the same language. Speech is defined as *natural* when the articulatory postures and gestures are appropriate for the particular talker. Helping those who are physically handicapped adapt to or compensate for their limitations as they seek to gain or recapture speech proficiency may thus be considered to be a commitment to discovering natural ways to achieve normal speech skills.

The palatometer was developed to help define normal and abnormal articulation functions more accurately and to discover natural ways to overcome speech abnormalities at the physiological level. First, it should be pointed out that the palatometer is simply a tool. Nothing more, nothing less. The usual way of thinking about tools is that they are invented to solve problems, but tools also shape the way we come to see the problems. Thus, the value of a tool depends on both the special characteristics of the tool and the understanding and skills a user brings to its operation.

Use of the palatometer rests on the premise that a picture is worth a thousand words. The palatometer portrays articulatory events in a spatial fashion easily assimilated by the relatively untrained human eye. By constructing a geometric representation of tongue actions in three-dimensional Euclidean space, the instrumentation provides an opportunity to approach speech disability from a motor skill framework. No longer need the speech clinician or the person who is handicapped be limited to auditory and phonetic impressions to discover, define, and modify articulatory deficiencies. The clinician can now help clients gain physiologically based percepts and concepts of speech production and modify speech skills rather quickly.

The ability to manipulate articulatory actions through palatometric processes adds a new dimension to the clinician's armamentarium. It provides opportunity to tap a deep pool of spatial information regarding imaging and other facets of motor skill learning that has been accumulating during the past decade but not yet used widely in speech pathology. Being able to manipulate spatial attributes of articulatory actions rather directly provides an opportunity to use converging acoustic and physiologic principles that throw new light on how speech skill is acquired and how it may be modified when it is deviant.

The material included in this book is not intended to be a compendium of knowledge in the area of motor skill development or a reference guide to research in articulation skill development. Rather, theories, concepts, and beliefs are presented as they are deemed by the writer to be useful in a proposed instrumental, physiologically based approach to teaching and learning speech articulation skills. The purpose of this book is to pave the way for the clinician to use the palatometer effectively and efficiently. The new approach described has been designed to help the clinician take full advantage of physiological and parallel acoustic information through palatometry and other tools that are becoming available for examining, assessing, and modifying speech motor skills.

One of the great lessons of modern science is that "common sense," "everyday experience," and "pure reason" may open the door to possibilities, but those possibilities are not trustworthy until they are proven. Genuine proof involves showing how beliefs are relevant to at least some well-grounded theories and practices, and the relevancy is established through accurate observations. The more directly and accurately observations can be derived, the more likely they are to be trustworthy. Measurement is the key to accurate observations. We cannot take for granted even those behaviors that seem to be based on our most common experiences such as speech until they have been objectively tested and measured. In this book such an effort has been made.

CHAPTER 1

SPEECH AS A
MOTOR SKILL

Broadly defined, *motor skill* refers to spatial and temporal proficiency in executing a motor task. More specifically, it means anticipating, timing, and executing graded motor responses rapidly, reaching physically defined action goals with a low error rate, and achieving action patterns with comparatively little wasted motion. Execution speed, spatial accuracy, and movement efficiency are each telling signs of skill level (Chase & Ericsson, 1982). For example, novices have low motor skill. Their movements tend to be slow, jerky, and erratic in goal achievement. Movement speed, accuracy, and efficiency will be examined in some detail as we seek to understand and apply principles of imaging and motor skill development to speech production, assessment, and modification.

Singing, throwing, typing, and talking are each distinctly different motor skills; yet, all of them have a number of things in common. They involve physical activities produced sequentially to meet specific goals of the person doing them, and they are performed with varying degrees of expertise. If basic movements are missing or erroneous, if action sequences are mismanaged, if timing of the actions is "out of synch," or if other disturbances divert the person's ability to reach the postures or perform the movements in any of these activities, the probability of successful performance is diminished. Motor skill thus means more than the ability to "do a motor task well." It has multidimensional facets, particularly when it is approached from a pathology or abnormality viewpoint.

SPEECH IN THE DEVELOPMENTAL PLAN

Even the simplest of utterances involves a whole series of temporospatial actions that are executed in elegantly coordinated and rhythmical movements. Before a child can embark on "cracking the speech code," the fact that there is a code to be cracked must be discovered (Wells, 1985). This discovery entails recognizing that arbitrary but conventional sound and movement patterns bring particular responses in attenders. Infants produce vocal sounds; mothers give *continuity* and *meaning* to the baby's utterances by the timing and aptness of their reactions to the sounds produced (Gilfoyle, Grady, & Moore, 1990). As Newsome (1978) puts it, mothers do not just reflect the baby's sound producing actions back to them automatically as physical consequences. Mothers process the vocalizations and action patterns through "a subjective filter of human interpretation." Some patterns are judged to be coherent and relevant to human communication. The caregiver is likely to echo those actions. The caregiver-refined vocal patterns are then mimicked by the child. These vocal patterns thus take on new meaning to the child and become part of its vocal repertoire. The temporal accuracy of this acoustic gestural match is impressive. Condon and Sander (1974) observed that frame-by-frame segmentation of acoustic boundaries in adult speech precisely matches similar frame-by-frame movement segments of an awake, active infant exposed to adult-produced speech sounds.

Robb and Saxman (1990) cite a series of studies that provide evidence that speech-like sounds and syllable shapes in infant preword vocalizations provide the rich soil from which words found in children's early words will grow. One of the most interesting aspects of developing vocal skill is that speech seems to emerge almost effortlessly from the usual day-to-day vocal and verbal exchanges. The master plan that sets the articulatory focusing process into motion is apparently functional early in life. It is partly inborn and partly acquired through experience.

Infants begin to express articulate words by being treated as if they already have the competencies. In early experiences the interpersonal and social aspects of communication predominate during speech development. The utterances of the child seem to mean more than it is able to express. Interactions and rhythmically executed episodes with mature talkers provide a framework within which children discover the motor principles and skills they will need to master fundamental speech articulation skills. This experience leads to the ability to control subtle changes in vocal tones, add articulatory "crispness" and emphasis to certain words, adjust the speaking rate, develop contrasts between momentary and prolonged breaks, add pauses in the speech output, and adjust the vocal output to transmit messages to listeners in noisy and quiet surroundings and in tense and relaxed circumstances.

MOTOR SKILL MATURATION

We will begin our search for a new approach to speech production and remediation through a broad look at motor skill maturation. The infant acquires the ability to sit up at about 6 months, crawl at 9 months, walk with support at 11 months, and walk without support at around 1 year of age. The infant also begins to produce true (continuous) vowels singly and in series at 4 to 5 months of age, a succession of vowels and consonants in marginal babbling at around 6 months, reduplicated and nonreduplicated syllables with true consonants in consonant-vowel (CV) babbling at about 9 months, and meaningful words at around 1 year of age (Stark, Ansel, & Bond, 1988). The well-recognized landmark skills of locomotion and many other basic motor skills thus arrive in tandem with those in speech. This parallelism suggests the presence of common ontogenetic functions in physical and intellectual attribute development. To examine this parallelism further, we will probe and compare locomotion and speech maturation processes more deeply.

During the early months of life, the infant expends considerable time and effort mastering rudimentary arm, leg, and body postures and movement skills. Movement in its most elementary form may be fruitfully viewed as modifications of basic body postures (Denny-Brown, 1960). Skills in achieving these postures expand as the baby's mobility repertoire grows. The infant learns many body control principles while it is limited to a supine posture. It then raises itself to sitting then standing positions, and the action possibilities and new skills acquired again expand in important ways.

Gaining voluntary control over basic body postures and orienting responses is a central feature of the infant's increasing versatility in position and movement possibilities. The motor skills appear to extend from innate, primitive motor functions that form the foundation from which skilled movement develops (Zelazo, 1976, 1983). Gallistel (1985) observed that the underlying mechanism of movements may be decomposed into three fundamental components: basic reflexes, oscillators or pacemakers that are the source of rhythmic signals, and feedback loops that provide servomechanism control. For example, the so-called scratch reflex of the cat has been decomposed into reflexive raising of the paw to the desired scratch point, rhythmic scratching movements, and feedback that enables self-monitoring and correction of the scratching action. That these basic motor constellations may persist although they are less apparent in neurologically intact, normally functioning individuals has been noted. Stress, for example, can evoke reflexive behaviors thought to have disappeared in infancy (Hellebrandt, Schade, & Carns, 1962). Clark (1982) and Leonard (1990) cited a series of writers who have demonstrated that interim structures for coordination emerge from reflexive actions that are present from early infancy.

The evolution of locomotion has been cited as an example of an automatically elicited action that may be traced from elementary neuromotor sequences. The sequences identified in early infancy appear to underpin later volitionally controlled walking and running actions. For example, babies exercised using the "walking reflex" have an earlier onset of walking than those not so exercised (Leonard, 1990). Given this coupling, Gallistel (1985) argues that basic reflexes, oscillators, and servomechanisms provide a built-in network system for later response programming.

Movement Stability-Mobility

Posture and movement have long been treated as two opposing facets of motor control. Posture has been viewed as an intrinsically organized system which develops to restore a structure's orientation automatically when it is disturbed. Movement has been conceived, in part, as a system developed to counter the effects of posture and static balance as segments of the body are displaced (Paillard, 1988). Hess (1943) was the first to clearly formulate the roles of posture and movement as interactive complementary components jointly involved in every self-induced action. He noted that movements include a *teleokinetic* component (telos = end) that dictates displacement toward a goal posture and an *ereismatic* component (ereisma = support) that provides both firm resistive support for launching the mobile segment and postural adjustment required to preserve the structure's orientation in the field of forces. Postural adjustment is thus as essential for efficient motor performance as the movement itself.

Massion (1984) extracted three characteristic features of goal directed actions that have been identified in recent studies: synergistic postural adjustments that anticipate predictable conditions for executing a movement, instantaneous adaptation to unexpected constraints, and variably preset movements that follow prior instructions. It is still unknown whether the motor commands are tailored to the mechanical requirements of the task by hardwired neural circuitry that tunes the system by local servoassistance loops or whether it is shaped by self-organizing, dynamically generated "coordinative" networks, as claimed by Kelso and Tuller (1984).

New motor skill learning provides an opportune time to identify integrated posture and movement principles. When a child is mastering a new motor skill, a combination of skeletal rigidity and muscle tone is used to maintain key structure positions (Turvey, Fitch, & Tuller, 1982). This stable posture allows the individual to explore possible movement strategies that can counterbalance the external and internal movement forces generated.

Learning to walk is a prime example of reciprocal adaptation in posture and movement forces. Walking is typically preceded by standing. The key to standing is the ability to balance the forces of gravity within the body in a steady upright posture. When that posture is achieved and equilibrium maintained, the infant is ready to begin experimenting with locomotion. Moving from the standing posture generates a new set of challenges. Among the most important is that the infant must now learn to cope with both a narrow, single foot postural base and instabilities that arise from the asymmetrical force that must be exerted to set the body into motion. New skills must be developed to maintain balance, extend stability of the body around its central axis, and gain volitional control of mechanisms that had heretofore been limited to reflexive neonatal stepping. In early walking efforts the stepping reflex appears to serve an important role. In cats, for example, reflexive flexing of the leg joints has been found to be activated by touching the dorsum of the paw. This triggers a lifting, swinging movement of the paw which carries it over obstacles and potentiates reflexive extension of the leg joints to complete the step (Forssberg, Grillner, & Rossignol, 1975). The potentiation and depotentiation of these reflex pathways by the cat's neural pacemaker sets the stepping rhythm.

The infant's early walking movements demonstrate a dominant, reflexively based, stiff-legged action that is accompanied by side-to-side swaying as the infant seeks to manipulate the body mass and accommodate the transfer of propulsion forces from one foot to the other. Like a sailor walking on a rolling deck through breaking waves and flying spray, the child's first steps are made with the feet far apart to provide a wide support base. The legs are held stiffly by a high degree of agonist and antagonist muscle coactivation during flexion. This stiffness serves to reduce the freedom of joint movement but still allows movements at the hip, knee, and ankle joints that are comparable with those of adults. Careful analysis of the stepping action shows each leg accelerating then slowing as reciprocal forces are actuated in balanced sequences (Smidt, 1990). One foot must always be in contact with the walking surface to provide independent weight-bearing support during a portion of each cycle.

As might be expected, the reciprocal transfer of energy in walking is at first halting and tentative as the infant seeks to stabilize and coordinate the multiple body segments around joint articulations. With walking experience comes increased joint mobility, postural and timing control, equilibrium, and movement variety. The achievement of these coordinated posture and movement skills is improved by motor and visual intersensory feedback, which integrates the movement components as the infant's drive to ambulate is realized. In this process, the child discovers that a given goal can be reached by diverse means. With practice, side-to-side and up-and-down movements diminish and forward progression becomes smoothly integrated and efficient. Motor skill is thus characterized by the discovery of flexible ways to use and integrate body postures and movement patterns.

From the foregoing, it is evident that mechanical efficiency is an important outgrowth of motor skill learning, and *fixation/diversification* is a fundamental process that underlies mechanical efficiency in movement (cf. Gentile, 1972; Rothwell, 1987, p. 2). Maintaining part of the body in a stable posture eliminates some of the degrees of movement freedom and helps stabilize the system (Turvey, Fitch, & Tuller, 1982). The price paid for rigid postures and body positions often adopted in early motor learning is clumsy, stereotyped actions. With experience, the mass-action style is modified. The individual learns to counterbalance reactive forces by controlled, flexible integration of postures and movements. A variety of stances and action patterns becomes available through different muscle combinations organized around different parameters of the intended movement (Berthoz & Pozzo, 1988). The degrees of freedom are thus gradually "unfrozen" as control over reactive forces is asserted through actions organized around the essential elements of the task. Movement sequences and reciprocal actions then become skillfully balanced.

Empirical evidence that mechanical efficiency is a key attribute in the motor skill mastery was provided by Sparrow and Irizarry-Lopez (1987). They required adult subjects to learn to crawl on their hands and feet at a rate of .76 meters per second on a motor-driven treadmill. As this task was mastered, improvements in efficiency were documented by a caloric test of the subjects' metabolic rate. The findings showed a 13.7% efficiency improvement from 3 minutes of practice per day across 20 days. The energy cost dropped as motor efficiency increased.

An important property of motor skill is that different postural control modes may be used to span a continuum of movements. Quadruped gait was described by Kelso (1982) as an example of this type of motor performance. As a horse increases its locomotion speed, it shifts from a walk to a trot to a gallop gait configuration. The abruptness of these shifts from one posture-movement synergy to another points to modular changes introduced to meet energy demands within specific rate-of-movement ranges. A similar shift is seen in the larynx as the pitch of a talker's voice moves from a low pitched, crackling "glottal fry" or "creaking" voice to the chest register then to the falsetto register. The creaking voice is characterized by a low, irregular pitch, sharply defined vocal tract resonances, and pairs of vocal fold contact sequences with very long closures between pairs. The pulse pairs usually evidence a small peak waveform followed by a larger one. If the smaller peaks are missing, the sound is heard as the vocal fry (Fourcin, 1981). In the chest register, the entire vocal fold vibrates essentially periodically. As the voice moves into the falsetto register, the bulk of vocal fold assumes a stable posture and vibration is concentrated along its inner margins. Thus the postural and moving components of the laryngeal actions change systematically as the pitch rises from register to register. The changes in moving tissue mass enable the vocal system to generate certain tones without excessive strain from muscular tension demands.

The above discussion isolates synchronized actions that appear to develop around basic, largely innate body postures and movements that are refined and generalized to satisfy the need for greater skill and differentiation in motor performance (Denny-Brown, 1960; Zelazo, 1983). Step-like changes in movement patterns illustrate the use of special motor programs to provide a range of responses within the mechanical capacity of an action system. This adaptive capacity highlights the inherent ability of the motor system to institute special actions that enable an individual to reach targeted goal positions and still maintain the integrity of the system. The functional differences also indicate that a relatively small change in one or a few control parameters can drive the system to another stable output pattern (Thelen, Ulrich, & Jensen, 1989). A key need in motor skill understanding is to discover precisely how the motor system is organized to facilitate smooth motor responses as actions shift from one qualitative mode to another. With such information one could use speech output characteristics to build theories of speech motor control in a way that is analogous to the use of phonetic transcription to construct theories of phonological competence (Folkins & Bleile, 1990).

Automatization also plays an important role in motor perform-ance. Practice of a developing motor action leads to automatization. Automatization increases efficiency by smoothing the action patterns and enabling the learner to experiment with variations in movement patterns and rates. For instance, in locomotion, skilled walking leads to running, swerving, dodging, and executing a wide variety of skilled maneuvers rapidly and efficiently. As the skills become integrated, sta-bilized, efficient, and automated, monitoring shifts to lower central control levels. This frees the person's attention for learning new tasks. By adulthood, differences in normal skilled actions are evident only in movement rhythms and amplitudes (Bernstein, 1967).

Speech and Oral Maturation

Speech development follows a course that almost parallels that of loco-motion. Newborn oral postures in crying, suckling, and swallowing are largely innate and reflexive. During early cry, the infant's legs kick, the arms slash, the head rolls from side to side, the eyes are tightly closed, and the mouth is widely open. With maturation, the crying movements become concentrated around the face, mouth, and larynx. Generalized body movements tend to subside. Balanced postures of structures with-in the mouth are added as the lips, jaw, and tongue become the center of vocal activities.

In the human newborn the tongue is closer to adult size than any other part of the body except the brain (Brodie, 1941). It almost fills the oral cavity. The newborn tongue is suspended from structures that are on the same horizontal plane as the tongue itself (see Figure 1-1). The resulting muscular forces are thus suited for infantile suckling-swal-lowing actions that draw the tongue forward to express milk from the nipple and pull it back to propel the food bolus from the mouth into the pharynx. This action has been likened to a plunger moving within a cylinder. This simple push-pull arrangement would not be suited for the series of dynamic postural adaptations and movements required in speech production.

As the child matures, space within the oral cavity is increased by rapid growth at the facial sutures, which are all oriented in a downward and forward direction (see Figure 1-2). The space for lingual maneu-verability is also increased by the descent of the tongue and hyoid bone within the facial complex, lateral expansion of the palatal alveolar pro-cesses, and eruption of the primary dentition. The capacity for new move-ments also increases via altered muscle orientations in the external suspensory system and internal refinement of the lingual muscles. For

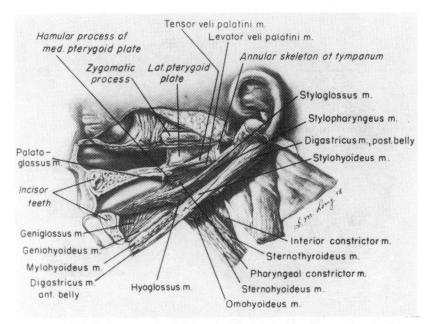

FIGURE 1-1. Dissection illustrating the anatomical relationships and suspensory musculature of the tongue, palate, and pharynx in the newborn infant. From Fletcher, S. G. (1958). *Hypernasal voice: Its relation to growth disturbance and physiological activity.* Unpublished doctoral dissertation, University of Utah, Salt Lake City.

example, the descent of the palate within the pharyngeal cavity converts the levator veli palatini and palatopharyngeus muscles into true elevators and retractors of the palate as the palate elongates. Descent of the tongue with respect to the base of the cranium and of the hyoid bone with respect to the vertebrae converts the styloglossus and hyoglossus muscles into elevators and depressors of the tongue. Lingual shaping possibilities also expand by parallel maturation of the intrinsic lingual musculature and alterations in lingual morphology. The tongue tip and blade show differentially rapid growth. Parallel nerve myelination prepares the tongue for the rapid volleys of neural stimulation needed to execute the intricate, delicately controlled postures, gestures, and action sequences demanded in speech articulation. Anatomical refinements thus multiply the potential for physiological maneuverability.

Biological evidence suggests that when new physiological capabilities arise, they operate through modulating and moderating previous ones rather than abolishing them (Reitman, 1965). Infants are presumed to discover the benefits of early elementary oral neuromotor patterns and add modifications from experiences they gain as primitive

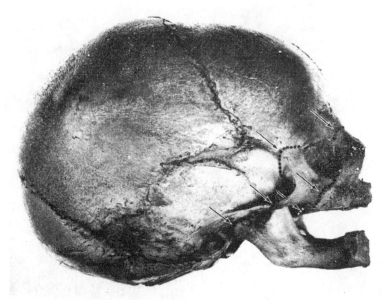

FIGURE 1–2. Facial bone sutures illustrating origin of downward and facial growth. From Fletcher, S. G. (1966). Cleft palate: A broader view. *Journal of Speech and Hearing Disorders, 31,* 1–13. Reprinted by permission.

movement sequences are executed in vocalizations. Children then derive strategies for executing and controlling more complex activities as they integrate and refine the more primitive reflex action patterns so discovered (Zelazo, 1976).

Primitive reflexes that could provide a foundation for speech articulation motor patterns include rooting, suckling and swallowing, motor reactions to sudden sounds, and visual fixation and movement tracking reflexes that enable infants to detect and mimic caregiver facial gestures. Other generally unnoticed oral reflexive patterns also seem to be preserved in speech. For example, Wassilieff (1886) reported that touching or stroking a baby's tongue elicits a spoon-shaped lingual configuration, characterized by an upraised ridge around its outer border (see Figures 1–3 and 1–4, from Strong, 1956). This basic, reflexively elicited posture which plays an important role in suckling activities is also found in the infant cry posture.[1] Wassilieff reported that a similar pos-

---

[1] This lingual stance also appears to be the basis for the linguapalatal valving in later speech production. Strong (1956) identified lingual contact around the outer perimeter of the palate as the common element in consonant sound production and traced it to special intrinsic lingual muscles that enable the spoon-shaped elevation of the tongue to be achieved. Evidence of the importance of this posture is found in the observation that lingual contact around the outer perimeter of the palate is the fundamental characteristic of /t/ sound production which is among the first intraoral sounds acquired in speech.

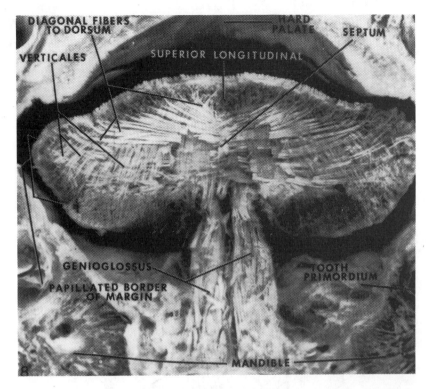

FIGURE 1-3. Coronal section of the tongue showing muscle fibers. Combined activation of the outer vertical and transverse fibers could result in the spoon-shaped configuration originally described by Wassilieff (1886). From Strong, L. H. (1956). Muscle fibers of the tongue functional in consonant production. *Anatomical Record, 126,* 61–79. Reprinted by permission.

ture could be elicited in adulthood by repeatedly touching, lightly stroking, or directing a stream of air across the tongue of the mature individual.[2] Such innate, genetically determined behaviors apparently become integrated with purposeful movement sequences in infancy. They are then expanded and refined as speech articulation skills are acquired.

As the oral cavity expands with downward and forward growth of the mandible and eruption of the deciduous teeth, the infant engages in a variety of oral exploratory movements linked with noise making activities. These activities help establish basic oral muscle control and sensory awareness of the tongue within the expanding oral space. Certain

[2] The spoon-shaped tongue posture is also found in the mature preparatory swallow just prior to release of the food bolus into the pharynx (Fletcher, 1970). In view of the many basic uses of this tongue posture, it will likely not be surprising to find it reappearing as the posture sought for speech skill development when palatometric modeling and shaping procedures are introduced.

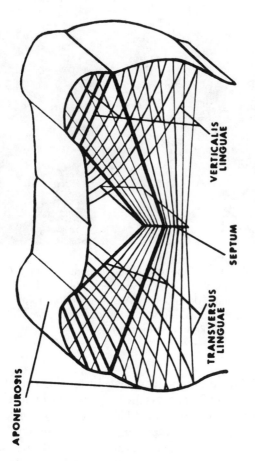

FIGURE 1–4. Schematic illustration of the intrinsic lingual musculature. Heavy lines indicate function of contracted muscles. From Strong, L. H. (1956). Muscle fibers of the tongue functional in consonant production. *Anatomical Record, 126,* 67–79. Reprinted by permission.

vocal patterns emerge repeatedly as rudimentary lip, jaw, and tongue postures are established in the isolated and occasionally combined sound elements of rudimentary babbling. The expansion of oral motor activities and controlled sound production during vocal play activities likely provide systematic preparatory experience for eventual emergence of specific articulation motor skills.

A major landmark in vocal development, as in locomotion maturation, is gaining the ability to shift back and forth between alternative postures in articulatory gestures. This lays the foundation for pacemaker control of rhythmical movement. The arrival of alternative articulatory postures and gestures in infant babbling also points to the important principle of *fixation/diversification* in motor skill development (cf. Gentile, 1972; Rothwell, 1987, p. 2).

Physical growth, as well as maturation, appears to play a role in motor skill fixation and diversification. This principle is illustrated in hand grasping. Initially, rapid finger growth is coupled with development of stabilizing wrist postures. The stabilized wrist in turn emancipates the pinching action of the thumb and fingertip, which is a central feature in controlled manual dexterity. It also facilitates independent movements of the fingers. Learning to use the wrist extensors to stabilize the hand thus frees the finger flexors to serve as prime movers in manipulating and exploring objects. An analogous pattern of development is found in the tongue. Initially the developing tongue is rather blunt ended. Even before birth, however, rapid growth of the tip and blade of the tongue is found. In early infancy, the continuing rapid growth of the peripheral part of the tongue is coupled with learning to stabilize the bulk of the tongue by activating its horseshoe-shaped outer ridge and pressing this ridge against the borders of the palate during sound production. Learning to *fixate* the jaw and bulk of the tongue in turn frees its tip and blade for the controlled alternating motions found in babbling and early words. Those skills then become available for later highly varied speech articulation sequences.

The emergence of stability and mobility functions is an essential part of speech skill development. Although early sound making is often viewed as nondirected, speech skill building starts with learning to stabilize the jaw and anchor the tongue along the outer, lateral margins of the palate. As described previously, this lateral lingual stability frees the tongue blade and root to produce alternative postures and reciprocal front and back articulatory gestures and action sequences required in consonant and vowel production (cf. Fletcher, 1973; Fletcher & Hasegawa, 1983; Fletcher, under review a & b). In essence, a reduction in the degrees of freedom in tongue movement emancipates certain portions of the tongue for precise articulatory actions. The integration of jaw stabilizing and mobilizing functions enables the child to move the distal parts of the tongue freely while the bulk of the tongue is stabilized laterally against the alveolar ridge and vertically by steady jaw positions. Operative coordination of stay-ability and move-ability thus define the articulatory postures of the tongue at any given moment. Dynamic interstructural stability allows a wide range of adaptive change in superimposed tongue tip and blade postures, gestures, and action sequences.

Phonological research suggests that at around 1 year of age children begin to incorporate the sound-making postures and gestures of vocal production into meaningful words. Expansion of the basic oral motor skills accelerates as children develop a "word-by-word look-up system" in speech production (Ingram, 1985). Sometime later in vocabulary expansion, the word-by-word look-up system becomes too cumbersome. The child then shifts to a phonology-based system. Phonetic properties permit words to be categorized, differentiated, and generalized as they are acquired and enable the child to handle the rapidly expanding lexicon efficiently.

Common characteristics are evident in the previous overview of locomotion and speech maturation. The child uses elementary neuromotor patterns as a foundation for learning to move structures into postures and positions required for ambulating and speaking. An important element in that development is learning special postures that reduce the degrees of freedom in movement and provide a firm postural base for new, more physiologically intricate activities (stable sitting and walking postures for locomotion actions, stable jaw and tongue postures for speech actions). The fixation-mobilization principles are applied as basic postures are acquired, then they enable coordinated reciprocal actions (crawling then walking in locomotion, babbling then reduplicated and nonreduplicated CV syllables in vocalization). Finally, the child gains speed, variety, and increased accuracy in connected motion sequences (running, swerving, and dodging in locomotion and anticipating, moving, blending, and combining articulatory sequences in speech). At the base of both ambulatory and phonatory systems is anatomical reshaping of structural form to fit emerging functional needs. During this process, new motor skills are acquired and integrated into new action sequences based on both innate and acquired neuromotor patterns.[3] The inborn patterns thus provide a substrata for

---

[3] Reflexes are innate neurological mechanisms that activate predictable postures and movement patterns. They are readily elicited during the first 6 months of life as the central nervous system matures. Reflexes are thought to help establish neural pathways and muscle functions that evolve into more controlled, directed movements that can be linked to mature actions as development unfolds. Gilfoyle and her associates (1990) describe the example of a baby who has experienced spontaneous rolling under the influence of righting reflexes learning. In this action, the infant reaches across the body with an arm or leg to trigger the automatic reactions. The reflexive response then activates

developing and refining controlled movement patterns in mature body gestures. Rhythmical, temporally, and spatially patterned movement sequences are then built on this firm foundation.

---

and sequences the rolling pattern. Later, the infant is able to initiate rolling volitionally and differentiate reaching components from automatic postural control components. The infant can then reach for a toy in a sidelong position. Reflexes may thus lead to development of more complex, purposeful movements.

CHAPTER 2

SENSORIMOTOR
FOUNDATIONS
FOR SPEECH

How could all of the vocal and other tasks involved in speech production develop within a single master plan? One possible answer to this question comes from the concept of a motor memory "schema." Schema theory revolves around the premise that motor skills develop from individual actions by a process of extracting core elements from motor experiences, discerning attributes that govern success in reaching action goals, deriving rules that dictate success in executing those actions, building a general plan or *schema* that encompasses the core properties of that information, and testing and refining the schema through continuing experiences in similar but not identical circumstances.

The concept of the schema was introduced originally by Head (1920) to explain body posture development and used by Lashley (1951) to account for serial ordering in speech production. It has been expanded and applied in many ways since that time.

THE SPEECH SCHEMA

A schema is presumed to be activated when information similar to its content is accessed. Once activated, the schema influences the processing of new information and provides a context for it. Bellezza (1987) has identified a number of properties that make the schema effective. The first of these properties is that the schema is *rule based*. This property enhances orderly information storage and retrieval. As a number of responses are executed within a single class of action, some are noted to be successful in achieving goals. Others are not. These perceptions are thought to be distilled, action restated, and used as the basis for rules that govern successful action patterns. Repeated applications of these rules provide an opportunity to discover both the context within which particular rules can be successfully applied and the relative success that can be expected as particular motor actions are used to achieve a given response goal. Properties of successful patterns are thus clarified through repetitions. These properties form the basis of generalized rules. The use of rules reduces the number of details that must be accessed when a response is activated. The rules are then tested and refined to verify their correctness and incorporated into the emerging schema. The schema is, in turn, used to organize and control motor actions in that class of responses.

The second property of the schema theory is that the greater the number and variety of experiences within a response class, the more *effective* the schema formulated will be. *Practice* is a core element in the developing schema. The more often a schema is activated, the more aptly it will function. This situation is illustrated by the use of natural numbers and the alphabet. Counting and alphabet reciting are so overlearned that they can be executed perfectly with each recall (cf. Bellezza, 1982, Chapters 3 and 5). Practice also smooths the way to executing novel movements. Shapiro and Schmidt (1982) used the scatter plot shown in Figure 2-1 to explain the role of practice as a basis for improving the ability to execute novel movements. They point out that if we think of each response as a point in a linear regression plot, the general trend will become apparent as the number of experiences, or points on the graph increase. The greater the number of related actions an individual has experienced, the clearer will be the relationships between input concepts and outcome actions.

The third property is *variability*. Schemas develop as a result of repeated experiences that are similar but not identical. Referring to Figure 2-1, varied experiences, particularly near the extremes of a response range, could help an individual perceive cause and effect relationships. In other words, variability would help define a clear central trend line as well as permissible differences in core features of the actions. The larger the "spread" of natural outcomes used to formulate a schema that represents a particular experience class, the more accurate it will be when it is used to generate novel responses. Thus, listening to many talkers produce the same sound many times and prac-

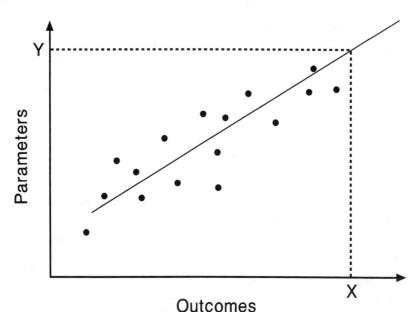

FIGURE 2-1. Graphical representation of the role practice plays in learning to execute novel movements. The upward sloping regression line represents emergence of the schema rule as a movement is learned. The dots within the graph represent individual subject responses produced under control of the central schema. The systematic rise of the curve illustrates that both the number of controllable parameters (Y) and possible outcomes (X) increase systematically with practice. Adapted from Shapiro & Schmidt (1982).

tice in attempting to match those varied model patterns may be expected to provide a more stable phoneme schema than one based on a single model pattern. This principle underscores the advantage of a wide variety of experiences and exposures as a schema is forged.

The fourth property in schema development is that items in schemas that represent more complicated objects or events have more information in them. They, therefore, emerge at a later period in the individual's maturational years. When more complex schemas are used, they also consume greater access and usually execution time than more primitive ones. Thus developmental order, central access time, and execution time are all functions of the *amount of information* contained in a schema. An example of this principle is found in comparing phonetic proficiency of children with normal and profoundly impaired hearing. Fletcher, Smith, and Hasegawa (1985) showed that children who are severely to profoundly hearing impaired are similar to their hearing peers as they produce a simple, nonphonetically differentiated "uh"-like vocal response. However, the children who were hearing impaired were slower than hearing peers in initiating counting responses and slower yet in digit naming reaction times. In other words, the experiential deficit of phonetic deprivation associated with a profound hearing deficit was associated with a systematic deficit in the time consumed in accessing vocal information and producing a phonetically based response. As the vocal tasks became increasingly complex phonetically, additional time was required to retrieve the appropriate patterns from central storage and generate the stipulated vocal output. Campbell and Keegan (1987) reported similar progressively longer reaction times among normal adults when they pressed a key as quickly as possible and simultaneously said "please," "pleasing," or "displeased." The findings from both studies would agree with a phonetic theory that conceives subprograms in the central speech program influenced by the phonetic content and complexity of an utterance.

The fifth property of the schema revolves around its *associations* and *meaningfulness* to the subject. Symbols representing meaningful events are those that can be represented in *mental images* that are drawn from *real-world objects* (Underwood & Schultz, 1960). This type of information is most easily accessed in memory. Parents recognize this. They help children build meaningful associations that can serve as the basis of speech motor schemata. A mother is most likely to vocalize when an infant vocalizes. Her next most likely response is to smile at, look at, or touch the infant. Vocal interchange is thus set in a *meaningful* context. The interaction patterns constitute a social system that facilitates growth of vocal communication (Freedle & Lewis, 1977). The frequency of experiences in normal childhood helps account for the fact that unusual or atypical responses require more time to process than those associated with common events in life (Bellezza, 1983).

Finally, schema development requires experiences with *discriminated* sensory and motor attributes that are identified and temporally differentiated in the contexts in which motor responses normally occur. This principle is illustrated by phonetic simplifications, sentence shortening, and assigning *names* to *things* in the child's perceptual world by caregivers as they strive to help children map their perceptual world onto the abstract sound system of speech. The requirement for discriminable stimuli dictates that only one schema can be active in memory at any given time (Mandler, 1979; Reddy & Bellezza, 1986).

VOCAL TRACT FUNCTIONS
IN SPEECH PRODUCTION

As suggested by many of the examples just discussed, the schema theory may be applied directly to speech production as we seek to conceptualize the physiological processes involved. The word "sound" is often used to refer to the segment sized units of speech. This is the basic unit around which phonetic textbooks are organized. "Rules" identify both how groups of sounds are modified as "bundles of distinctive features" (Jakobson, 1938) and principles that govern the underlying articulatory gestures. The premise of the following discussion is that internally and externally perceived movement sensations and experiences are used to build and constantly update central schemata. These schemata are thought to contain the rules and other information that underpin speech production.

The vocal schema outlined in Figure 2–2 contains a wealth of presumed information about vocal patterns in one's language. The speech sounds, as elements in the vocal schemata, are presumed to arise from the auditory, oral, and visual sensations surrounding articulatory postures, gestures, and action sequences. These sensations are processed in parallel as they enter the person's perceptual field. Each sense has special properties and characteristics that help meet the individual's communication needs and intents. A number of these attributes will be briefly reviewed, highlighting those aspects that are uniquely pertinent to speech perception and production.

Perhaps because x-rays have been the principal objective means of assessing tongue positions within the oral cavity, articulatory positions and movements have typically been described from a lateral, midsagittal orientation. This has limited the perspective on consonant sound production and at the same time fostered the belief that during vowels "none of the articulators come close together" (Ladefoged, 1975, p. 11).

Studies spanning the last decade have shown that vocal tract descriptions based on midline tongue configurations diverge in important ways from acoustic observations (Wood, 1979), listener perceptions (Borden & Harris, 1984, p. 109), and tongue movement sensations (Lindblom & Lubker, 1985). An important element has been missing, especially in vowel descriptions. In the present discussion of vocal tract functions and sensations special attention will be given to how actions along the lateral borders of the mouth might be included in the sensorimotor schema.

Concepts from developmental anatomy can help us understand many of the normal and abnormal functions of the human body. Information about where cells originate, how they migrate to their location in the body, and the source of their nerve supply is particularly helpful in our efforts to conceptualize the integrated neural and muscular framework of speech production.

There is something almost magical in the way embryonic cells follow an obviously well coordinated, synchronized plan to prepare for special activities such as speech reception and production. Cells subdivide, move past others streaming along common pathways, converge

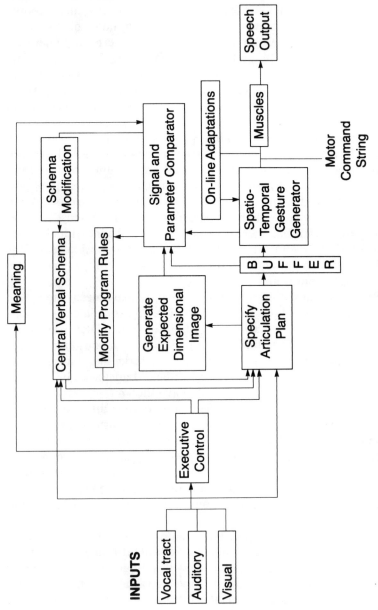

FIGURE 2-2. Schematic illustration of how inputs from the vocal tract and from auditory and visual sensations could be used in the development of a central verbal schema for speech articulation.

at predetermined locations with cells from other origins, and there form structures which when activated will perform special tasks smoothly and harmoniously. Muscle cells, for instance, become highly oriented muscle fibers with well-defined anatomical origins and insertions. This process begins with a small number of founder cells that originate in dynamic mesenchymal tissues (Holtzer, Sasse, Horwitz, Antin, & Pacifici, 1986). They then migrate along set pathways to the site of the mature muscle. Upon arrival, premuscle masses form then expand within a restricted and predictable cell lineage and begin the process of splitting into individual muscle primordia. As they do so, separate cells fuse into multinucleated muscle fibers. Connective tissue and tendons needed to move body structures being formed arise separately and become attached to the muscles secondarily. As soon as the rudiments of the muscle fibers are organized, they become capable of weak contractions that are integrated in a functional neural circuit for coordinated actions. The sequence of actions is tightly dictated and controlled. For example, if sensory nerve fibers are prevented from interacting with the muscle fibers at a critical developmental stage, muscle spindles do not form (Zelená, 1957).

Over the years, many methods have been devised to study embryonic development. One of the most valuable has been the use of *vital dyes*, or trace markers, that allow cell movements to be tracked or located through computer-based *imaging* at critical points in the developmental process. Through such studies, a clear picture has emerged showing how head and neck structures evolve through a cascade of closely integrated events to form the "speech mechanism."

One of the early signs of the developing speech mechanism is the arrival of four *branchial arches* (see Figure 2–3) that appear when the human embryo is about 4 weeks old. Within the next week most of the facial structures become individually distinguishable. Among the most conspicuous landmarks is the stomodeum formed between an expanding forebrain and the *mandibular arch*. The upper face, which includes the nose, upper lip, and maxillae, develops from primitive tissue above the stomodeum. The oral and nasal cavities are subdivisions of the stomodeum.

Development of the tongue presents an interesting example of the critical role that cell migration plays in *epigenesis*, or progressive growth and development within body regions. The lingual muscles do not develop from the same tissues as those of the facial and jaw muscles. Rather, they develop from cell primordia that originate in the occipital myotomes. These cells then journey to the mandibular arch by passing around the primitive digestive tube (which will later become the pharynx) then push into the mandibular branchial arch just inside its inner (endodermal) lining. Some cells continue on to the inner surface of the

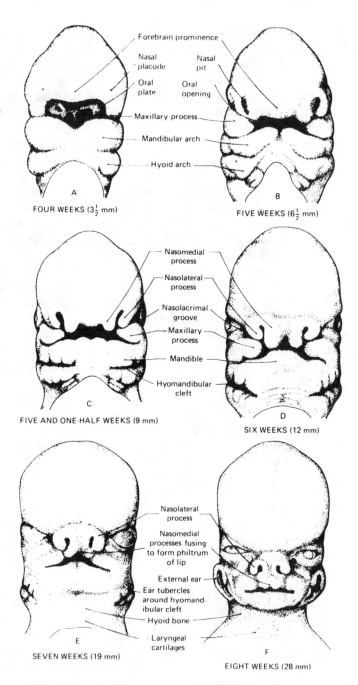

FIGURE 2-3. Formation of the face from the 4th to 8th week of embryonic development. From H. Morris, (1942). *Morris: Human anatomy* (10th Ed.), (p. 27). Philadelphia, PA: Blakiston.

mandible and begin immediately to form the genioglossus muscle. Other primordial lingual cells halt their movement and begin to subdivide to form the *lateral lingual swellings* along the inner walls of the mandibular arch. A third group of cells pushes into the back, upper edge of the first branchial arch and forms a median swelling, called the *copula*. The main part of the tongue body develops from the lateral lingual swellings. These swellings expand medially into the stomodeal cavity as they grow. Ultimately the swellings from each side meet near the midline and fuse together to form the forepart of the tongue. The copula becomes the tongue root. A small pit known as the *foramen cecum* (a hole that ceases) and the circumvallate (encircled valley) papillae identify the border between the parts derived from the first and second branchial arches. The foramen cecum is actually the vestige of a tube that extends from the pharynx to the thyroid gland in the early embryo. Growth and differentiation within the tongue is rapid, but it is not completed until after the infant is born. Postnatal growth along the outer margins of the tongue changes it from the stubby, rather blunt-ended structure of the newborn into a longer, more slender, and mobile organ of the mature individual. Maturation provides a tongue that is better suited to the intricate movements of sound production than that of the infant.

Shortly after the tongue begins to form along the lower walls of the stomodeum, the embryonic palate appears as swellings along the upper, inner stomodeal walls. By the time these swellings are noticeable the primordial tongue already fills most of the stomodeal cavity. The bulky tongue in the middle of the cavity causes the developing *palatine processes* to be temporarily diverted downward. They form initially as vertically oriented plates along each side of the tongue (Figure 2–4). It is thought that when the lingual muscles become functional, their primitive contractions cause the tongue to be lowered. This then triggers a rapid upward and inward migration of the cells within the palatine processes. This brings them to a horizontal position and splits the stomodeum into nasal and oral cavities. Shortly thereafter the palatine plates are joined by the downward growing nasal septum to separate the nasal passageway into two chambers. In the process of growth, the palatine shelves first contact each other. They then join with the simultaneously developing premaxillary process that forms within the outer facial primordia. The three structures then fuse in a front-to-back sequence, like a zipper closing space between two pieces of cloth. Cleft palates result if the cell movement is blocked during a critical time in this zipping process. Submucous cleft palates are explained as a depletion of the cell movement energy within the dynamic myoblast (muscle generating) unit before mesodermal infusion is fully accomplished (see Walker & Fraser, 1956). As illustrated in Figure 2–5, innervation of the

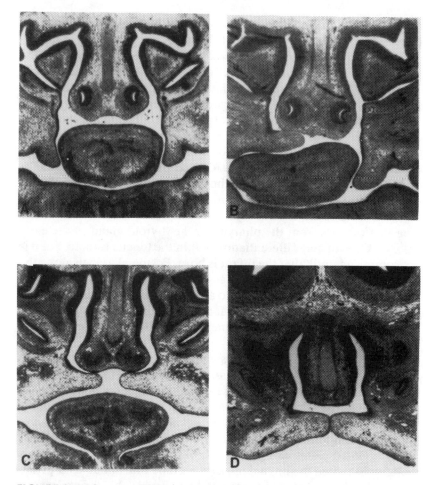

FIGURE 2–4. Cross sections of the embryonic palatine plates at the level of the nasal septum illustrating their movement from a vertical to horizontal orientation. (A) shows both plates in a vertical position on each side of the tongue. In (B), one plate has shifted, and in (C) both plates have shifted to the horizontal plane. As shown in (D), the space between the plates is soon bridged by the palatal growth. Soon after that, nasal septal growth completes separation of the two nasal cavities. After Walker & Fraser (1956).

oral and facial structures reflects their multiple origins. Sensory and motor innervation for structures that develop within the first branchial arch, the branchial groove between the first and second arches externally, and the pharyngeal pouch which separates them internally is from the trigeminal nerve. It serves facial and oral sensations and motor innervation to the muscles of mastication, tensor tympani, tensor veli palatini, and anterior belly of the digastric. The facial, stape-

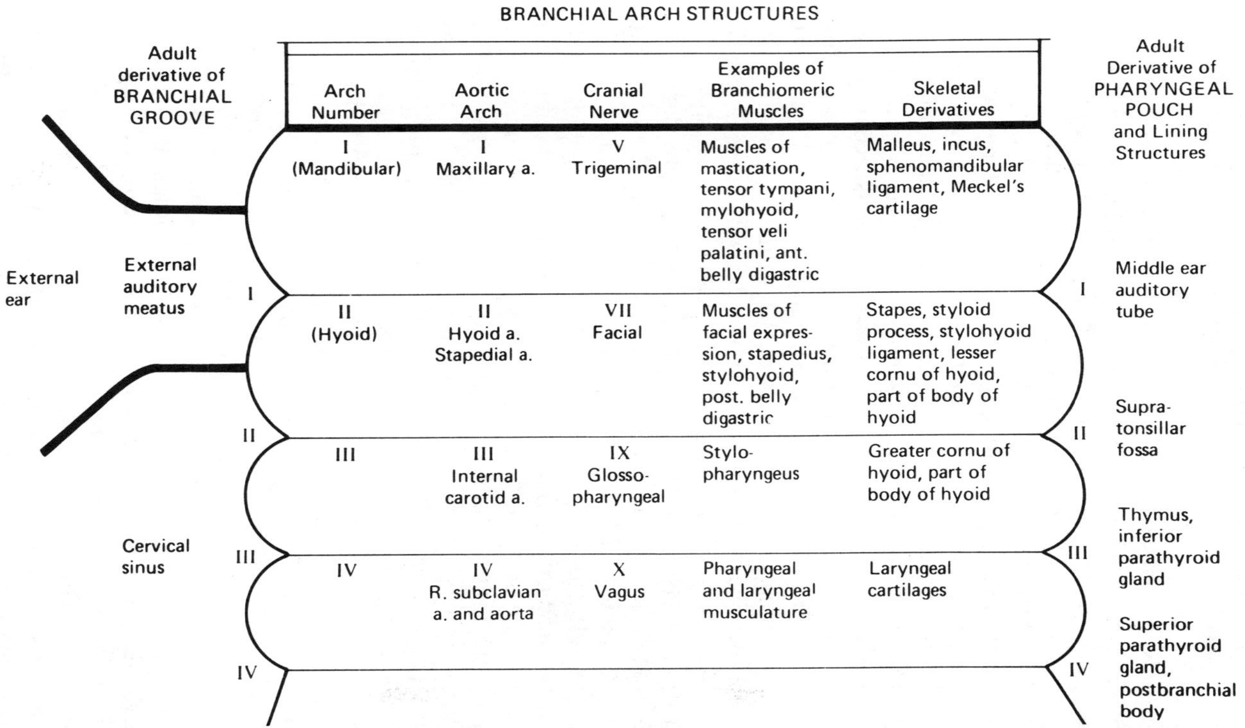

FIGURE 2–5. Facial, oral, and pharyngeal derivatives from the branchial arches and grooves and from the pharyngeal pouch. From Carlson, B.M. (1988). *Patten's foundation of embryology.* (5th Ed.), (p. 536). New York: McGraw-Hill. Reprinted by permission.

dius, stylohyoid, and posterior belly of the digastric muscles all originate from cells that migrate upward from the second branchial arch. The glossopharyngeal nerve provides sensations to cells and cavities that develop within and around the third branchial arch. The structures which develop from this arch include the upper pharyngeal wall, root of the tongue, and the stylopharyngeus muscle. The remaining pharyngeal muscles along with those in the larynx are from myoblastic cells from the fourth branchial arch. Sensory and motor innervation for these muscles and the overlaid cavity surfaces is from the vagus nerve.

The near proximity and interlinking relationships between structures derived from the branchial arches and clefts fosters the richly integrated movements and action patterns demanded in speech production. Delicate control over the muscle system is accomplished through a clearly differentiated neural substructure. Even structures formed in near proximity to each other may be served by different nerves. For instance, each of the three muscles that originate from the styloid bone (see Figure 2–6) is supplied by a different nerve. The styloglossus is innervated by the hypoglossal (XII) nerve, the stylohyoid fibers by the facial (VII) nerve, and the stylopharyngeus by the glossopharyngeal (IX) nerve. The combined stress from the three muscles stimulates formation of the styloid bone.

The genioglossus muscle forms the bulk of the tongue. Its fibers fan out from their origin just behind the symphysis of the mandible and insert into the undersurface of the tongue in a broad arc along its full length from apex to root (see Figure 2–6). The genioglossus muscle has two major functions. Those fibers that attach along the posterior margins of the tongue draw its root forward. The fibers that enter the tongue from the genial tubercle of the mandible arch in an upward then forward direction to insert at the tongue apex. When this part of the genioglossus is activated, it tends to pull the tongue backward in the mouth and draw the tip down. It may be evident that simultaneous activation of the fibers connected to the tongue root and apex would cause the tongue to arch upward as its root is advanced and its tip pulled back. The resulting high, rounded, tongue posture is the typical stance seen during production of the /i/ vowel. As might be expected, different degrees of contraction across the three divisions of the genioglossus muscle are linked with specific changes in vowel acoustic formant frequencies (Fujimura & Kakita, 1979). When all of the muscle fibers contract simultaneously and in constant proportion, the formant pattern converges toward the high, front point vowel, /i/. This effect is consistent with the notion that the /i/ may function as an optimal vocal tract length-calibrating signal in vowel comparisons (Lieberman, 1975; Nearey, 1978). Activation of the fibers in the central region of the tongue may function to counteract the upward rise of the tongue and

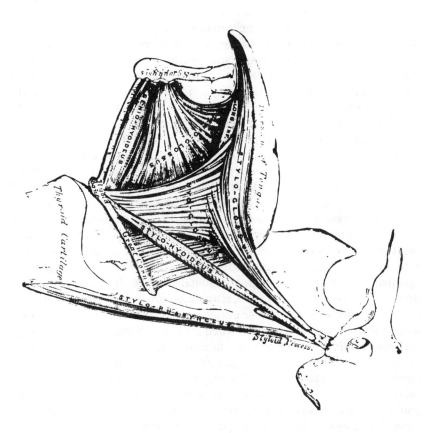

FIGURE 2–6. Extrinsic muscles of the tongue seen from the left side. From Goss, C. M. (1954). *Anatomy of the human body by Henry Gray* (26th Ed.), (p. 1262). Philadelphia: Lea & Febiger. Reprinted by permission.

contribute to its precisely controlled height during intermediate vowel production.

The other muscles that enter the tongue from external origins are used to counterbalance the genioglossus and establish tongue posture control within the oral cavity. For example, finely balanced, reciprocal contraction of the styloglossus, stylohyoid, and posterior digastric muscles pulling rearward and the genioglossus, geniohyoid, and anterior digastric muscles pulling forward enable tongue placement to be finely controlled along the front/back continuum. The supra- and infrahyoid (*sternohyoid, omohyoid, thyrohyoid, mylohyoid*) muscles play important secondary roles in tongue postural actions. They adjust the location of the hyoid bone upon which the tongue rides.

The intrinsic muscles of the tongue develop as later subdivisions of the extrinsic muscles. Their smaller size, well-endowed neural supply, and orientation within the major anatomical planes enhances the roles they serve in precisely controlled tongue movements. One set (*transversus linguae*) spans the tongue from side to side, another set (*longitudinalis*) extends from the front to the back in upper and lower layers, and the third set (*vertical lingualis*) are vertically oriented.

The transverse fibers originate from each side of the tough, fibrous lingual septum. The septum originates along the tongue midline when the primordial lingual processes meet and fuse during embryogenesis. The muscle fibers then extend laterally to insert into fibrous tissue along the outer margins of the tongue. When unopposed, these fibers would round the tongue along its horizontal axis. This action is important for creating a tongue shape that allows it to be raised within the palatal vault and clear food remnants from the mouth during late swallowing activities. The longitudinal rounding is not often seen in speech. The Spanish /ɲ/, which requires linguapalatal contact along the relatively unused center of the palatal vault, is an exception to this rule. More commonly, actions of the transverse muscles are carried out in combination with other muscles. For example, when they are activated in conjunction with the middle set of genioglossus muscles, the result would be a lowering of the central part of the tongue and an upward raising of its outer borders. This function is likely the major source of lateral linguapalatal valving actions during sound production. Activation of these muscles could also be used to create the long, midline channel found during all vowels. The groove is always deeper and narrower toward the back of the tongue. The difference is most pronounced in front high vowels produced in a labial consonant context (Stone, Shawker, Talbot, & Rich, 1988). As might be expected, lax vowels have shallower grooves than tense vowels.

Strong (1956) described a special set of short-fiber transverse muscles that travel outward and upward within the outer margins of the tongue. These fibers could be particularly helpful in fine-tuning and differentiating the place and pattern of linguapalatal contact during vowel and consonant sounds. Control over the tongue contact location could also be enhanced by hyoglossal muscle activity. The hyoglossus consists of a relatively thin sheet of muscle tissue that originates along the upper margins of the bone and inserts into the tongue along its lateral margins. Its action could thus help counterbalance transverse muscle action and enhance lateral linguapalatal contact control.

As indicated, two sets of intrinsic muscle fibers extend along the longitudinal axis of the tongue. One set (*longitudinalis superior*) is located immediately under the lingual surface. This muscle originates at the tongue root close to the epiglottis and inserts at the tongue apex. In the central part of the tongue, it develops into a triangular mass that is above the transverse and vertical intrinsic muscles (Abd-El-Malek, 1939). This more massive central construction suggests that the muscle likely plays a major role in interior tongue postural stabilization. For example, in cooperation with the transverse muscles it could facilitate alternating front-back linguapalatal articulations in words such as "talk," "caught," and "keating."

The other set of longitudinal lingual muscles (*longitudinalis inferior*) is located in the lower part of the tongue between the genioglossus and hyoglossus muscles. Its fibers extend from the tongue root to its apex, blending with parallel fibers from the styloglossus. Thus, reciprocal activation of these muscles would appear to counterbalance the forces generated by the superior longitudinal fibers thereby enabling finely controlled raising and lowering of the tongue blade and dorsum during sound production. The function of the vertical intrinsic fibers is less clear than that of the others. They could help to flatten and broaden the tongue shape. They could also help stabilize the medial part of the tongue during lateral linguapalatal contact actions.

Examination of the lingual sensory nerve supply points to a rich kinesthetic and tactile system for monitoring the train of neural events culminating in articulator contact position and movement sensations. Muscle spindles have been identified in all extrinsic and intrinsic human lingual musculature (Bowman, 1968; Cooper, 1953). The ganglia are distributed throughout the tongue with two thirds in its anterior half (Fitzgerald & Alexander,1969). The superior longitudinal muscle spindles are particularly dense in the front third of the tongue (Cooper, 1953). Those in the transversus muscle are most dense in the midregion, toward the lateral borders. The special central structure enables the receptors within the tongue to respond to both the degree and rate of muscular stretch (cf. Hardcastle, 1976). Since the muscles traverse the tongue in a network of transverse, longitudinal, and vertical fibers, the embedded spindles form a substratum for highly discriminative movement monitoring and action control across an exceptionally wide range of static and dynamic responses (Bowman, 1971). The lingual neural supply and distribution appears to ensure keen sensorimotor control in monitoring and regulating the postural and action status of the tongue.

A rich tactile neural supply is also present in the tongue and other parts of the oral cavity. As with the spindles, the tactile nerves are most dense toward the front of the mouth. Their density then decreases progressively toward the rear (Grossman & Hattis, 1967). Light touch is sensed by diffuse, interweaving terminal filaments that branch from myelinated nerve fibers and penetrate into the base of the epithelial membrane (Hardcastle, 1970). Krause end-bulbs and Meissner corpuscles below the free nerve endings respond to deeper touch and localized deformations of the tongue surface. Fine filament periodontal receptors with richly varied terminal endings (Seto, 1972) contribute exquisite sensitivity to even delicate contact with the teeth (Scott & Symons, 1974).

Stimulation of oral tactile sensors evokes potentials along a short-latency, fast-acting pathway that parallels the spindle afferents and converges on the same cerebrocortical neurons (Bowman & Combs, 1969). Precise tonotopic representations of tactile stimulus locations are retained as this information is relayed to the central nervous system. The tactile neural responses reach the cortex with a latency only slightly longer than that of the spindles. The importance of the tactile information is highlighted by the fact that the cerebellum receives tactile but not spindle afferents from the tongue, and the volume of thalamic and cortical tissue devoted to tactile representation is considerably larger than that for the spindles. The tactile-kinesthetic makeup of the tongue is thus capable of providing exquisite sensitivity to central and lateral lingual position, movement, and contact information during static postures and dynamic speech articulation gestures and actions. Guided by the intelligible speech motive, all relevant sensory signals — tactile, proprioceptive, and exteroceptive — can thus be united, compared, and integrated within a central schema directed, motor control program.

AUDITORY SENSATIONS

Audition has been recognized as the common gateway to speech production. The auditory system has four major components each of which has special design characteristics that influence perception of acoustic information received and contribute to speech production. The auricle or *pinna* of the external ear collects vibratory information from the outside world and channels it through the external auditory canal to the tympanic membrane. Phase differences between sounds arriving at the tympanic membranes of the two ears (see Figure 2–7) are used to locate sound sources in space and help the listener follow conversations between more than one talker. The shape of the auricle helps isolate the direction of noise arriving from the environment and enhances high frequency sound reception from in front of the head. The concha and external auditory canal parts of the outer ear act as bandpass filters, enhancing frequencies in the 2 to 7 kHz, mid- to high-frequency range. The pinnae and auditory canals filter out much of the back-

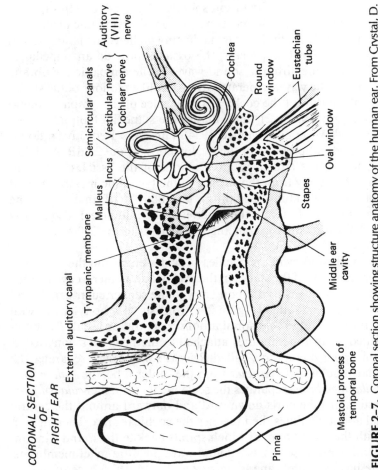

CORONAL SECTION
OF
RIGHT EAR

FIGURE 2-7. Coronal section showing structure anatomy of the human ear. From Crystal, D. (1980). *Introduction to language pathology (2nd ed.)*. London: Whurr Publishers Ltd. Reprinted by permission.

ground noise and aid perception of the softer, high-frequency consonants as the acoustic signals are relayed to the middle ear.

The tympanic membrane and three ossicles in the middle ear
transpose the acoustic signals into mechanical energy and relay them
to the inner ear. The tympanic membrane is a sophisticated sound
transducer that vibrates as a unit in response to low frequencies and as
subparts in response to high frequency sounds. Its tension can be finely
tuned to increase sensitivity to soft sounds or relaxed to help suppress
unwanted noise. The mechanical energy from the tympanic membrane
is relayed through the middle ear via the tiny malleus, incus, and stapes
ossicular bones. In this process, the ossicles provide an impedance
match between the airborne sound waves at the tympanic membrane
and the hydraulic waves generated by piston-like motions of the stapes
in the oval window of the cochlea. The surface of the tympanic membrane is approximately 21 times that of the stapedial footplate in the
oval window (Wever & Lawrence, 1954). This 14 to 1 effective ratio increases the sound pressure at the oval window about 23 dB. An additional 2 to 3 dB is added by lever actions of the ossicles. The concentration of energy from the surface of the tympanic membrane and
ossicular mechanical leverage thus adds about 26 dB intensity to the
sound as it is transferred to the inner ear. The middle ear also acts as
another bandpass filter enhancing frequencies in the 200 to 2000 Hz
range (Zwislocki, 1975).

The oval window in the cochlea provides entry into the inner ear.
Vibratory motions of the stapes in the oval window enter a cavity called
the vestibule, which is a common entry to the semicircular canals and
the cochlea. The cochlea (Figure 2–8) consists of a bony cavity with
three fluid-filled tubes that spiral around a central pedestal. The tubes
are created by two membranes attached to the pedestal's bony ledge.
The thin upper membrane, called *Reissner's membrane,* separates the
vestibular tube or *scala vestibuli* from the center tube, the *scala media.*
The *basilar membrane* separates the scala media from the *scala tympani.*
The vestibular tube curls downward and outward around the central
pedestal about 2½ times then reaches the cochlear apex. There it con-
nects with the scala tympani which spirals back to the round window.
The round window serves as a sound wave pressure relief membrane.

The basilar membrane is narrow and stiff at the base of the cochlea where sound enters. As it spirals around the modiolus, it becomes wider and thinner. This structural variation plays a primary role
in auditory frequency analysis as sound traverses the cochlea. The
membrane resonates to high-frequency tones as sound enters the cochlea and low-frequency tones as the traveling wave approaches the
cochlear apex. The *Organ of Corti* is seated on the medial surface of the
basilar membrane (Figure 2–9). It is the sensory organ of the auditory

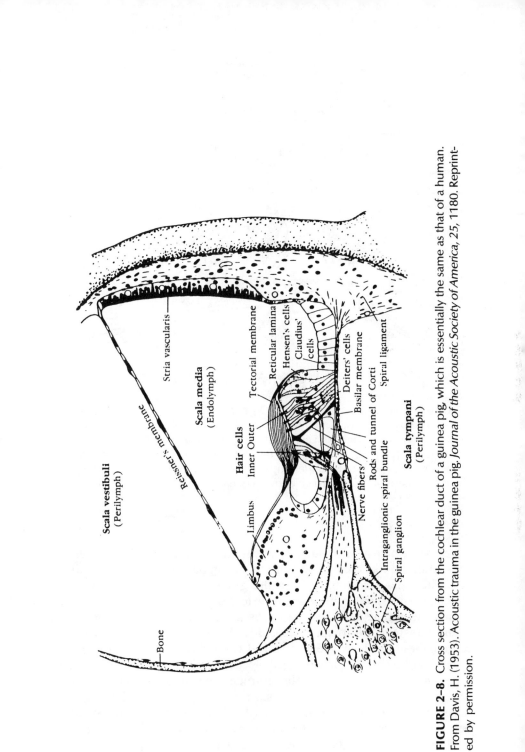

FIGURE 2–8. Cross section from the cochlear duct of a guinea pig, which is essentially the same as that of a human. From Davis, H. (1953). Acoustic trauma in the guinea pig. *Journal of the Acoustic Society of America, 25,* 1180. Reprinted by permission.

Tectorial membrane

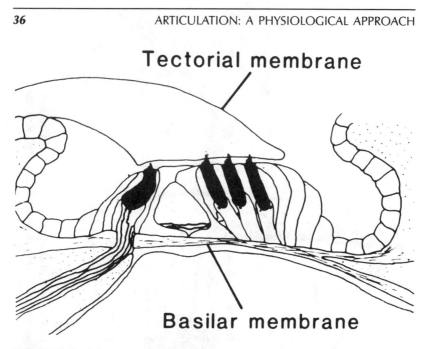

Basilar membrane

FIGURE 2-9. Schematic diagram of the Organ of Corti. Four rows of hair cells are surmounted by the tectorial membrane. The pivoting of the Organ of Corti from basilar membrane movements causes a shearing force that deflects the outer hair cells. The inner hair cells are thought to be bent by fluid movement between the tectorial membrane and the underlying hair cells. From Hudspeth, A. J. (1985). The cellular basis of hearing: The biophysics of hair cells. *Science, 230,* 745–752. Reprinted by permission.

system with three rows of outer hair cells and a single row of inner hair cells. Stiff, rod-like cilia are attached to the upper surface of each hair cell. The outer cilia terminate in the gelatinous tectorial membrane attached to the spiral lamina. Shearing forces are generated between the basilar membrane and these hair cells as the membrane resonates to sound transmitted through the cochlea. Angular displacement of the cell bundles transduces the mechanical vibrations of the basilar membrane into Fourier frequency-coded electrochemical nerve impulses. It is thought that the inner hair cells protrude unencumbered into the surrounding fluid (Hudspeth, 1985). Their activity is dictated by the length, mass, and hydrodynamic drag of the cilia that extend across the space between the tectorial membrane and are bent by fluid moving. The presence of hair cell impulses can be measured as changes in the electrical potential of the cells. The hair cells are most sensitive to frequencies that vary inversely with the lengths of the hair bundles. Low-frequency stimuli deflect the long, massive bundles but leave the short bundles relatively undisturbed. Conversely, high frequency stimuli bend the short hair bundles.

The spectral analyzer functions of the basilar membrane are derived from traveling waves that focus energy at different points along its length. Low frequencies excite motions nearer the apex of the cochlea, higher frequencies deflect the membrane near its base. Hair cell potentials within the cochlea evidence some fine tuning as energy from nearby cells is suppressed through lateral inhibition during the energy transfer from the basilar membrane to the hair bundles. The outer hair cells are innervated almost exclusively by efferent fibers which feed tiny muscles. When these cells are strongly stimulated, the muscles act to raise the auditory threshold thereby effectively suppressing the responses of the auditory system to the incoming sound waves. The frequency response of associated afferent fibers is also broadened (Art & Fettiplace, 1984). The outer hair cells thus help to suppress responses to loud noise and perhaps sensitize, or "tune," the system to certain broad acoustic patterns in speech.

The cochlear Fourier separation of complex sounds into component frequencies is retained as neural energy is excited in auditory cranial nerve fibers. This information is relayed via the central auditory pathways to the auditory cortex in the temporal lobe of the brain. From there it is transmitted to other centers of the brain where the message is decoded.

The fact that speech-relevant acoustical processing takes place in the cochlea does not necessarily mean that the peripheral auditory system reacts differently to speech sounds than other sounds. Rather, human speech likely develops in a way that takes advantage of the special characteristics of the auditory system (Goldhor, 1985).

How is information about changes in the vocal tract recaptured from the acoustically derived message? Traditionally, constant relationships have been sought between vocal tract shapes and consequent acoustic spectra. It was assumed that similar shapes produce similar spectra (cf. Hockett, 1960). It may be evident from these descriptions of acoustic processing in the auditory system that this explanation faces a particular problem. The signals emerging from the cochlea differ significantly from those arriving at the ear. They also differ from patterns derived through acoustic spectral analysis techniques that have been developed to study speech.

Speech spectrograms display many properties that are not perceptually relevant to a listener and seem to obscure other properties that are both important and perceptually meaningful (Klatt, 1982). No single shape or spectrum, nor any particular sequence of shapes or spectra, can be found that is invariantly related to the speech sounds or sound sequences (Porter, 1987). Direct phonetic representation is too often missing. This situation has led to an alternative viewpoint: Phonetic constancy is a product of standard articulatory movements conveyed by changes in articulator positions and vocal tract shapes. Information related to the articulatory interpretation of phonetic constancy will be presented in the upcoming discussion of the vocal tract. At this point, it is sufficient to note simply that in this viewpoint the auditory system provides a means of accessing dynamically coordinated movements that are naturally periodic or oscillatory (Kelso, Saltzman, & Tuller, 1986; Kelso & Tuller, 1984). Explicit identification and definition of the implied effects of articulatory actions on the acoustic spectra and how this information emerges from the cochlea is now being sought. Current emphasis is on ways to recapture phonetic information manifested by movement rates of change (velocities) and relative acoustic energy phases that reflect *changes* in vocal tract shapes rather than absolute sizes or shapes of the structures and cavities.

As pointed out by Porter (1987), currently favored dynamic action models of speech articulation imply two important auditory consequences. First, they incorporate the commonly assumed ability to distinguish messages by using actions to produce distinctive acoustic contrasts that reflect changes in articulation space and time. Second, they provide a means of conveying messages through acoustic signals that retain information about the relative rates of change in articulator positions that may be independent of absolute positions in oral space and time. Such observations have led the search for the origins of speech sensations to include a focus on the special ways the auditory system transforms spectral shapes, intensity profiles, and temporal relationships from vocal tract functions into auditory sensations.

VISUAL SENSATIONS

When all sensory systems are available to guide movement, vision is used and trusted most (Posner, Nissen, & Klein, 1976). In speech, visual information is normally used to verify auditory sensations, particularly in difficult listening conditions (Fletcher, 1983b; MacDonald & McGurk, 1978; McGurk & MacDonald, 1976; Summerfield & McGrath, 1984). The natural correspondence between visual and auditory information about speech has been attributed to their common physiologic ties to articulatory gestures (Studdert-Kennedy, 1984). Visual and auditory sensations may, in fact, be interchanged to optimize energy expenditure during phonetic learning and speech perception (Lindblom, 1983).

Information about visual perception, shape recognition, and cognition has accumulated rapidly during the last decade as a result of converging investigations by researchers in a number of disciplines

(Biederman, 1986; Pinker, 1988; Stevens, 1987). In the current most accepted conceptualization, visual sensory information is treated as a hierarchical representation of structures, objects, or organisms. The brain receives visual information in coordinate frames from images on the retina. The location of visual stimuli in space is mapped in pinpoint projections from the retina to the posterior parietal cortex of the brain (Anderson, Essick, & Siegel, 1985). The resulting form can be regarded as a composition of parts. Each part is described in terms of how its cross-section varies as a function of its position along the object's axis in the foveal field of view (Binford, 1971). The persistent problem of how to separate a complex surface shape into component parts has been solved in part by considering silhouettes outlined in two-dimensional images. The procedure involves identifying points along the silhouette where parts intersect (Hoffman & Richards, 1984). The object image is then derived by examining the intrinsic geometry of its surfaces. The structure may also be depicted as a graph whose nodes correspond to parts or properties of the structure with its spatial relations established by linking the nodes at the edges.

As illustrated in Figure 2–10, the relative sizes of parts, colinearity of points or lines, curvilinearity of arcs, symmetry, parallelism, and how axes join in space (Biederman, 1986; Marr & Nishihara, 1978) have each been identified as possible primitive components in visual perception. Neisser (1963) showed that the contrast between straight and curved edges enables a letter, such as Z, to be perceived faster when it is embedded in a field of curved distractors, such as C and Q, than when it is among letters with straight segments, such as N and W. Visual perception is biased toward symmetry (King, Meyer, Tangney, & Biederman, 1976), and the degree of symmetry is distinctively perceived (Pomeranz, 1978).

Binford (1981) suggested that the major function of eye movement is to determine coterminous edges. This belief was supported by Perkins (1983) who found that when vertices formed a central angle in a polyhedron, the surfaces were almost always interpreted as meeting at right angles as long as none of the angles were less than 90°. This bias was even stronger among subjects with less exposure to carpentered (right-angled) environments than Westerners (Perkins & Deregowski, 1982). Vertices with three segments, such as a Y and an arrow, and their curved counterparts are important in determining volumetric or planar components. An infinite degree of variability exists in aspect ratio, degree of curvature for curved components, and departure from parallelism for nonparallel components. Variations over two or three levels across four of the components can capture the essence of a broad range of shapes, however (Biederman, 1986). The ratio is the most important variation.

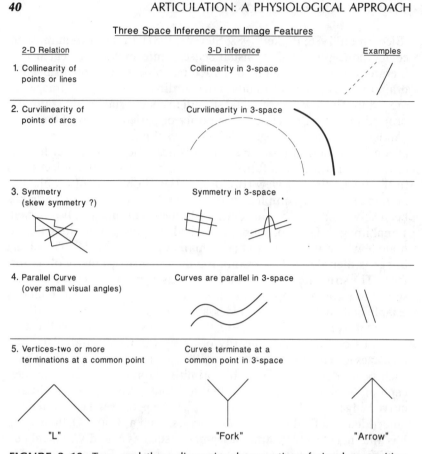

FIGURE 2-10. Two- and three-dimensional properties of visual recognition. From Biederman, I. (1986). Recognition by components: A theory of visual pattern recognition. *The Psychology of Learning and Motivation, 20,* 9. Reprinted by permission.

Attention plays a special role in all three avenues of speech perception. A single feature can often be detected with no effect from the number of distracting items in the visual field although target detection time increases linearly with the number of distractors. The ability to maintain attention despite sometimes conflicting features has led to the theory that a human can attend all positions in a visual display simultaneously and with unlimited capacity for a single feature (e.g., blue points representing sensors *or* sibilant groove width in a palatometric video display). It is important to note, however, that when a pattern is defined by a series of features, the visual system can only examine one of them in a display at a time (Treisman & Gelade, 1980).

The ability to rotate three-dimensional shapes mentally suggests that the visual system is able to manipulate images in a continuous manner using an internal representation of a seen object which captures salient part-whole relations (see Shephard, 1981). Biederman (1986) hypothesized that the largest, most diagnostically relevant component, such as the fuselage and wing on an airplane, provides primal access in recognizing a complete object. Objects furnishing more diagnostic component combinations would be identified more rapidly than simple ones. He also notes that the principles of Gestalt psychology suggest that if the components of an object can be recovered in noisy or perturbed conditions, they should be recognizable through functions such as contour restoration. Errors are explained as originating in the mapping of perceptual input onto a schema based on regular primitives. Slight irregularities are coded as the closest regular neighbor of that form. An additional code is added to represent an irregularity. This process was described by Bartlett (1932) in his "schema with correction." Biederman (1986) showed that when contours of an object are deleted in such a way as to remove the prime components, the object is virtually impossible to identify. The subjects in his study were still able to recover objects in which the contour deletions retained recoverable components, but the process required additional time, and the image had to be present.

Research has shown that for accurate "homing in" on a target the predominant benefits of visual perception are contributed during the final phase of a movement (Magill, 1989). That is, visual feedback may not be as important during the early part of a movement but may be critical during the later parts. This hypothesis was tested by Moore (1984) by varying visual feedback during the initial 25%, 50%, 60%, 65%, and 100% of a 400 millisecond aiming response. She found that the magnitude of error did not increase when vision was not available during the first half of the response, but under all other conditions, accuracy decreased dramatically when vision was blocked during the last half. These findings were replicated in a later study by Beaubaton and Hay (1986) who added conditions in which vision was blocked during the terminal part of the response. Again, vision was not crucial during the initial movement but was strongly affected by accuracy in its final phase.

This discussion suggests a number of stringencies that may be applied to use vision to its maximum potential in palatometric training. These stringencies include seating the subject so the gaze is focused easily on movements in the central part of the retina, using the concept of colinearity to establish contact-nocontact boundaries in the lingua-palatal contact patterns generated during sound production, focusing attention on only one articulatory feature within the action field at a time, centering prime attention on final-phase movements as a targeted posture is approached, referencing the action location to known landmarks such as the dentition and the palatal arch as part-whole relationships are established, and tying the visually extracted information directly to parallel oral sensations.

SENSORY INTEGRATION AND MOTOR PROGRAM SPECIFICATION

The schema model of speech assumes that auditory, vocal tract, and visual sensations are extracted in parallel and linked together to define articulatory gesture perception at every level of representation from linguapalatal contact to the geometry of sound production. As portrayed in Figure 2–2, this information is acquired and integrated under the talker's executive control. In other words, it is previewed and sifted. What is retained depends in part on the individual's inherent ability to discern important elements in an action pattern, in part on the current stage of development, and in part by interest at the moment.

Some general principles may be stated regarding the integration of auditory, oral, and visual sensations in speech production. First, although it is possible to carry out articulatory movements in the absence of either auditory or visual feedback, noticeable degradation in movement precision may be expected when external feedback is unavailable, particularly in complex maneuvers. Second, the amount of degradation seems to be related to the movement duration. Very fast, ballistic-like movements, as in stop consonant production, seem to be affected less by lack of feedback than those of longer duration, such as the vowels. Third, tactile/kinesthetic and visual feedback play potentially parallel roles in articulatory movement perception and in guiding articulatory trajectories toward targeted positions. For instance, initially palatometric feedback may be used along with oral sensations to establish a stable lateral linguapalatal contact preparatory posture for an upcoming articulatory task. The resulting stability afforded by the lateral contact posture subsequently enables the talker's prime attention to be focused on the intricacies of articulation. This situation in turn enables movement adaptations to be introduced rapidly and accurately to fit the phonetic demands of the system at the moment. Depending on the length of time available, these two functions could be activated in an oral and auditory and/or visual feedforward or feedback manner as particular tasks are repeated and schemata accuracy refined. Feedback information would be expected to serve a particularly important role in both activating and homing-in functions during some open-closed loop combinations.

How individuals move from executive control to the central verbal schemata is age dependent. Bruner (1964) suggested that as children mature they move from reliance on motoric information to sensory or perceptual codes and finally to the speech symbolic code[1]. In this linkage, it is possible to distinguish the *idea* behind an utterance from the *plan* used to carry it out in executive control functions. When stimulating conditions are such that an utterance is motivated (the idea), a schema (the plan) is retrieved from the memory of previous utterances. The schema includes a long-term memory record of past utterances with syntactic, morphological, and phonological rules used to organize its execution. In the schema, articulation movements performed and consequent communication results are intimately associated with speech goals stored in a motor memory bank. Lexical memory is applied to retrieve appropriate words that meet the specific communication goals of the talker.

Dual coding theory (Clark & Paivio, 1987; Paivio, 1971) provides an interesting viewpoint that is relevant to speech perception and ultimately to speech production. This theory splits the "central verbal schema" into separate verbal and nonverbal symbolic processing systems (see Figure 2-11). Verbal-related representations, called *logogens* by Morton (1979), are organized around vocal properties with rules derived from a language context. These abstractions bear little resemblance to the things they stand for. They are exemplified by phonemes that can be isolated or combined in a variety of ways to generate new meaningful units. The meanings for these entities are determined by central associations with other events and by their temporal or serial order (e.g., "John hit" differs from "hit John"). Temporal constraint is demonstrated by an inability to verbalize more than one sound or word at the same time. We cannot say "John" and "hit" or even [n] and [t] at exactly the same moment in time.

Nonverbal representations provide the other half of the dual code. These representations draw heavily from visual and vocal tract sensations. Their principle elements are called *imagens*. The distinctive property of imagens is that they are stored as integrated, continuous, analogue or holistic patterns in visual or oral space. Imagens may be thought of as a hierarchical collection of parts. They are rarely recombined, but do occur as nested elements in other imagens. For example, an imagen for "nose" is nested within a "face" imagen and includes a

---

[1]If development of phonetic categories follows concept formation, the developmental sequence described would suggest that individuals could have more difficulty in ferreting out the crucial information in visual articulatory displays derived from spatially encoded information than from naturally perceived articulatory gestures.

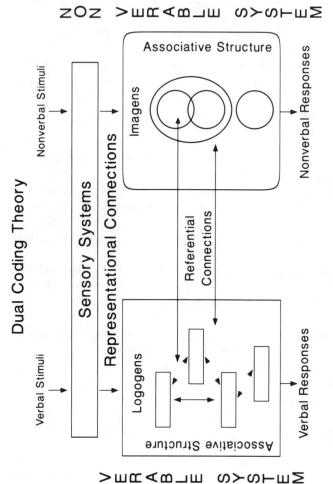

FIGURE 2-11. Verbal and nonverbal processing. Clark, J. M. & Paivio, A. (1987). A dual coding perspective on encoding process. In M. A. McDaniel & M. Pressley (Eds.), *Imagery and related mnemonic processes* (p. 7). New York: Springer-Verlag. Reprinted by permission.

"nostril" imagen. The continuous, analogue property of an imagen is illustrated by smooth spatial restoration of the whole when parts are missing. For example, we recognize a person from a glimpse of the face and can readily imagine spatial changes such as a smile or frown within a facial image. Imagens also have a synchronous or parallel property not present in logogens. Complex concepts that require many words to describe, such as a person with a "bloody nose," can be pictured by a single imagen. Finally, imagens are not arbitrary. They retain some of the object's perceptual properties and are therefore isomorphic with the things they stand for.

Multiple referential connections develop between the verbal and nonverbal systems as a consequence of increasingly complex experiences with objects and their names. The cartoon-like puzzle figures developed by Gibb (1985) and used to study novel English word learning (Gibb, 1985; Kiernan & Swisher, 1990) provide an example of the utility of these interconnections. Such between-systems connections activate joint verbal and nonverbal processing, sometimes in coordinated and complementary rather than *retroflex* fashion, as in imaging words and naming pictures. Most of our reactions to words and objects are composite or aggregate representations activated by direct external stimulation, with responses that spread to internal associative and image pathways. For instance, the word "nose" can activate a "part of the body" verbal identity or a "boxer with a bloody nose" image. By the same token, an image of a pseudopalate showing linguapalatal contact around its entire outer border could activate a "stop consonant" phonetic identity to a clinician or "standard posture" to a subject experienced in palatometry. To a more sophisticated clinician, the stop consonant percept would also include the notion that this stance or posture represents only a brief moment in a moving articulation sequence hinged at the lateral palatal shelves.

The verbal and nonverbal processes are bidirectional. For example, initially the abstract word "fiscal" could be transformed into the associated word "money." Later, the person may recall either the word "money" or a visual image of money. One of the basic notions derived from this bidirectionality is that individuals can move easily and accurately back and forth. Visual articulatory images and oral gestures could thus presumably be interchangeable and in the process common elements could be extracted to guide and ultimately govern speech development and production.

After sensory information activates executive control, an appropriate schema is selected from central memory to specify an *articulatory plan.* In this plan, movement strategies are set into play with special motor programming functions that incorporate phonotactic and syntactic rules. Grammatical and phonological encoding are added to provide lexical form as the rules are applied in utterances (Levelt, 1989). Specific phonetic and articulatory movement strategies, adapted to fit the individual talker's unique physical attributes, are also added to the plan. Perkell (1979) notes for instance that subjects with deeper palates generally have greater changes in linguapalatal contact and tongue height during speech than those with shallower palates.

The notion of *coordinate structures* will be introduced at this point to help us understand how complex movement patterns can be executed without overwhelming the encoding and response system. The coordinative structure concept was introduced by Bernstein (1967) and Greene (1972) to solve central storage and working space problems.

Rapid, continuous movement in activities such as speech production suggests the need for a motor control system with subsystems that would allow lower level organizations to control individual movement components. That remarkably complex processing tasks imputed to the brain can be performed by lower neural structures is indicated by such observations as those reported by Sechenov (1863/1965). He catalogued the complex adaptive behavior of a decapitated frog. After the frog had recovered from the shock of its head being cut off, it adopted a normal standing posture and leaped away from noxious stimuli with a jump that was proportional to the intensity of the stimulus. If the animal were suspended and pricked on the stomach, the leg ipsilateral to the prick would knock the offending instrument away. If acid were applied to the same skin, the leg would wipe at the stimulated area. If that leg were now amputated, the same defensive actions would be executed by the contralateral leg. The processes involved in performance of such responses are seen as intrinsic properties of the coordinative structure that embodies them (Easton, 1972). Relegating the details of an action to a lower level of coordination reduces the load on higher neural centers. The coordinative structure system is conceived as a multistage function in which each level controls the level below it thereby systematically reducing demands on executive control.

The Articulation Program

Following the basic coordinative structure concept, specific articulatory postures are viewed as controlled at the peripheral level by biomechanical properties and mechanical possibilities of the articulators (Ostry & Munhall, 1985). One of the notable advances in physiology understanding is the growing appreciation of the need for large neuron populations to control complex muscle functions (Henneman, 1990). Muscles must be capable of developing a wide range of tensions quickly and exactly. To do this, combinations of a large assortment of contractile units finely graded in size are available. The smallest cells in each pool supply muscle fiber groups that conduct impulses slowly, fatigue little, and develop small tensions. Progressively larger motoneurons innervate stronger motor units that conduct impulses more rapidly and fatigue more quickly (Henneman & Mendell, 1981). The intensities of the total inputs impinging on cells with different excitabilities then determine which ones are fired and what combinations result. Stronger inputs discharge successively bigger motoneurons, adding larger increments of tension to the total muscle force exerted. A particular cell in this fixed hierarchy fires only if all the lower ranking cells in the pool discharge with it. Total muscle tension is, therefore, controlled with maximum precision, and sustained strong contraction is retained longer and at a higher level because of the greater fatigue resistance of the smaller motor units in the active population. In emergencies, or special circumstances, this rank-ordered control process can be overridden.

The anatomy of the vocal tract provides a highly constrained, three-dimensional framework for coordinated articulation movements. Tract variables associated with a particular set of articulatory gestures are again conceived as organized within structured tiers, such as the lips and the tip and body of the tongue. Browman and Goldstein (1987) have shown that these tiers may be modeled by separate dynamic equations which represent integrated movements within an articulatory gesture. Concurrent gestures are then synchronized under the spatial and temporal control of the system. Once movement is begun, positions are normalized and timed for specific consonant-vowel gestures by minimum and maximum positions within normal movement ranges. This approach abandons the concept that linguistic units are abstract mental entities. Instead, lawful regularities with observable parameters are expected to govern the articulatory structure of speech (Nittrouer, Munhall, Kelso, Tuller, & Harris, 1988).

In the coordinative structure concept, phonological contrast is realized as stable spatiotemporal functions of articulatory gestures. Löfqvist and Yoshioka (1981) observed that laryngeal and oral articulatory gestures are precisely coordinated with respect to the aerodynamic requirements of speech production. For example, peak glottal opening occurs earlier during fricative sounds than during unaspirated stops. It is systematically delayed with respect to stop implosion duration during aspirated stops. Post aspirated stops have larger glottal openings than their preaspirated and unaspirated cognates. Similarly, Wood (1986) reported that in production of the rounded vowel [y], larynx depression complements the lip rounding. Moderate lip rounding, a prepalatal tongue position, and a depressed larynx are all used to differentiate the [y] from its near neighbor [i]. Tongue blade elevation reinforces the larynx depression effect. All of these observations presuppose the operation of a sophisticated speech motor control system.

Nittrouer and her associates (1988) produced evidence that the intersegmental organization of articulatory gestures is a function of the utterance being produced. Phonetic segments may therefore be specified by parameters such as the time period between flanking vowels rather than simply by articulation targets that can change with the context of an utterance (Tuller & Kelso, 1984). This allows the gestures to overlap in varying degrees at all organization levels by regulating the relative timing of movements associated with any stable segment. The Nittrouer et al. data (1988) suggested further that intersegmental articulatory gestures vary "systematically and discretely as a function of the exact utterance being produced" (p. 1660).

There has been a tendency in past descriptions of central speech motor plans to expect them to prescribe all or most of the articulatory details. Developments in motor control theory have made this viewpoint less attractive. As described in Fugimura's iceberg model (1986), commands in the articulatory plan are now thought to involve only *context free* or *invariant* aspects of motor execution. The gestures themselves include the pathways through which articulators move in vocal tract space to execute specified utterances. Studies of actual speech production show clear commonalities under different modes of execution. Kent and Moll (1972) observed, for instance, that articulatory movements of the tongue are highly regular in form even when they serve different phonetic goals. For example, the tongue body movement between [i] and [ɑ] was shown to be essentially unaffected by the presence or absence of an intervocalic consonant.

Context-dependent neuromuscular implementation of an articulation program is accomplished by the highly self-regulating neuromuscular system as the articulatory plan is implemented (Gallistel, 1985). This mechanism is an important consideration. It is thought to work as follows: The higher central nervous system levels of the motor system preset the lower centers for movement in terms of movement parameters and sequences. Final tuning then takes place as the planned movement is executed (Marteniuk & MacKenzie, 1980). Without context-dependent processes, a different motor program would be required for each execution. This requirement would produce an immense drain on information-processing resources in motor planning (Levelt, 1989).

Special spatiotemporal articulatory parameters are added at the speech-planning stage to ensure that vocal tract goals are achieved. For example, lateral linguapalatal fixator postures could be specified at the planning stage to ensure lingual stability and control during rapidly executed, reciprocal articulatory activities. Provision must also be made to adapt conflicting and blending gestural requirements across sound sequences and add pitch and loudness qualities to the utterance. After such contingencies, the articulatory plan is relayed to the muscles where the actions are tuned by the neuromuscular system as they are executed.

The articulatory plan is likely not relayed to the musculature sequentially as gestures are generated. As suggested by Levelt (1989), the plan is probably stored in a temporary articulation buffer to be retrieved later in successive inner speech chunks.[2] Also, the motor commands would likely not be identical each time a sound sequence is spoken. No two movements are exactly alike. If certain movements are hampered, the action does not cease. A general plan appears to be specified then adapted to fit the current articulatory goal as it unfolds (see Fletcher, under review, b).

The verbal schema concept includes upgrading the developing central speech schema as an inherent function of executing the articulatory plan. As it is retrieved from the buffer to execute a stipulated set of articulatory gestures, an expected dimensional image or "perceptual trace" (Adams, 1971) of the motor outcome is thought to be produced. This image is relayed to the signal and parameter comparator. In the comparator, expected articulatory properties are matched with what we hear, see, feel, and discern from evidence of listener-perceived meanings. Discrepancies between expected and actual results, or consequences, are then evaluated qualitatively and quantitatively and perceived shortcomings fed back to the central speech schema memory to be rationalized. The articulatory gestures in the schema and motor programs defining the action sequences are then updated and elaborated to bring expected and actual outputs into congruence for future utterances.

Articulatory postures are considered to be the ultimate primitive units established and coordinated in speech. Combinations of the postures into articulatory gestures provide the dynamic basis of speech production (Nittrouer, Studdert-Kennedy, & McGowan, 1989). Browman and Goldstein (1987) have shown that the coordinated gestural movements of the articulators can be characterized using dynamic equations. Phonemes and their identifying articulatory features are formed as abstract products of the postures, gestures, and action sequences as articulatory routines are established.

Phonological development is seen as a process of diversifying articulatory routines to encompass an increasing number of contrasting

---

[2]See also Miller (1956) for a discussion of speech "chunking" and McNeil (1987) for further consideration of the role that inner speech may play in articulatory planning. The idea of chunking is that grouping sounds, or written representations of sounds, into larger and more meaningful sets (words or sentences) would enable the items to be recalled and/or manipulated more easily in motor memory. The capacity of short-term memory is thought to be about seven chunks.

sounds. This process occurs in parallel with learning phonotactic constraints that limit where sounds may occur within words.

In young children, the speech schema seems to develop from the bottom up: from body sensations, to imagery, to abstract concepts (Bellezza, 1987). Speech skills are acquired globally then abstract rules including articulatory features are derived (Macnamara, 1972). To crack the speech code, youthful learners likely form general hypotheses about uses that utterances might serve in interpersonal communication. They then experiment with different vocal patterns to test their hypotheses (Wells, 1985). Through this process, sublinguistic oral postures merge into prephonetic gestures and subsequently into structured articulatory sequences with recognizable words in spoken language. In the central schema, separate actions become subsumed under a general plan that coordinates them with little overt attention by the talker.

THE TALKER

Perception and production skills do not develop in isolation. Many facets of phonetic discrimination appear to be inborn. Phonetic recognition matures gradually as the child actively scans incoming sights and sounds in the environment and discerns systematic relations between words heard and seen on the face of the talker. The talker's primary aim is successful communication. To this end phonetic choices and sequences are directed by the needs of both the talker and the listener. Perceptually determined constraints on articulation such as postures, gestures, and rhythmic cues that facilitate segmentation of words in an utterance are remarkably pervasive in the production process (Cutler, 1987). Meanings are then assigned to the composite phonetic output.

There is considerable evidence that initially the child does not get a complete picture of the word he or she has begun to learn (Ingram, 1974; Macken, 1979; Menn, 1982). The child cannot always distinguish similar words from each other, and unfamiliar words tend to be heard as familiar ones. These fuzzy concepts bias tests of word recognition and increase the difficulty of ascertaining what the child's understanding really is and what roles vocal experiences play in verbal meaning as we seek to track progress in the developing lexicon.[3]

The child's ability to assign meaning to words seen and heard is typically well ahead of the ability to manipulate articulatory gestures

---

[3]"Lexicon" denotes "a collection of stored, accessible, memorized bits of information about sounds and meanings of words, and/or their component meaningful parts" (Menn, 1982, p. 8.)

and achieve phonetic contrasts in sound production. The talker's primary aim is successful communication. To this end, phonetic choices and sequences are directed by both the desires of the talker and the needs of the listener. Perceptually determined constraints on articulation such as rhythmic cues that facilitate segmentation of words in an utterance are remarkably pervasive in the production process (Cutler, 1987). Menn (1982) has observed that as early as 15 months of age a child may not even attempt to say words with "adult sounds" he cannot produce. Fortunately, this reticence to try difficult-to-produce words is normally short lived. Schwartz and Leonard (1982) showed that the avoidance of sounds the child perceives to be difficult can be demonstrated experimentally in children who have fewer than 50 words (near the onset of speech), but not in older children. This example provides a clear illustration of the tenet that recognition may precede articulatory production by many months.

Menn (1982) suggests that avoidance of the more difficult articulatory patterns indicates that two forms may be stored centrally for each word: a recognition form and a production form. Macken (1979) traces the sound recognition to phonetic production sequence as follows: The child first recognizes sounds in a word but cannot produce them well. The input representation has developed but not the output skill. Through practice, the child begins to bring production into line with the target pattern. Children may still fail to gain skill in producing particular words or sets of words, however. Menn suggests that this failure may be traced to difficulties in either of two stages of correct sound production skills. In the first stage, trial-and-error attempts are thought to be used to match a sound sequence. For each sound some children succeed; others fail. Success depends in part on factors such as the clarity of the adult model, how often the sound is experienced in the environment, how salient the sound has become to the particular child, as well as the physical complexity of the sound. The accidental aspect of integrating all of these potential sources of error in phonetic learning could account for the variability across children in acquiring adult sounds. The general order of phonetic development across children clearly indicates, however, that most children follow a rather "natural" order of sound acquisition. This suggests that the order is largely based on physiologically governed ease of production.

The second stage of sound acquisition involves perceiving the essence of articulatory successes and extracting generalized "rules" that can be tried in new situations. A trial-and-error success does not always lead to a rule, however. A child may try dozens of sound patterns before he or she captures the essence of imbedded successes (Menn, 1982), or a rule may emerge rapidly. Additionally, the rules that are formed may not always be adequate. A child may accept an early rendition of a sound even when it is not accurate. Macken (1979) suggests that such maintenance of an old mispronunciation may indicate that the child has replaced his original input representation gleaned from adult standards with a new one based on his own input. He assumes incorrectly that his internalized schema for the sound is now correct. In this instance, the expectation may bias perception, stifle self-monitoring, and retard rule modification for a time. On the other hand, since the acquisition of speech is a problem-solving task, children often go off by themselves to practice new sounds (Weir, 1962) or whisper new words or sounds to themselves (Leopold, 1939). In the usual process, these and other strategies enable the child to gradually increase the number of articulatory parameters that are manipulated freely and the number of values each parameter can be assigned. The new strategies, in turn, allow the child to recall stored articulatory patterns for words in their canonical form and plug these values into the articulatory output. The richness and accuracy of this information in the central articulatory program thus dictates both the range of possible phons that can be produced intelligibly in words and how to link the articulatory gestures together in polysyllabic sequences.

Older individuals with well-established schemata appear to approach learning tasks from the top down (Norman & Bobrow, 1976). They are presumed to use past experience to generate a model or template that dictates how feedback should be heard, seen, and felt when articulatory movements are performed correctly (Sage, 1984). Only when discrepancies are sensed is the central program altered. Feedback seems to be used to check the output until acceptable responses are established or re-established (Summers, 1981). Mature talkers thus appear to build new concepts with a minimum amount of sensory input by using mnemonic structures stored in memory schemas (Pressley, Borkowski, & Schneider, 1987). Simple verbal rehearsal declines markedly with age while the use of special strategies, such as elaborating word meanings in new sentences, increases with linguistic experience (Ericcson & Simon, 1983).

Phonetic percepts and actions demand a *form* that differentiates articulatory dimensions from mere representations of spatially oriented sensations and externally perceived configurations. For a phonetic label to be appropriately applied, the actions must have common properties that group oral, auditory, and visual sensations together in equivalent forms. The descriptions must also be sufficiently detailed to distinguish specific actions within phonetically differentiated events. It is not sufficient for talkers to learn which articulatory cues are properties of a prototype sound. They must also learn what articulatory variations can be tolerated within phonetic categories. Because of this stringency, training routines must include a range of articulatory samples, preferably from different speakers, that represent normal as well as natural articulatory variations within the phonetic categories being learned. Once differentiated, the oral, visual, and auditory sensations can yield stable phonetic percepts by being repeatedly encountered in words heard from different speakers and produced in different contexts.

A pool of special strategies that enables talkers to adapt quickly and accurately to unique speaking conditions takes time to develop. The use of the most efficient strategies is only occasionally found in young children (Pressley & Levin, 1977).

The availability of efficient, automatically applied articulatory strategies frees talkers to concentrate their attention on utterance meanings. One of the sources of phonetic meaning is posited to be articulatory distinctions found to be relevant and useful. These distinctions are thought to be registered in the developing articulatory schemata that code and preserve relations between oral sensations and auditorily and visually derived spatial patterns. During maturation, the percept thus becomes as much a function of what the individual knows about articulation as it is of the spatial properties of the oral sensations and associated feedback.

McCarty and Hamlet (1977) sought to determine to what extent phonetic judgments correspond with actual physiologic events. They first used electropalatographic procedures to document how two adult speakers normally produced the consonants [t, d, s, z, n, l, ʃ, r, j, k, g] followed by the neutral vowel [ʌ]. They then repeated the procedure with the subjects producing the same CV syllables in two different ways. In one case, the consonants [t, d, s, z, n, l] that were normally produced with linguapalatal contact just in front of the alveolar-palate ridge were articulated with a retracted or retroflexed tongue position. The other sounds, which were normally produced with contact behind the alveolar ridge, were spoken with contact on the ridge. In other words, the normal alveolar and palatal place of articulation was reversed for the two sets of sounds. In each instance, the speakers attempted to have the syllables sound normal for an English speaker. In the second experimental condition, the speakers produced common distorted versions of the sounds, such as lisping sibilants and dentalized stops while still retaining the phonetic identity of the consonants. The normal, articulation reversed, and distorted syllables were then replayed to 10 listener judges who had had at least one course in phonetics. They were asked to mark a plus on the score sheet if they thought the consonant they heard had been produced with anterior linguapalatal contact or a minus if nonanterior. Judgments were identified as correct when the place identified agreed with the physiological data. The mean number of incorrect judgments when the syllables were produced normally was 2.8. When the articulation place was reversed, the mean incorrect judgments rose to 16.5 errors. It dropped to 5.7 for the syllables in the distorted articulation category. The investigators concluded that the large number of errors in the second category indicated that the actual place of articulation was not accurately perceived. When the syllables sounded normal, the judges apparently assumed that the articulation was normal and scored them accordingly. These findings also suggest that during the formative years phonetic concepts would likely depend heavily on articulatory confirmation of auditorily perceived differences.

Separated into its most primitive features, the speech percept can be thought of as a series of *oral images* that in total define the *essence* of contrastive articulatory gestures. The necessary articulatory images would not be expected to be fully constructed upon first exposure to a spoken word. In usual circumstances, accurate production would be expected to evolve as articulatory postures, gestures, and action patterns in words are sensed orally, auditorily, and visually. The images would become progressively elaborated in the course of continuing experience with manipulating the elemental postures and gestures and observing outcomes as words, phrases, and sentences are produced and repeated in different contexts. Palatometric displays may thus be thought of as providing one form of spatially relevant images that could aid a learner in perceiving articulatory change as movements are underway. They also provide a means of helping the learner evaluate the degree of success attained as actions are developed through mimicry. Ultimately, success is defined by the extent to which articulation patterns produced duplicate articulatory characteristics of mature speech *and* the output fits listener perceived phonetic patterns of normal talkers.

CHAPTER 3

EXPOSING THE ARTICULATORY SYSTEM

A tacit belief in speech training is that "to teach a speech sound target one should 'know' how the sound is made" (Klein, Lederer, & Cortese, 1991, p. 559). Efforts to achieve that goal face three major barriers: (a) most of the information about speech production is concealed within nonvisible parts of the vocal tract; (b) a one-to-one relationship does not exist between what we hear and what is actually happening within the mouth during speech production; and (c) untrained ears don't hear the same thing as trained ears, and trained ears tend to hear what the listener expects. True, impressions can be checked by careful comparisons across observations by different phoneticians, but such observations are subjective and must still be checked objectively.

Special technology, such as moving picture and video recordings, has helped increase the validity and objectivity of open-mouth observations. Other technologies have been developing rapidly that may be used to check beliefs about unseen articulatory actions. Some of these will now be briefly reviewed to provide insight into the scope of technology becoming available for objective speech observations.

Zemer (1985) observed that as new technology and procedures evolve, the reports describing their functions and usefulness seem to progress through four stages. At first, results are evaluated in anecdotal descriptions. As the new modality becomes established, it tends to be touted as superior to all others. In the third developmental phase, technological shortcomings begin to emerge and a backlash occurs. Finally, as the instrumentation and usage procedures mature, their effectiveness and utility are assessed realistically.

In the past, the most common way to try to overcome the barrier of phonetic subjectivity in speech studies has been through acoustical observations. Increasingly powerful acoustical analysis procedures have rewarded this effort. They are reaching their mature stage of development. The search for physiological procedures is now underway to verify the accuracy of predictions from acoustic inference to physical speech functions. The use of x-rays has played a major role in these efforts.

X-RAYS

X-ray was discovered rather serendipitously in 1895 by Wilhelm Konrad von Roentgen. The following account by a *McClure's* magazine reporter (Dam, 1896) describes the discovery:

"Now, professor, will you tell me the history of the discovery?"

"There is no history," Roentgen replied. "I have been for a long time interested in the problem of the cathode rays from a vacuum tube, as studied by Herz and Lenard. I had followed theirs, and others researches [sic] with great interest, and determined, as soon as I had time, to make some researches of my own. I had been at work for some days when I discovered something new."

"What was the date?"

"The eighth of November."

"And what was the discovery?"

"I was working with a Crookes tube covered by a shield of black cardboard. A piece of barium platinocyanide paper lay on the bench there. I had been passing a current through the tube, and I noticed a peculiar black line across the paper."

"What of it?"

"The effect was one which could only be produced, in ordinary parlance, by the passing of light. No light could come from the tube, because the shield which covered it was impervious to any light known, even that of the electric arc."

"And what did you think?"

"I did not think; I investigated. I assumed that the effect must come from the tube, since its character indicated that it could come from nowhere else. I tested it. In a few minutes there was no doubt about it. Rays were coming from the tube which had a luminous effect upon the paper. I tried it at greater and greater distances, even at two metres. It seemed at first a new kind of invisible light. It was clearly something new; something unrecorded." (pp. 412–413)

This new ray, given the symbol "x" for an unknown quantity, immediately became a powerful tool for understanding biological structure and function. Its use took on new significance as ways to measure different shapes and postures portrayed in radiographic images evolved. Particularly accurate and structurally detailed descriptions were found to be possible from full size, single frame, "still"[1] x-rays.

In the same year as Roentgen discovered x-rays, 1895, the first motion picture was described. Within a few months, x-ray and cinematography technologies were combined in cinefluorography. Still x-ray procedures have since been used to study steady-state speech functions and postures (Russell, 1928; Scheier, 1898). Cinefluorographic procedures have evolved for information about fleeting actions and movement patterns that characterize speech (Fletcher, Shelton, Smith, & Bosma, 1960; Moll, 1960; Subtelny, Pruzansky, & Subtelny, 1957).

Although x-ray provides a powerful means of probing speech production, two major problems have prevented its potential from being fully realized. The first is that it converts three dimensional functions into two-dimensional images. This limited perspective has led to some important misconceptions about speech articulation properties. For example, the commonly held belief that vowels are produced without contact between the tongue and palate is directly attributable to lateral-view, midline x-ray descriptions.

The principal reason that the budding interest in x-rays for speech studies waned rather rapidly is the accumulating evidence of radiation risk. An x-ray beam consists of a stream of radioactive photons. Images are obtained by directing the stream of photons toward a specific area of the body. Body tissues absorb the photons in varying degrees. The image is a record of the relative number of photons absorbed compared with those that complete the transit through the tissues and change the photon-sensitive videofluoroscopic screen or chemicals on the surface of an x-ray film. The kilovoltage (kV) and milliamperage (mA) levels of the radiographic system are adjusted to regulate penetration through the structures being examined. For speech articulation studies, the settings are adjusted so that the muscular articulators absorb more photons than the more open vocal tract areas but less than the bony structures. Normally the kV and mA levels are set so that bone will absorb virtually all of the photons. Bony structures are then represented by clear areas on the x-ray plate after the film is chemically processed. Soft tissues are displayed in different shades of grey depending

---

[1]The use of the word "still" simply means that the person maintains a steady-state position of the structure being examined during the period of time when the x-ray is being taken. In speech, this is usually achieved by prolonging the sound.

on their thickness and opacity. Since all of the shades of grey represent special properties of the structures exposed, computer-based procedures can be used to enhance the images and maximize soft tissue differentiation within selected structures. Open vocal tract passages allow the photons to pass through unimpeded. They are black on the processed film.

Laminography, or *tomography*, is a special type of x-ray procedure used to examine structure and function within a limited body layer. Laminograms are obtained by locating an individual or part of the body between a moving photon emitter and a moving x-ray plate. The depth of focus is set so that only structures a certain distance from the emitter are in focus. The plate and beam movements blur information from structures above and below the selected narrow focus (e.g., 1 cm) plane. The resulting laminograms are particularly useful in situations where information is needed about functions that are normally concealed by surrounding structures. Because of the need to maintain the structure imaged at a constant distance from the laminographic beam focus, this technique is appropriate only for postures such as those during sustained vowels in which organ positions can be maintained in the same position during more prolonged time periods.

The use of x-ray microbeam technology is among the latest developments in radiographic observations. It was introduced specifically to reduce radiation exposure in speech articulation studies (see Fujimura, Kiritani, & Ishida, 1969; Kiritani, Itoh, Imagawa, Fujisaki, & Sawashima, 1975; Nadler & Abbs, 1988). Reduced radiation is accomplished in microbeam x-ray by using a high acceleration voltage (150 kV) with a low current (1mA) target focus. An electromagnetic beam deflector with a pinhole aperture is then used to form a narrow beam of about 10^7 photons per second reaching the detector. The emerging photon beam is aimed under computer control at gold pellets attached on the tongue or other articulator surface. The shadows cast by the pellets as the photons pass through the subject are detected by an ultraefficient scintillation counter. A computer then locates the beads within the X-Y field. A number of points can be imaged in parallel. Tissue absorption is low, because it is necessary only to image the pellets, not soft tissues.

Awareness of the fact that radiation contamination damages tissues, and the residuum from natural and unnatural radiation sources accumulates throughout the lifetime of the individual have led to increasingly stringent prohibitions on the use of any x-ray device. The general dictum is that if equivalent data can be obtained through other means, they should be used.

ULTRASOUND AND MAGNETIC RESONANCE IMAGING

Another promising way to study speech positions and actions is through ultrasound technology (Keller & Ostry, 1983; Kelsey, Minifie, & Hixon, 1969). This technology involves generating an ultra high-frequency (1.5 to 10 megaHertz [mHz]) sound by passing a voltage through a piezoelectric crystal. This signal is then used to probe differences in body structure and function, with no apparent adverse effects.

Ultrasonic transmission through body tissues is defined by the formula $z = pc$, where z is the medium's acoustic impedance, p its density, and c its sound propagation velocity. Higher frequencies increase resolution but have less penetrating power. By carefully controlling the settings, rather subtle differences in tissue can be detected.

The basic principle of ultrasound imaging is that some ultrasonic energy is reflected back toward the transducer whenever the impedance changes during transmission of the beam. Thus, each time the beam passes from one medium to another with a different impedance some energy is reflected back. This property has been used to discriminate between individual muscle layers in the tongue (Figure 3–1) as well as to identify the distance from the submental transducer to the tongue surface (Shawker, Sonies, & Stone, 1984).

Transmission of the ultrasonic beam through air spaces is negligible for frequencies greater than 1 mHz; therefore all energy is reflected back toward the crystal transducer when the wave arrives at a tissue-air interface. The distance from the transducer to the beam reflection source is calculated by measuring the time between the ultrasound burst and the large echo from the tongue surface, assuming an average soft tissue sound speed of 1540 meters per second (m/s) (Goss, Johnston, & Dunn, 1978). By using different scan angles from a transducer located below the mandible and just in front of the hyoid bone, shapes and positions of structures such as the tongue and lateral pharyngeal walls that border the vocal tract can be defined with a measurement error of less than 1 millimeter (mm) (Kelsey, Minifie, & Hixon, 1969; Stone, Shawker, Talbot, & Rich, 1988). Data for three-dimensional tongue movement models may be obtained by using multiple scanning procedures (Watkin & Rubin, 1989). Imaging the vocal tract itself is precluded, however. The air passageway above the tongue blocks the ability to image the palate from the submental transducer location. Nor can the position of the tongue blade and tip be identified since an airway exists between the floor of the mouth and the undersurface of the tongue. Structures such as the hyoid bone and mandible are also not imageable, because their irregular shapes reflect the sound away from the transducer.

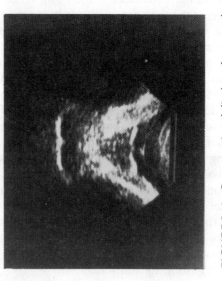

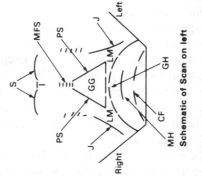

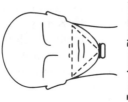

Transducer Placement

S, Tongue Surface; GG, Genioglossus; GH, Geniohyoid; MH Mylohyoid; MFS, Median Fibrous Septum; LM, Lateral Muscles; J, Jaw Inner Aspect; PS, Paramedian Septum; CF, Cervical Fascia.

Schematic of Scan on left

FIGURE 3–1. Cross-sectional display of tongue shape and muscle locations from ultrasound measures at a midtongue location. From Stone, M., Shawker, T. H., Talbot, T. L., & Rich, A. H. (1988). Cross-sectional shape during the production of vowels. *Journal of the Acoustic Society of America, 83,* 1586–1596. Reprinted by permission.

Magnetic Resonance Imaging

Magnetic resonance imaging (MRI) is another rapidly developing technology. MRI is based on the magnetic properties of atomic nuclei with an odd number of protons and neutrons. In biological studies, such images have been most easily generated from hydrogen protons (Pykett, 1982). Ordinarily, atoms behave like small, individual magnets without any general charge. They generate their small magnetic field around an electrically charged nucleus as the protons rotate like a spinning top around their own axes. When the atoms are placed within a strong static magnetic field, their dipoles reorient themselves in either a parallel (with the field) or antiparallel direction. They are not perfectly aligned, however, so the magnetism causes them to precess, or wobble, as they spin. This induces an oscillating voltage in a receiving coil which is amplified, filtered, and recorded as a magnetic resonance (MR) signal.

A second signal must be applied for the MR signal to be viewed. This is done by applying radiowaves (RF1) perpendicular to the constant magnetic force at a frequency in harmony with the atom's precessing activity. This resonant energy is absorbed by some of the lower-energy dipoles which shifts them to higher antiparallel states. These states change the net magnetization vector from the original vertical (Z axis) to a transverse (X-Y) "tilt." The degree of tilt depends on the intensity of the constant magnetic field and the time when the second signal is applied. After the RF1 force is terminated, the energized dipoles tend to return to equilibrium at tissue-specific T1 and T2 relaxation rates. As they do, a second radio frequency signal (RF2) is generated which is also picked up by the receiver coil antenna. Images are derived from interpreting the signal for density and spatial relationships. The temporal repetition time (TR) identifies the time lapse from the termination of one RF1 to the next one. T1 (spin-lattice or longitudinal relaxation time) refers to the time required for the proton spins to relax and realign with the external magnetic field. T2 (spin-spin or transverse relaxation time) identifies decay of the transverse X-Y component produced by interactions among the dipoles. By varying the radio frequency pulse conditions, the T1 or T2 weightings can be emphasized. This permits images of different appearances and informational content to be produced (Easton & Powers, 1986; Pykett, 1982).

In the MR images, structures with high hydrogen or water density are displayed in white. Empty cavities are black. Intermediate density structures are indicated by shades of grey. Bone centers are white because of their hydrogen-laden fatty marrow. The tongue and soft palate are white because of their plentiful blood supply and saliva-coated surface. Cartilage and cortical bone are relatively devoid of water; therefore they emit a low signal intensity and appear as black bands in the image. Muscles, which emit intermediate intensity signals, are grey. MRI data can thus yield important information on the general structure and cavity shapes such as tongue positions and pharyngeal cavity size.

Earlier MRI speech studies were handicapped by slowness and poor structural contrast (e.g., Baer, Gore, Boyce, & Nye, 1987), but progress in MR imaging has been rapid. The progress has recently accelerated through the introduction of echo planar imaging. Planar imaging is similar to laminographic radiology in that observations are restricted to a narrow (3 to 5 mm) strip or line of spin within the field. Ultrafast repeated scan, rapid gradient-echo imaging technology (see Wehrli, 1990) is then added. This combination has solved the major problems that have limited the use of MRI technology.

Figure 3-2 shows midsagittal images of the vocal tract recently obtained by Lakshminarayanan, Lee, and McCutcheon (1991) with a 4-second imaging time interval (TE = 10 ms, TR = 33 ms). The 4-second time span was short enough for the subject to sustain the vowels comfortably. It was long enough for the repeated recycling procedure to generate the high resolution images shown. An earlier study had demonstrated that accurate midsagittal tongue-palate distances could be obtained through MRI measures (McCutcheon, Lee, Lakshminarayanan, & Fletcher, 1990). The resolution currently attained is sufficient for direct measurements of the entire vocal tract in a steady-state position. It appears reasonable to assume that eventually the state-of-the-art will permit such images during real-time vowel and consonant studies.

Another promising MRI use is to study temporomandibular joint (TMJ) stucture and function (Helms, Richardson, Moon, & Ware, 1984; Schach & Sadowsky, 1988). In these displays the auditory meatus is shown as a rather large black area, the central marrow of the condyle as white, the articular cartilage and cortical condylar bone as black, and the muscles and bilaminar zone of the disc as grey. The disc itself is black. Thus, ll of the major landmarks are differentiable.

Possible biological side effects or complications from use of MRI with people are rather uncertain at this time. During the past decade, epidemiological evidence has indicated that electromagnetic field effects may influence living cells in a number of ways but no harmful side effects have been reported from the scan. The images it produces are similar to those from x-ray computer tomography (CT), but they do not have the ionizing radiation. Proof of possible detrimental effects is difficult because electromagnetic forces are so pervasive, emanating from such diverse sources as powerlines, household appliances, computer monitors, and microwave ovens. Some evidence suggests that EMFs

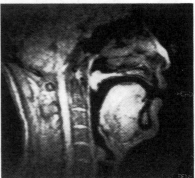
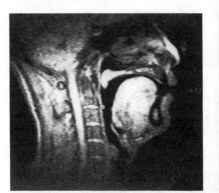
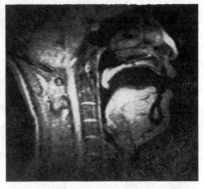
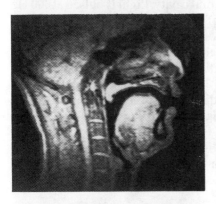
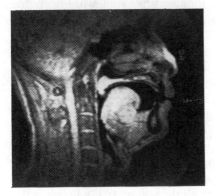

FIGURE 3–2. MR images of the vocal tract during sustained (4 sec) production of [ɪ, ɛ, æ, ɑ, ʊ] in the hVd words (a) *HEED*, (b) *HEAD*, (c) *HAD*, (d) *HOD*, and (e) *WHO'D*. From Lakshyminara-yanan, A. V., Lee, S., and McCutcheon, M. J. (1991). MR imaging of the vocal tract during vowel production. *Journal of Magnetic Resonance Imaging, 1*, 71–76. Reprinted by permission.

may have an effect only within a narrow range of exposure or temperature or strength or orientation of the particular field. It has been shown that the magnetism may interfere with the operation of a cardiac pacemaker (Pavlicek, Geisinger, & Castle, 1983). Patients wearing devices such as aneurysm clamps and orthodontic bands with ferromagnetic properties may also need to be excluded from certain studies (New et al., 1983, Schach & Sadowsky, 1988). Otherwise, the possibility of risk remains cloudy.

GLOSSOMETRY

The glossometer is another new device that promises to help fill the void left by the demise of x-ray procedures. It uses paired light-emitting diodes (LED) and photosensors to establish the distance between the tongue and palatal vault within the oral cavity. Light is pulsed at 100 Hz in rapid sequence from a series of narrow-beam LEDs mounted in small ($2 \times 3 \times 6$ mm) boxes at equidistant points along the midline of a pseudopalate (Figure 3–3). The light is scattered when it strikes the tongue surface. Some of the light reflects back to a photosensor mounted beside each LED (see Figure 3–4). The amount of reflection is approximately proportional to the distance between the tongue and the photosensor transducers, but is highly nonlinear across certain portions of the range. A lookup table is used to convert the photosensor voltages to a linearized value that is an approximate analogue of the inversely squared distance between the tongue and transducer. Use of multiple sensors enables a broad surface of the changing tongue shapes to be sensed and displayed.

The reflective properties of the tongue differ somewhat from one person to another; therefore, the glossometer transducer values must be calibrated for each user. This calibration is done by comparing the voltages generated with the user's tongue touching lightly against the lingual surface of each sensor assembly and with the tongue restrained at a known distance from the assemblies by a "tongue spacer." The spacer is worn only during calibration procedures. It consists of a molded plastic frame with an open center. Stiff, stainless steel wires mounted along the outer borders span the spacer's central opening. When the spacer is snapped over the glossometer pseudopalate, the wires prevent the tongue from rising above a certain height within the palatal vault (e.g., 188 mm from a transducer near the high point of the vault), but allow emitted and reflected light to pass freely between the tongue surface and the paired emitter-sensor assemblies. The calibration data obtained under these conditions is stored in a computer file to avoid repeating the routine during every data collection or training ses-

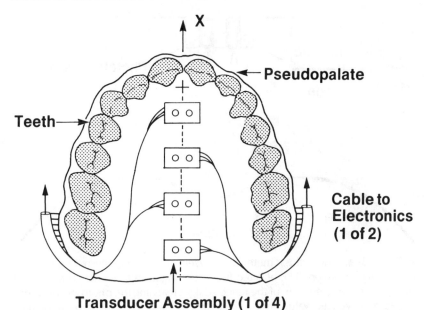

FIGURE 3–3. Glossometer transducer assemblies mounted along the pseudopalate midline surface.

sion. During use of the glossometer, data are acquired, processed, and used to generate real-time video displays at the 100 Hz rate during ongoing speech activities.

The ability to measure distances using paired LED-photosensor assemblies had been used for some time in industry before its first use in speech by Chuang and Wang (1978). Since then, the technology and procedures have been fundamentally modified and improved by Fletcher and his colleagues to arrive at an effective, practical experimental and clinical speech tool (Fletcher, 1982; Fletcher & Hasagawa, 1983; Fletcher, McCutcheon, Smith, & Smith, 1989; McCutcheon, Smith, Stilwell, & Fletcher, 1982; Smith, Fletcher, & McCutcheon, 1986).

The report by Fletcher, McCutcheon, Smith, & Smith (1989) summarizes progress to date in developing and using glossometric measures to assess tongue postures and shapes. The examples given show how a glossometer may be used to measure tongue-palate distance, calculate tongue shapes and postures within the oral cavity, and provide visual feedback for modifying tongue placement and movements during speech production. The results in both assessment and training applications are encouraging. For example, Figure 3–5 illustrates changes in the tongue position and shape during vowels spoken by one of six children who are severely to profoundly hearing impaired. Data were collected before and after daily glossometric training sessions spanning a rather brief, 3½-

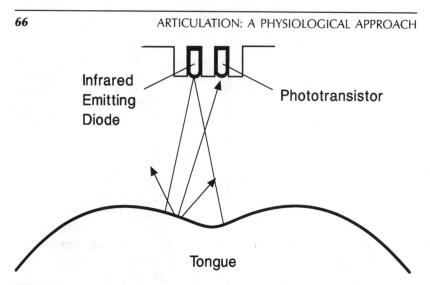

Infrared Emitting Diode

Phototransistor

Tongue

FIGURE 3–4. Single glossometer emitter/sensor assembly illustrating incident infrared light from an LED reflected from the tongue surface back to the paired photosensor. The intensity of the reflected light reaching the photosensor is converted to a voltage value from which to calculate the tongue-pseudopalate distance.

week period (see Fletcher, Dagenais, & Critz-Crosby, 1991a). It may be seen that prior to the training this girl used the same tongue posture for all vowels. The glossometric plots following the training showed changes in both the tongue and its position within the oral cavity. When the posttraining tongue positions were ranked by height, they fit the expected [i, u, æ, ɑ) vowel order. It should be noted that although these changes are physiologically impressive, speaking remained laborious and general intelligibility low. Such discrepancies provided the impetus for seeking the more rigorous, motor skill theory-based training approach currently described. Much still remains to be learned about how to use the glossometer most effectively alone and in combination with other instruments to achieve its potential more fully in diagnostic and training routines.

PALATOGRAPHY

Palatography is a technique for graphically registering tongue contact against the palate, alveolar ridge, and inner margins of the teeth. As indicated in Marchall's (1988) review, palatography has long been used to study speech production both clinically and experimentally. The first objectively documented actions of the tongue were made with deformable materials placed in the mouth. For example, in 1803 an

English physician and naturalist, Erasmus Darwin, placed a thin sheet of aluminum foil in his mouth, produced a vowel, then attempted to describe how the foil was deformed during the sound production process. It was quickly realized that more information could be gleaned about speech production by coating the surfaces of the articulators with a material that would be removed by the warm, moist tongue during speech production. This led to the palatographic observation procedures described by an English dentist, J. Oakley Coles (1872a, b).

Dr. Coles became interested in acquiring greater understanding of speech physiology from his work with individuals who had palatal clefts. He was particularly disturbed with his inability to describe the physiology of erroneous sound production more accurately in order to help cleft palate and deaf talkers improve their speech. After thinking through the problem, he devised the following approach, now referred to as *direct* palatography (Coles, 1872):

> I determined on the following plan of ascertaining more accurately the physiology of speech. I took an impression of my upper jaw, extending to the posterior wall of the pharynx, and thereby including the soft tissue and fauces; also an impression of the lower jaw, with the tongue in a state of repose. These I had engraved to one stone, with a drawing of the lips below.... A number of these I had printed. Then my trial began. The mode I adopted at this stage was to make a mixture of gum and flour, and paint over the whole of the hard and soft palate and the surface of the teeth of my upper jaw. I then sharply articulated a letter. On the upper jaw where the tongue had come into contact, the flour was removed and deposited on that part of the tongue which had touched it. These localities were at once faithfully transcribed on to the engraved plate with red paint. (pp. 110–111)

Coles produced three-dimensional topographical "plates" to portray the place and area of linguapalatal contact during the 26 letters of the alphabet. The patterns were sketched from both palatal and lingual orientations. Lip opening was also included for each letter (see Figure 3-6). The plots detailed contact patterns, including the size and locations of apertures through which the phonic stream was channeled during sibilant sound production. The following comment by a discussant, Mr. Charles C. Tomes, in response to Coles' presentation shows the already firmly entrenched belief that lingual contact was not to be expected during vowel production: "It is quite certain that the contact with the upper teeth is not essential [during vowels], and being not essential, is objectionable in a diagram used for teaching" (Coles, 1872, p. 118). This historical evidence of misunderstood functions of linguapalatal contact during vowels has had a surprisingly robust life.

Pretraining

Posttraining

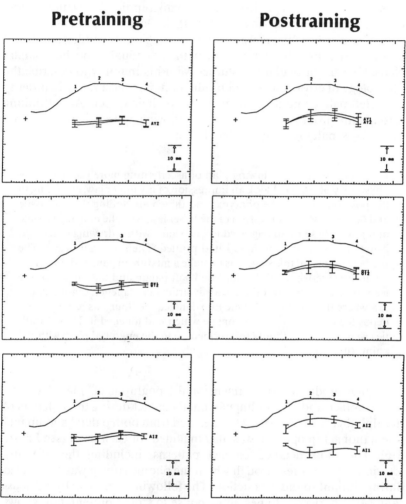

6 Months Post

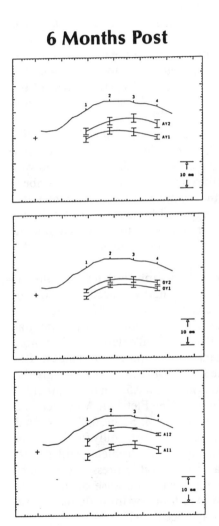

FIGURE 3-5. Tongue position and shape before and after a 3½-week period of glossometric vowel training given to a young girl who was profoundly hearing impaired. From Fletcher, S. G., Dagenais, P. A., Critz-Crosby, P. C. (1991a). Teaching vowels to profoundly hearing-impaired speakers using glossometry. *Journal of Speech and Hearing Research, 34,* 943–956.

A few years later, Grützner (1879) described a somewhat different palatographic procedure. He removed excess saliva from the subject's palate, coated the tongue with a Chinese red rouge, had the subject produce a sound, then used a mirror to examine the color transferred from the tongue to the palate. The resulting contact patterns were plotted in two-dimensional displays. Information concerning palatal vault height, slope steepness, and palatal shape details were thus ignored. Ways to correct this oversight have since been described through using a stylus to etch contour lines on a stone model of the palate at specific depths from the occlusal plane of the teeth (see Bloomer, 1943; McCutcheon, Hasegawa, Smith, & Fletcher, 1981). As yet, this type of information has not been applied rigorously in speech articulation studies, however.

In 1877, Kingsley described a procedure now called *indirect palatography*. He used a pressure molded, removable rubber plate to register and explain palatographic contact patterns. After the target sound was spoken, the plate was removed, and the chalk removal pattern described. This procedure was adopted as the standard way of documenting articulation in the emerging "Experimental Phonetics" field (cf. Rousselot, 1901). Essentially the only major change in indirect palatometric procedures since that time has been substitution of a metal or thin plastic material for the rubber plate.

An inherent problem of indirect palatography is that fabrication of a well-fitting plate, or *pseudopalate,* is a lengthy procedure. Nagging problems have also persisted concerning possible artifacts from the pseudopalate used to register the articulation patterns. Even one that fits perfectly takes up some space within the oral cavity and alters normal sensory feedback to some extent during speech production. Research on these topics has indicated that if the pseudopalate fits the natural palatal contours closely and is less than 0.5 mm thick, articulation is essentially undisturbed (Flege, 1976; Fletcher, McCutcheon, Wolf, Sooudi, & Smith, 1975; but see Hamlet & Stone, 1978). Lingual feedback also appears to be sufficient to compensate fully for the loss of tactile information from a thin pseudopalate. Problems still persist because of the time consumed in taking the oral impressions and fabricating an essentially perfectly fitting device. Because of this, most palatographic studies have been limited to a few individuals "whose articulation may not be typical" (Ladefoged, 1957, p. 765).

Ladefoged (1957) suggested circumventing palatographic problems by simply using an atomizor to deposit material, such as a carbon dust-chocolate mixture, directly onto the palate and inner surfaces of the teeth. Intraoral photography was then recommended to assess lingual contact directly following sound production.

The principal limitation of both direct and indirect palatography is that the image represents the maximum contact pattern. All of the move-

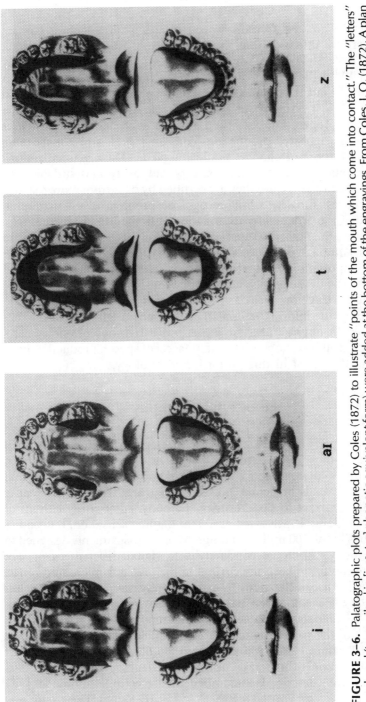

FIGURE 3-6. Palatographic plots prepared by Coles (1872) to illustrate "points of the mouth which come into contact." The "letters" produced (transcribed in [i, aɪ, t, z] phonetic equivalent form) were added at the bottom of the engravings. From Coles, J. O. (1872). A plan for ascertaining more accurately the physiology of speech. *Transactions of the Odontological Society of Great Britain, 4,* 189–217.

ment details are lost. Certain aspects of articulation such as contact force may be inferred from the total area of linguapalatal contact (Moses, 1940; Straka, 1965), but it is not possible to ascertain precisely when and how the force is exerted from such displays. Variability as a function of a talker's motor skill and of the phonetic content of sound sequences is lost in static palatographic displays. Additionally, the time required to prepare for, elicit, and analyze utterances of a particular sound across repeated productions consumes such a prolonged time span that important changes could intervene. Thus, generalizations across repetitions must be drawn very cautiously and still be considered questionable until they are certified by data from more dynamic procedures. Finally, a long-recognized problem of palatographic data is that the articulatory information is limited to events that take place within the oral cavity and sounds that involve observable tongue contacts. Although contacts of the tongue against the palate and teeth provide important insight into speech production principles, they are still only part of the speech act. Despite these limitations, the unique ability to portray how speakers actually produce sounds, the phonetic relevancy of the information obtained, the meaningfulness of the patterns even to novices, and the portent of a rigorous physiologically based conceptualization of important facets of speech production have maintained interest in this promising technology.

Electropalatography

The human body may be thought of as an electrolyte solution confined within a leathery sack (Bruner, 1967). The tough envelope of skin usually offers high resistance to electrical current passage. When that protective cover is breached, however, even tiny voltages may cause substantial current to flow through the body. Alternating current of about 1 milliamp is perceived as a faint tingling sensation. It becomes dangerous in the 100 milliamp range. Modern instruments designed to use the body's electrical conductivity to signal different events are therefore careful to keep the current in the low, *safe* microamp range.

The first use of electricity for palatography was described by Schilling (1930). He embedded paired electrodes in a celluloid pseudopalate. Linguapalatal contact detection required contact with both members of the pair. This requirement limited his observations, and those of Kuzmin (1962) who also used the dual electrode method of contact detection, to bilateral symmetrical articulation patterns. In 1968 Shibata (1968) described a modified dual electrode approach. One member of the pair carried a 5000 to 15,650 Hz signal. The circuit was completed when it was contacted along with a nearby output electrode.

The signals from the output electrode were processed then fed into a sound spectrograph to produce a time series display of the contact pattern. A computer-controlled version of this palatographic system was described by Fugii (1970). Figure 3–7 shows a "palatospectrogram" of [ata].

In 1964, Kydd and Belt described a "continuous palatography" system which used 12 stainless steel electrodes mounted on the lingual surface of a pseudopalate to detect lingual contact. Each electrode functioned as a negative pole in a direct current (DC) oral battery analogue. The tongue with saliva as an electrolytic agent served as the positive pole. When the moist tongue touched an electrode, a small current

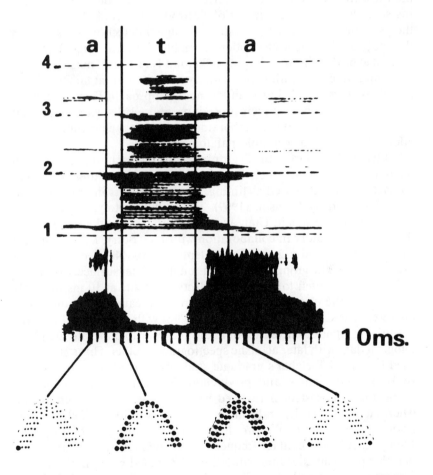

FIGURE 3–7. Palatospectrogram of the nonsense word "ata" spoken by a male Japanese talker. From Fugii, I. (1970). Phoneme identification with dynamic palatography. *Annual Bulletin* (Research Institute of Logopedics and Phoniatrics, University of Tokyo), *4*, 67–73. Reprinted by permission.

was generated. This current was amplified and used to activate lights on a readout panel. Motion pictures were made of the display for frame-by-frame articulatory pattern analysis. In a later system, the readout panel was replaced by a multichannel recording system (Palmer, 1973). One channel recorded the acoustic event, another recorded time in 1-second intervals, and the other 12 recorded linguapalatal contact. This system was used by Harley (1972) to study tongue contact area, timing, and laterality in vowel and consonant sound spoken by six American English talkers. Personal communication with the original investigators indicated that two major limitations had plagued their research. First, DC "body current" inter-electrode salivary bridging severely limited the number of electrodes that could be placed on the pseudopalate. Second, adjusting the signal detection threshold on the individual contact electrodes to enable the faint lingual contact current to be discriminated from background electrical "noise" was difficult and time consuming, particularly across different talkers. These problems eventually led to abandoning the approach. They were, however, gracious in sharing their procedures and results with the present author when he visited their laboratory in 1966 at the beginning of his efforts to develop a workable palatometer.

Fletcher's goal from the beginning of his research was to develop a palatographic system which would yield precise measures of lingual contact placement as well as timing. His early efforts in that direction were described by Johnson (1969). The initial prototype system was planned when he was in Utah and later fabricated at the Los Alamos Scientific Laboratory in collaboration with J. G. Berry, J. S. Levin, and M. Kellogg. It used a 2-volt DC potential across 48 electrodes on a pseudopalate. The ground contact was on its palatal surface. Computer software was written to sample the electrode status at 10 ms intervals and display the electrode contact pattern on a cathode ray tube. The data were listed on a printer (see Figure 3-8) with parallel 100 Hz synchronizing signals relayed to an audio recorder to correlate the physiological data with later acoustic spectrographic plots. This system was used by one of Fletcher's graduate students, Berry (1971), in a thesis study of consonant sound production. Fletcher and his associates found that this system performed well in areas of the pseudopalate where electrode density and contact frequency was low. DC electrolysis bridging posed a particular problem in the anterior region of the palate where articulation contact frequency was high. It was hypothesized that this problem could be reduced or eliminated with an alternating current circuit. Another of Fletcher's graduate students fabricated a single channel prototype model to test this hypothesis (Greer, 1970). The results were positive.

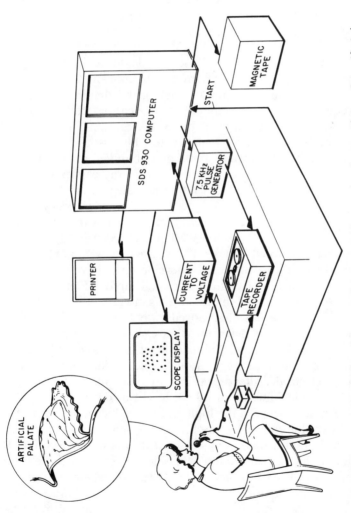

FIGURE 3–8. Schematic drawing of instrumentation fabricated at the Los Alamos Scientific Laboratory. From Berry, J. K. (1971). A study of lingual-palatal contacts during the production of selected consonant sounds. Unpublished master's thesis, University of New Mexico, Albuquerque, NM. Published by permission.

In 1970, Fletcher moved to the University of Alabama in Birmingham. There he made arrangements with R. Steel, an engineer at the Southern Research Institute, to fabricate a 48-electrode "palatometer" that sampled lingual contact data at a 100 Hz rate under computer control (Fletcher, McCutcheon, & Wolf, 1975). The system was later expanded to 96 channels to increase measurement precision and a 32 channel, 200–5000 Hz parallel filter bank was added (Smith, McCutcheon, Hasegawa, Christensen, & Fletcher, 1980). The filter bank output and supporting software were used to produce digital sound spectrograms relating articulatory and acoustic events.

A special instrument, called DYTAPS, was designed later to provide simultaneous side-by-side, split-screen glossometric (midsagittal sideview) and palatographic images from a clinician and a client talker. This device was used in articulatory modeling and shaping routines to teach vowel and consonants sounds to a 3½-year-old child who was profoundly hearing impaired (Fletcher & Hasegawa, 1983).

A final problem faced by Fletcher and his associates was that because the electrode lead wires were tightly bundled as they passed from the mouth to the palatometric circuitry, stray capacitance and inductance introduced some cross talk and transients in the signal. Saliva on the pseudopalate and subject-to-subject differences in body and lingual conductivity caused additional signal variability. This situation caused some channels to be "stuck on" because they were too sensitive. Others remained "stuck off" because they were not sensitive enough. This problem was resolved by developing an in vivo automatic calibration routine (see McCutcheon, Smith, Kimble, & Fletcher, 1983). The pseudopalate was placed in the subject's mouth and moistened by the tongue. The tongue was then moved away from the pseudopalate and an average value was determined for each electrode in the noncontact condition. Next, the maximum contact level was established by having the subject move the tongue around the pseudopalate and touch it against each electrode. After repeating the contact versus non-contact procedure levels four times, a threshold level was determined by calculating differences between the high and low values multiplied by a bias sensitivity value chosen by the clinician. When this procedure was followed, recalibration was rarely required during data collection. It was later found that the calibration values derived could be stored in a computer file and used in other sessions with the same subject.

For further information about the development and characteristics of other electropalatographic systems the reader is referred to Hardcastle (1972) and Marchal (1988).

CHAPTER 4

HIERARCHIES WITHIN PHONETIC ELEMENTS

During speech production, phonemically specified utterances are presumed to be interpreted by the language phonological component that generates allophones. They are then fed phrase-by-phrase into a neurological encoding system, which times, integrates, and coarticulates the allophones to produce the dynamic speech movement stream. The *spread of features* is conceived as a way to avoid abrupt articulation changes and transitional sounds that would otherwise occur as articulatory actions move from feature bundle to feature bundle. Feature spreading adjusts the elements within phonetic boundaries. It does not make the segments continuous. It simply allows adjacent sounds and gestures to be accommodated to each other. This *accommodation* takes two forms. When adjacent sounds are produced with a similar articulation, they are combined. For example, [d] followed by [θ] becomes [ḏ]. When sounds have nonconflicting articulation sites, the actions proceed in parallel. For example, during articulation of the word "cry" the tongue tip is not involved in the [k]. It is therefore free to move toward the [r] posture as the [k] is produced. This smooths sound-to-sound transitions. The listener recovers message meaning by mental gymnastics which include "segmenting" and "phonemicizing" the utterance.

SEGMENTATION AND COARTICULATION

Descriptions of how actions are integrated across the elements of speech production begin with the intuitive concept of a *segment*. When we listen to someone speaking, we hear a succession of qualitatively and temporally distinct sounds or segments. But when we examine acoustic or articulatory displays of the same utterance, only the qualitative differences survive. Temporal discreteness is no longer present. Different gestures are seen to be underway simultaneously with no apparent segmental boundaries identifiable in either the acoustic or articulatory records. This speech characteristic led Hammarberg (1976) to conclude that "segments do not exist outside the human mind." We simply impose them on the acoustic signal in the process of speech perception. Daniloff and Hammarberg (1973) explain that we do this by using "invariant, ideal, uncoarticulated target forms" (p. 240). These forms, or phonological features, were suggested to contain all of the information needed to identify the canonical phonological segments and no more. The coarticulation entities were thought to be conceived "when a segment is produced in isolation in a sustained manner, or when the sound is produced in a context assumed to be minimally coarticulatory" (ibid. p. 241). The notion that the articulators are continually moving into position for other segments over a stretch of speech is the central function described by the term *coarticulation*. Coarticulation is thus conceived to be the adjustment of idealized segments resulting from influences exerted on them by neighboring segments. It does not mean the overlapping or coproduction of separate segments. They never appear in connected speech. Rather, the essential properties of the segment are timeless. One segment terminates at the beginning of the next one.

Fowler (1980) challenged the previously outlined coarticulation assumptions on two fundamental grounds. First, the concept of distinctions based on canonical forms introduces a mind/body problem, which vastly complicates the concept of a segment. It requires repeated translations from psychological-to-physical and physical-to-psychological functions. Second, the separation imposed between canonical and actualization forms implies the untenable assumption that the acoustic data are insufficient for the conceptual categories we perceive.

The concept of nonexistent physical segments is directly challenged by both historical concepts and phonetic transcription studies. Anderson (1974) notes that during early phonetic history much effort was devoted to using phonetic transcription to produce "a complete and faithful record of the physical event it describes" (p. 4). In this encyclopedic task, phoneticians sought to document the neurological, physiological, and aerodynamic events of sound production "so that no physical property of the speech event would escape unnoticed." This work led to the concept that spoken sounds represent a sequence of discrete, homogeneously characterizeable, atom-like segments with predictable transitions that follow general physiological laws. The validity of the segment abstraction was based on the observation that a beginning set of principles could be identified from which coarticulatory actions could be deduced and movements reconstructed. Anderson observed that such segmental structure descriptions have been "the basis of virtually every result of note that has ever been obtained in the field of linguistic phonetics or phonology" (p. 6).

The concept that all biological activities are performed by coordinated structures (cf. Easton, 1972) has recently been applied to coarticulatory phenomena. Significant properties of coordinated structures are that they are self-executing once they are formed, generate equivalent movement classes, tend to have smaller actions nested within larger ones, and are often cyclical. Speech seems to show each of these properties. For instance, self-execution is found at all speech levels. In breathing, subglottal pressure is maintained at a nearly constant level by self-acting responses despite gradual depletion of air in the lungs (Lieberman, 1967). The self-acting quality is also indicated by the fact that similar vocal output occurs over a range of subglottal pressures by increased tension in the adductor muscles and decreased tension of the abductors (Wyke, 1974). In articulation when the jaw is prevented from reaching its usual posture, lip (Folkins & Abbs, 1975) and tongue (Fletcher, under review, a) elevation is virtually instantaneously increased to compensate for the jaw restriction. When tongue structure is surgically removed, equivalent lip actions have been found to be instituted spontaneously to enable talkers to recapture phonetic goals (Fletcher, 1988).

Many examples could be cited to illustrate nested articulation actions within larger ones. A pertinent example of this is seen in the role played by lateral linguapalatal contact. The contact steadies the bulk of the tongue, provides a fulcrum that magnifies tongue-palate valving forces for air pressure buildup within the oral cavity, and adds biomechanical leverage for rapid, precise articulate speech movements. The nesting of consonant movements within vowel gestures has also been frequently described (Butcher & Weiher, 1976; Farnetani, Vagges, & Magno-Caldognetto, 1985). This effect is greatest when the vowel is [i], which has the most extensive linguapalatal contact.

Finally, the dynamic actions of speech are intrinsically rhythmical and the rates and phases of their periodicities may be identified in particular subcomponents coupled within the system. Thus, reality of speech segments appears to be well grounded from both an historical viewpoint and more recent recognition that speech exhibits all of the properties associated with coordinative structure systems.

VOWELS AND CONSONANTS

The phonetic elements of speech are divided into two basic sound classes in all traditional phonological considerations: vowels and consonants. The acoustic differences between these sound classes may be clarified by examining how they appear in spectrographic displays. The nonsense sentence *"Measure why that possum views a boy will Ruth each awful gay cushion young Joe now heard"* shown in Figure 4-1 will be used to introduce consonant-vowel contrasts. This sentence is from Fairbanks (1960). It samples each phoneme of the English language at least once and was recorded as the words were spoken by a male talker with a General American dialect. He was careful to have no pauses or exaggerations during his utterance of the sentence.

Time is represented in the spectrogram by vertical tick marks at 0.1 sec intervals across the horizontal axis of the graph. The vertical axis identifies the acoustic frequency in cycles per second (cps), now more commonly labeled in Hertz (Hz). The term *spectrum* refers to the distribution of energy within acoustic frequency bands or ranges. The 0 to 5000 Hz range shown in Fairbanks' spectrogram covers a practical band width for speech. Acoustic energy within the trace is indicated by the darkness of the plot; white areas identify moments in time when the energy was below the instrument's sensitivity. The vocal fold vibration rate or *fundamental frequency* (F_o) of the speaker's voice is represented by the fine vertical lines or striations that appear periodically across the traces and by the dark bar scrolled horizontally near the baseline of the graph. This talker's F_o ranged from about 80 to 115 Hz. To estimate the F_o, just count the number of vertical lines within a 0.1 sec time period (represented by tick marks below the spectrograms), then multiply the result by 10. A 100 Hz fundamental frequency of the voice would be indicated by 10 vertical lines during a 0.1 sec time period. The *voice bar* should also be near the 100 Hz baseline.

As a vocal tone passes through the cavities of the vocal tract, certain frequencies in its spectrum are suppressed. Others match the resonant characteristics of the vocal tract and are amplified. Acoustic intensity is indicated by the darkness or prominence of the traces; therefore the amplified frequencies appear darker on the spectrographic display. Pauses with little or no noise are shown as white

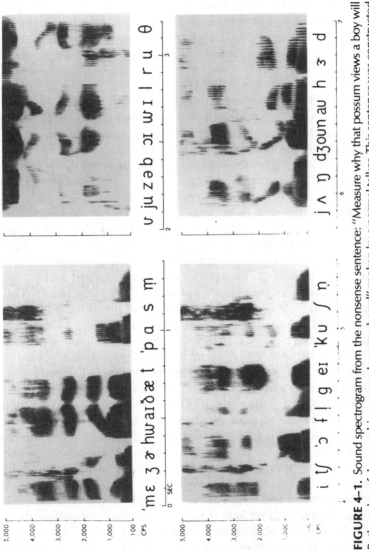

FIGURE 4–1. Sound spectrogram from the nonsense sentence: "Measure why that possum views a boy will Ruth each awful gay cushion young Joe now heard" spoken by a normal talker. This sentence was constructed to sample each phoneme of the English language. From Fairbanks, G. (1960). *Voice and articulation drillbook* (2nd Ed.), (p. 2). Copyright 1960 by Grant Fairbanks. Reprinted by permission of HarperCollins Publishers.

spaces in the display. Vowels generally are higher in intensity than consonants; therefore, their patterns are darker than consonants in the spectrogram. Now let us examine the acoustic characteristics of the vowels. First inspect the traces for the [i] in *each* (at 4.1 sec in the graph). Immediately above and merging into the voice bar at the bottom of the spectrographic display of the [i] is a band of acoustic energy representing a vocal tract resonance centered around 300 Hz. This is called the *First Formant* (F1). A gap is shown above the F1. The *Second Formant* (F2) then appears at around 2300 Hz and the *Third Formant* (F3) at about 3000 Hz. Compare these formant levels with those of the [ɑ] in *possum* (at 1.0 sec). Note that the voice bar shows a slight drop in the speaker's F_o as the articulators move from [*p*] to the steady acoustic output for the [ɑ]. At the same time, the first and second formants rise to steady 730 and 1090 Hz levels. Both the consonant-vowel (CV) formant transitions and the resonance frequencies are used by listeners to identify the vowel spoken.

The formant differences between the [i] and [ɑ] vowels show how the vocal tract is *tuned* as an adjustable resonator to produce vowel contrasts. Noise generated at the larynx and other sound sources is molded into specific vowel and consonant sounds as it is resonated and articulated on its journey through the vocal tract. The [i] and [ɑ] are called *pure* vowels, because their formants are relatively steady. This steadiness contrasts with the formant patterns of the diphthongs, such as [aɪ], [ɔɪ], and [eɪ], that appear at 0.5, 2.5, and 4.75 sec in the spectrogram. During the diphthongal vowels the articulators move from one position to another. This movement creates marked changes in the acoustic spectra. For example, the tongue moves from a low back position within the oral cavity for the [a]-like onset of the [aɪ] diphthong to a high front position during the [ɪ]. This movement is mirrored by a strong rise in the second acoustic formant. The diphthongs differ in how much movement is involved in their production. Comparatively little change is shown in the spectrum of the [eɪ] diphthong which begins and ends with positions close to those of the [ɛ] and [ɪ] pure vowels.

Although sound spectrograms do not represent the acoustic qualities of speech exactly as we hear them, they provide information about many of the features we find meaningful. The F1 and F2 levels are especially helpful in vowel differentiation. What has been called *vowel height* is inversely proportional to the frequency of the first formant. *Vowel backness* is directly proportional to the difference between first and second formants (Ladefoged, 1975). We also use momentary pauses to help segment sounds and phrases. These pauses are evidenced by gaps in the voice bar at the bottom of the spectrogram.

A brief pause, called a *pseudosilence*, is shown just before the noise burst for the [p] in *possum*. The pseudosilence reflects the time consumed during breath pressure buildup within the oral cavity for the explosive production of the [p]. Presence or absence of noise during this time differentiates voiceless and voiced sounds.

Consonants are identified by turbulence as the phonic air stream passes through apertures along the phonic tract, by abrupt release of air impounded behind articulators, and by the presence and timing of voicing. The frictional turbulence produced by forcing air through a groove between the tongue and the palate during production of the two voiceless sibilants, [s] and [ʃ] is shown at 1.1 and 5.1 sec in the spectrograms. Notice that both of these consonants have their major energy concentrated in the high frequencies. The principal resonances of these sounds, indicated by darker areas in the plots, center at about 2600 Hz during the [ʃ] and 4100 Hz during the [s]. These differences reflect the larger resonance cavity in the front of the mouth during the [ʃ].

Consonants often have voiced and voiceless *cognates*, which differ only in voicing. Otherwise their production patterns are essentially identical. For example, the [d], [g], [z], and [ʒ] are voiced cognates of [t], [k], [s], and [ʃ]. They differ by voicing but their articulation patterns are otherwise similar.

The *voiced stop* [b] at the onset of *boy* and the voiceless affricate [tʃ] at the end of *each* (2.4 and 4.2 sec) are identified by short periods of vocal fold vibratory sound alone or pseudosilence before noise bursts. During this time, air is impounded behind an articulatory constriction. It is then released abruptly to produce the stop burst or continuously during the fricative part of the affricate. The puff of air that accompanies the abrupt stop sound release is often indicated by a sharp noise burst in the spectrogram. The talker who spoke the sentence in Fairbanks' spectrograms produced stops with less intense sound bursts. This sound is indicated by spaces between the formants at the acoustic onset of the stops produced.

Spectrograms may also be used to identify *coarticulatory* conditioning effects from neighboring sounds. For example, the rather prolonged pseudosilence between the voiceless [t] at the end of *that* and the [p] at the beginning of *possum* suggests that this talker replaced both the [t] and [p] by a single glottal stop gesture. Listeners knowing that speakers use such articulatory simplifications or coarticulatory shortcuts when adjoining sounds share the same articulatory feature simply add them as the words are heard. They are usually not even aware that the particular sounds are missing in the utterance.

Notice how the starting spectrum of the [i] at 4.25 sec and the ending spectrum of [ʊ] at 5.0 sec were influenced by the preceding and following consonants. Such transitional phenomena have been used to explain why vowels are often described functionally as forming a "syllabic peak" in the central or nuclear part of words. From the same orientation, consonants are described as non-central or marginal in the syllable. Syllables can be produced without a consonant but not without a vowel.

VOWEL ARTICULATION

Vowels reflect relatively slow, global changes in the vocal tract shape. Perkell (1969, p. 61) suggested that vowel articulation likely is accomplished mainly by the larger extrinsic lingual musculature,and consonant articulation by the smaller intrinsic ones. This difference in muscular involvement permits vowel and consonant movements to overlap as they are produced. Fowler (1980) sums up such observations in the following statement:

> Taken together, these observations and extrapolations from them indicate that true co-production occurs in speech, and that the capacity for co-production derives from an adaptive property of speech ... the two classes of articulatory gestures, consonants and vowels, are products of different (coordinated) neuromuscular systems. (p. 129)

Stevens (1975) hypothesized that vowels may be differentiated in part by the degree of vertical contact between the tongue, the palate, and the teeth. This hypothesis was initially rejected by Perkell (1979) on the basis of static palatographic comparisons of the [i], [ɪ], [æ], [ʊ], and [u] vowels. In a later dynamic palatometric study, Fletcher (1989a, 1990) found that most vowels are distinguishable through anterior-posterior contact differences along the lateral borders of the palate. His findings also showed that the contact patterns could neatly distinguish diphthongal vowels from glide /j, w/ and liquid /r, l/ consonants that also have moving articulatory actions.

The high front tense [i] vowel, as in "beeb," is characterized palatometrically by extensive contact along the lateral borders of the palate (see Figure 4-2). During production of its near neighbor, the high front lax [ɪ] vowel in "bib," the contact is farther back and more lateral. Fewer sensors are touched. The area contacted (number of sensors touched) becomes progressively less during the midfront vowel [ɛ] and the low front [æ] (see Fletcher, under review a, b). It may be seen that when the front vowels /i, ɪ, ɛ, æ/ are arranged by the amount of linguapalatal contact, their order parallels that found in traditional phonetic descriptions based on perceived "vowel height" and "frontness." Among the back vowels, only [u] and [ʊ] exhibit significant linguapalatal contact. Lip rounding serves an important role in distinguishing front and back vowels in the English language.

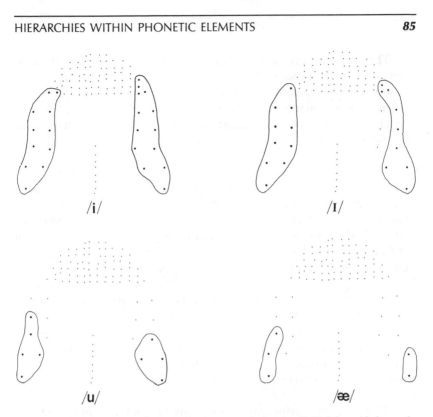

FIGURE 4–2. Contrasting linguapalatal contact during the [i], [ɪ], [u], and [æ] vowels.

In a recent study, Fletcher (under review, a) compared lateral linguapalatal contact during production of 14 English vowels spoken by six normal 7-year-old children. He found that all vowels except those produced with the tongue in a "low" central or back position (ɑ, ʌ, o) may be differentiated by the degree of lateral linguapalatal contact. Moreover, when the vowels were ordered by their contact magnitude and pattern, their distribution coincided rather closely with those reported in past vowel phonetic descriptions, based on tongue midline "height and place" percepts. The vowels were also found to cluster into three main groups, ordered by contact place and magnitude. The group with greatest linguapalatal contact consisted of the high and midfront vowels [i, eɪ, ɪ] and the high back vowel [u]. The [u] ranked below the others in its group in both contact place and magnitude. The second group included the midfront vowel [ɛ], the diphthongs [ɔɪ] and [aɪ], the rhotic vowel [ɜ], and the [ʊ]. The location of the diphthongs in the center of this group is explained by their movement from a low back tongue position at the diphthong onset to a high front position at their offset. Their *average* contact thus placed them with the midvowels.

The final vowel set consisted of low vowels. The /æ/ headed this list even though it exhibited contact only on the back outside corners of the pseudopalate. It was followed by [aʊ], [o], and /ɑ/ which rarely or never evidenced any contact. Thus, the traditional vowel order based on perceived "vowel height" and "frontness" could be at least in part an outgrowth of talkers' experiences in discerning the degree and place of linguapalatal contact.

The data from this study of 7-year-old children were also plotted by the percentage of sensors contacted row-by-row across the pseudopalate (Figure 4–3). When this was done, other important attributes of linguapalatal contact emerged. The vowels were still distinguished by systematic differences in the magnitude of lingua-alveolar contact from the front to the back rows. This ordering of the data showed, however, that the most common and consistent site of contact was on the back half of the palate. This observation supports the assumption that the postero-lateral margin of the palate serves as a primary anchoring region used by speakers to stabilize the tongue as specific vowels as well as consonants are spoken. It also supports the concept that postero-lateral linguapalatal contact may function as a pivotal fulcrum area for maintaining control of anterior tongue actions during the precise, physically demanding maneuvers involved in front and back consonant articulation.

These findings concerning lateral linguapalatal contact may be summarized as indicating that such contact helps stabilize the tongue, contributes directly to vowel differentiation through tongue placement contrast, and facilitates fine motor control and precision in lingual consonant articulations. These conclusions are consistent with the importance given to tongue shapes and positions within the oral cavity from phonetic introspection and auditory observations.

Verbrugge and Rakerd (1986) cited a series of previous studies which have shown that when a vowel is coarticulated with surrounding consonants to form a syllable, the movements to and from the targeted vowel posture serve as strong predictors of the vowel spoken. This observation suggests that the acoustic imprint may contain movement-specific information about facets of articulatory actions within the oral cavity, such as linguapalatal contact sequences that lead to the desired target configurations.

Fletcher applied a principal components analysis to identify basic processes underlying vowel differentiation. Two major factors emerged. The first component identified the palatometrically measured place and area of linguapalatal contact as the principal source of vowel identity. By itself this factor could explain about 70% of the contact variance. The second factor loaded most heavily on the maximum minus the

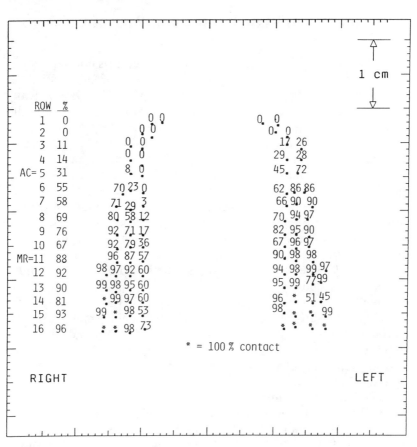

FIGURE 4–3. Percentages of the 96 sensors contacted during production of different vowels.

minimum number of sensors contacted. This factor represented the difference between the greatest and least number of sensors contacted as the vowels were spoken. It captured dynamic movement as a central function in vowel differentiation and specifically separated the diphthongs from the pure vowels. Together, the two factors extracted from the principal components analysis accounted for almost 90% of the contact variance. Vowels can thus be differentiated rather accurately by lateral linguapalatal contact place, magnitude, and dynamic change. These findings again provide impressive evidence that linguapalatal contact plays a central role in vowel production and differentiation.

Tongue and Jaw Positions in Pure Vowels

A number of writers have observed that jaw lowering is normally counterbalanced in speech by compensatory tongue elevation. Fletcher (under review, c) hypothesized that if the jaw were systematically lowered during production of a high front /i/ vowel, at some point the distance between the jaws would exceed a talker's ability to compensate fully by lingual supershapes. This hypothesis led to the prediction that as lingual compensatory capability is challenged and its compensatory limits passed, linguapalatal contact will begin to shift posteriorly, and the area contacted will drop. Based on the previously established relationship between linguapalatal contact and vowel production, the hypothesis further predicts that as the tongue loses contact with the palate, the vowel heard will change from /i/ to /ɪ/ to /eɪ/, to /ɛ/, and finally to /æ/.

These hypotheses and predictions were tested by Fletcher (under review, c) in a study of [i] vowels spoken by the six normal 7-year-old children described earlier. The children were first asked to say "EE" five times as clearly as possible with the teeth held 3 mm apart by a mechanical device.[1] The jaw was then lowered 2 mm and five more vowels were elicited. The procedure of jaw lowering in 2 mm steps and soliciting repetition of a 5-vowel set was continued until the child could tolerate no further jaw opening. During this process the subjects were repeatedly urged to continue to try to make the "EE" vowels sound as normal as possible no matter how widely their mouth was opened.

The vowels produced under these conditions were recorded and replayed to 26 phonetically trained listeners who transcribed the vowels they heard. The transcribers were advised that the vowels would initially be [i] but might change as the test progressed. It was emphasized that they should transcribe each vowel as they heard it, not what they expected to hear or thought the child was trying to say. They were not informed that the children were always trying to produce the same vowel.

The data from the listener transcriptions were pooled across reponses, and scores were derived for the percentage of times i, ɪ, eɪ, ɛ, u, ʊ, or æ were identified. Other vowels were rarely heard. The results from the data analysis showed that jaw lowering beyond an interincisal space of about 18 mm caused a systematic change in the vowel perceived from the /i/ to /ɪ/, to /eɪ/. Sometimes the vowel change progressed to /ɛ/ and finally /æ/ as the interincisal distance expansion continued beyond the lingual compensatory range of some subjects. The findings thus supported the hypothesis that linguapalatal contact

---

[1]The Burnett TMJ device is manufactured by Medrad Technology for People, Pittsburgh, PA.

along the outer margins of the palate is linked with vowel perception as well as production.

Tongue Midline Shape

Findings from previous investigators (Fletcher, 1989b; Harshman, Ladefoged, and Goldstein, 1977) have shown that vowel articulation can also be differentiated by midline tongue postures. As indicated in the midline tongue profiles of Figure 4–4, midline plots reveal systematic lowering and retraction of the tongue body as the vowel changes from the high, front /i/ to the low, back /ɑ/ vowels. These tongue positions were noted to be similar to those proposed in Lindblom and Sundberg's (1971) two-dimensional model which identified the /i, ɑ, u/ vowels as maximal distortions of a neutral vocal tract. /i/ represented maximum change in the palatal region, /u/ in the velar region, and /ɑ/ in the pharyngeal region of the mouth. Other vowels were described as being intermediate in place and degree of distortion. Further analysis of their data by Harshman et al. (1977) uncovered two major factors that could explain the contrasting tongue shapes (see Figure 4–5). The first factor focused on changes in tongue height at the front of the mouth and forward movement of the tongue root. The second factor was associated with upward and backward tongue movements.

Thus, we have two potential ways to explain vowel differentiation physically: differences in tongue contact along the lateral borders of the vocal tract and differences in lingual midline postures and shapes. It may be that talkers manipulate each of these parameters separately to achieve specific phonetic goals. It seems more likely, however, that they manipulate them jointly with tradeoffs to facilitate adaptation in different speaking situations or to compensate for individual variations in oral morphology and/or physiology. Perhaps talkers use contact along the lateral borders of the oral cavity to differentiate the vowels broadly and to stabilize the bulk of the tongue in both vowel and consonant sound production. Midline tongue shaping and contact along the anterior and posterior borders of the palate may then be manipulated to accentuate contrasts in vocal tract configurations and fine tune the acoustic output. The relative contribution of each of these articulatory dimensions, the specific role that jaw position may play in each, and possible variations in the weight individual talkers assign to tongue and jaw positions and actions deserve careful evaluation in future studies.

Vowel Development

The observations just discussed support and extend previous observations of skills underlying vowel production. Such findings pave the

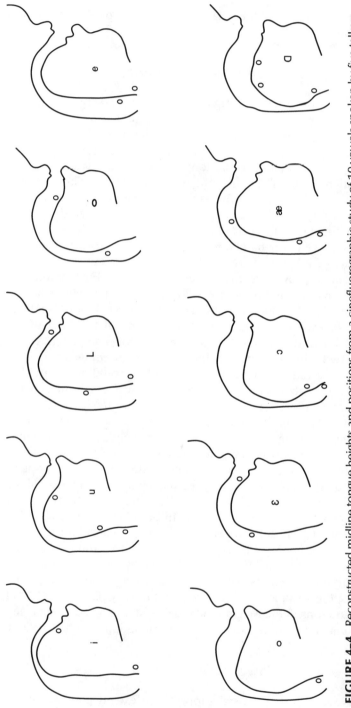

FIGURE 4–4. Reconstructed midline tongue heights and positions from a cinefluorographic study of 10 vowels spoken by five talkers. The zeros alongside the tongue position indicate locations where a noticeable difference was found between the reconstructed and original data. From Harshman, R., Ladefoged, P., & Goldstein, L. (1977). Factor analysis of tongue shapes. *Journal of the Acoustical Society of America, 62,* 693–707. Reprinted by permission.

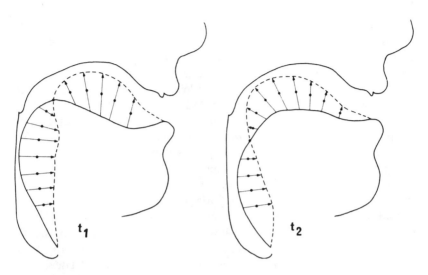

FIGURE 4-5. Plot showing the source for the two sets of constants, t_{i1} and t_{i2}, identified by Harshman, Ladefoged, and Goldstein (1977) from cinefluorographic measures of tongue positions in 10 vowels spoken by five talkers. From Harshman, R., Ladefoged, P., & Goldstein, L. (1977). Factor analysis of tongue shapes. *Journal of the Acoustical Society of America, 62*, 693-707. Reprinted by permission.

way for grouping vowels into "natural" classes dictated by articulation processes. The search for these touchstones of vowel differentiation may be facilitated by the concept that the earliest sounds of speech are likely to develop from comparatively simple, easily acquired articulatory gestures. Mastering elementary gestures would then pave the way for acquiring the more difficult (more physically complex) articulation skills.

Based on these descriptions of vowel production, we may predict that vowel development in speech will usually begin by acquiring an initial contrast between linguapalatal contact and no contact (e.g., high vs. low tongue postures). This contrast would be expected to be followed by gaining control over contact place (front vs. back) and magnitude (extent of medial contact spread) contrasts. Vowel differentiation through dynamic movement (rhotic, diphthongal vowels) would then be expected to emerge as the final articulatory skill mastered during vowel acquisition.

Articulatory information to test this predicted vowel development order is not yet available, but findings from some preliminary acoustical studies seem to support the generalizations outlined. Bickley (1984, 1986) examined the emergence of high front (i, ɪ), high back (u, ʊ), and low central or back (ʌ, ɑ) vowel changes in words spoken spontaneously by fifteen, 14- to 24-month-old normal children tested at 1- to 3-month intervals. One of the long debated issues concerning early childhood sound making is whether it is appropriate to use an adult speech-based phonetic system to transcribe sounds produced by infants and young children (Winitz, 1969). At times, sounds produced by young children fit the adult standard model. At other times they do not.[2] To avoid problems from differences between child and adult sounds and variability in childhood articulation, Bickley (1984, 1986) used word recognition rather than phonetic transcriptions to describe the sounds. For example, all pronunciations of the word "ball" were assumed to include [ʌ] or [ɑ] vowels. She also chose to ignore differences in vowel tenseness within a class. This permitted her to focus attention broadly on the acquisition of high versus low and front versus back vowels. Her data showed that a high-low vowel distinction was consistently acquired before front-back distinctions. In no instance did any child establish tongue placement contrast before tongue height.[3] These findings support the general vowel developmental order postulated on the basis of linguapalatal contact.

These observations suggest that there is a vowel acquisition order that may be traced to natural oral sensations and motor control. In this context naturalness is defined by ease of sound production and speech sequencing in a framework of increasingly complex maneuvers. An articulatory action would thus be judged to be more natural than another if it appears earlier in the development sequence.

Much of the data reviewed has indicated that speech obeys the general rule that motor skill development is guided by movement efficiency and conservation of energy. Since the goal of speech production is speech perception, a second force comes into play. To permit a person to converse easily and naturally in a variety of speaking situations, sound development must also be dictated by sound contrast. This tenet is supported by studies such as that conducted by Lieberman (1980) who studied longitudinal changes in vowels produced by five children from 16 weeks to 3 years of age. He found a gradual and consistent change toward adult-like vowels from the earliest stages of babbling into meaningful sentences. Examination of the formant plots in his paper indicates that the vowel space expansions developed initially from changes in the F1 domain. This is consistent with the fact that the first formant is particularly sensitive to changes in lip and jaw opening and tongue height which are the most visible aspects of speech produc-

---

[2]See Smith (1973) for an enlightening discussion of the role that early sound approximations play in emergence of standard articulation.

[3]A possible explanation for the early emergence of the high-low contrast may be that tongue height is linked rather closely with the degree of mouth opening. The early learner can therefore draw from both visual and oral cues in developing a tongue height concept whereas the front-back concept must be gleaned strictly from auditory and oral sensations.

tion. Later changes then reflected developing control of front versus back tongue postures, evidenced by an expansion of the F2 range. During the second year of life, Lieberman found that the children he studied developed a full [i, ɑ, u] vowel triangle with integrated high-low and front-back contrasts. He noted further, however, that temporal distinctions between the vowels were acquired later than those reflecting articulator positions as the children transferred vowel production skills into meaningful words and connected speech utterances. The earlier vowels had formant patterns that resembled those in common words, but their durations were too brief (80 to 100 msec) to meet language standards. As might be expected, the implied developmental order indicates that phonetic contrast, which leads to phonemic contrast, follows motor control development rather closely. Clear tense-lax contrasts were not apparent in Lieberman's vowel plots until after the subjects were about 3 years old. And those achieved at that time were still primarily limited to the high front [i] and [ɪ] vowels.

Vowels in World Languages

The sounds of world languages may be expected to follow the energy conservation and phonetic/phonemic contrast principles tentatively identified in speech development. By and large, languages would thus be expected to adopt vowels that are most easily produced and make best use of oral space for phonetic contrast. If so, the frequencies with which different vowels occur across languages could provide a metric to help document a natural vowel hierarchy that could be used to predict natural speech sound emergence and test assumptions about phonetic contrast and vowel oral space utilization.

Data for these purposes have been provided by Maddieson (1984) who compared the content and structure of phonological inventories within a representative sample of the world's languages. Using the conventional parameters of vowel height, backness, and lip rounding, he found that vowels in the midrange were slightly more common than high vowels (40.5 vs. 39.0%) and low vowels (20.5%) substantially less common. The front vowels were slightly more frequent than back vowels (40.0 vs. 37.8%) and considerably more frequent than central vowels (22.2%). Central vowels were usually low (75.1%). Unrounded vowels were considerably more common than rounded vowels (61.5% to 38.5%). Whether specific vowels were rounded depended on their frontness. Front vowels were usually unrounded (94.0%); back vowels were usually rounded (93.5%).

The vowels /i, ɑ, u/ located at the corners of the conventional vowel triangle were most widespread. Of the 314 languages surveyed, 91.5% had an /i/, 88.0% had an /ɑ/, and 83.9% had a /u/. The high incidence of

/i/ and /ɑ/ supports the assumption that visually perceived lip and jaw openings and tactually perceived linguapalatal contact versus no contact serve as basic core elements in vowel differentiation.

The emerging /i/ versus /ɑ/ contrast would be expected to be followed by contact place (front vs. back) contrasts. Maddieson's data also support this prediction. Twenty-four fewer languages had /u/ than /i/. Maddieson felt that lower acoustic intensity could be the major factor in the relative disfavoring of the /u/; however, visually perceived lip rounding during the back vowels could also counterbalance loss of acoustic and tactile information during their production. The mid-vowels /ɛ, o/ complete the set of most common vowels in world languages. They are diametrically contrasted by linguapalatal contact with no lip rounding in /ɛ/ and lip rounding without linguapalatal contact in /o/.

As the number of vowels in a language grows, the probability increases for time (long vs. short or medially extensive vs. nonextensive) contrasts to differentiate them. No language with only 3 vowels includes time contrasts, and only 14.1% of those with 4 to 6 vowels do so. Furthermore, 24.7% of those with 7 to 9 vowels and 53.8% of those including English that have 10 or more vowels use vowel length contrasts. Vowels tend to be produced with the tongue in a higher position when they are lengthened or tensed. This discrepancy could be a rather straightforward function of time required to achieve greater linguapalatal contact positions in tense vowel contrasts. Other properties such as nasalization, pharyngealization, and breathy voice not used to contrast English vowels will not be reviewed.

The Diphthongs

As might be predicted by physiological effort, diphthongs are less common than pure vowels in world languages. The most common diphthongs, that is, those that occur in more than two languages, show a distinct preference for postures that begin or end with a high vowel. This trend cannot be explained by distinctiveness since vowels such as /eɪ/ with short trajectories through vowel space are as common as those like /aɪ/ with long trajectories. Perhaps the amount of sensory feedback from linguapalatal contact serves as the common reference in vowel differentiation.

Disner (1984) found evidence in Maddieson's survey of vowel systems in 314 languages that supported a general dispersion theory. This theory holds that vowels will tend to be evenly and optimally distributed to maximize contrast within available phonetic space. A specific prediction of this theory is that five major regions along the

TABLE 4-1. Vowel hierarchy implied by emergence of phonetic features during speech development, frequency occurrence in world languages, and control of linguapalatal contact parameters.

Phonetic Feature	Articulatory Control
Height	Linguapalatal contact magnitude
Frontness	Contact forwardness
Back	Contact backness ± lip rounding
Length	Length of contact steady state
Tenseness	Mediolateral contact extent
Diphthongal	Extent of contact change

periphery of vowel space — high front, high back, mid front, mid back, and low central — will be filled with at least one vowel. This theory contributes helpful insight in our current efforts to derive a natural vowel hierarchy based on oral space utilization, but fails to explain diphthongs.

A Vowel Hierarchy

A proposed vowel hierarchy drawn from the child developmental studies and language phonetic distribution observations cited is shown in Table 4-1. Both sets of data support a physiologically based interpretation of vowel acquisition.

CONSONANT ARTICULATION

Consonants are differentiated by articulation place, manner, and voicing. Their noise sources differ by the different ways in which sound may be generated as the air stream moves through the vocal passageways (Figure 4-6). Semivowels are produced by moving the articulators rapidly from one vowel-like posture to another. Fricatives result when the phonic stream is channeled through constricted passageways. Stops are generated by building up air pressure behind places where a passageway is completely blocked then suddenly opened. This produces an explosive sound burst. Examination of the articulatory gestures that produce consonant noise reveals a systematic developmental order growing out of lawful physical relationships. This order can be described in part as a function of linguapalatal contact place and pattern (see Figure 4-7).

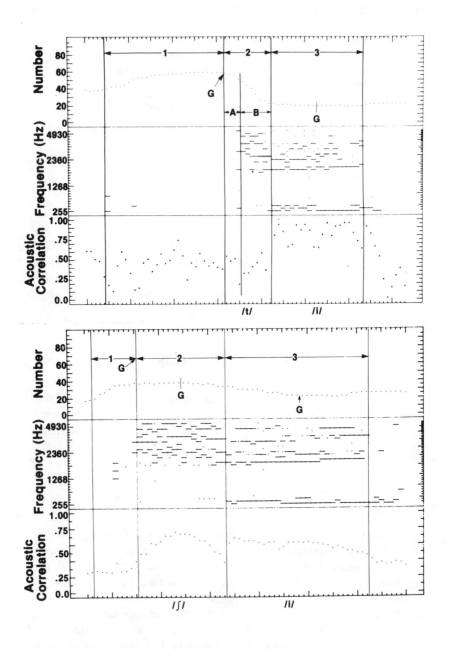

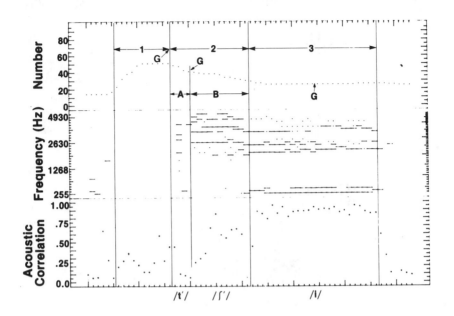

FIGURE 4–6. Computer generated plots of "tee," "she," and "chee" spoken by a normal 14-year-old male. The middle and lower portions of each plot show sound spectrographic and acoustic correlation changes that coincide with tongue contacts. The vertical lines separate the utterances into three time segments: (1) the period of increased linguapalatal constriction, (2) consonant sound production, and (3) vowel sound production. The partial vertical lines segment the consonants into linguapalatal release preceding (A) and following (B) the acoustic period of consonant sound production. The "G"s identify the frames selected to represent the stop, sibilant, and vowel portions of the words. Note that during the "tee" the contact changes progressively as the action moves from the [t] to the [ee]; whereas the contact changes little from [sh] to [ee] in "she."The contact during "chee" shows a linguapalatal release onset similar to "tee" with a plateau for sibilant sound production during the [ch]. Thus, the affricate represents a smooth blending of movement from stop to sibilant postures. From Fletcher, S. G. (1989a). Palatometric specification of stop, affricate, and sibilant sounds. *Journal of Speech and Hearing Research, 32,* 736–748. Reprinted by permission.

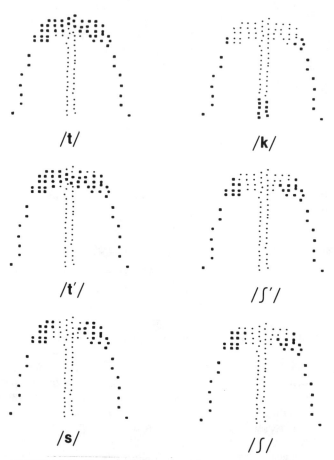

FIGURE 4-7. Linguapalatal contact during production of the /t/, /k/, /s/, and /ʃ/ consonants and the /t'/ and /ʃ'/ phases of the /tʃ/. The squares represent sensors contacted 80% of the time during repeated utterance of each sound by a 14-year-old male talker with normal speech. The dots identify uncontacted sensors. Fletcher, S. G. (1989a). Palatometric specification of stop, affricate, and sibilant sounds. *Journal of Speech and Hearing Research, 32,* 736–748. Reprinted by permission.

Glides and Stops

The glide sounds provide a bridge from vowel to consonant articulation. Glides are produced by rapid movements between vowel-like postures. The movements are so rapid, however, that the vowel identity is lost. For example, [j] is executed by placing the tongue near an [i] vowel posture then releasing the contact rapidly by lowering the tongue. During the glide the channel through which the air stream passes is never narrow enough to produce frictional noise. The noise that is generated appears in consonant-like fashion at the margins rather than in the central or nuclear part of words.

The stop sounds are characterized by complete stoppage of the air stream within the vocal tract. During production of the front stop the lateral borders of the tongue are tensed to produce a spoon-shaped configuration. The elevated outer edges of the tongue are then moved into contact with the palate around its entire outer periphery. The linguapalatal contact thus produces an anteriorly sealed cavity which blocks the flow of the phonic stream. The spoon-shaped tongue posture is reminiscent of a similar shape found in infant crying and swallowing (Fletcher, 1974; Strong, 1956; Wassilief, 1886). It is important to note that during production of the front stop sounds (i.e., [t, d]) the constriction is not simply at the anterior border of the alveolar ridge. Rather, intraoral containment of the phonic stream is achieved by bringing the outer border of the tongue against the entire peripheral border of the palate. Sound is then produced by building up air pressure behind this extensive intraoral obstruction then abruptly releasing it to generate the rather sharp sound burst of the stop sounds.

As illustrated in Figure 4–6, the sound production process may be separated into three divisions. During the initial action the tongue is brought to a preparatory articulation posture. This action is identified palatometrically by a systematic increase in the number of sensors contacted by the tongue as it moves into the preparatory posture. This position is maintained for a short time during which air pressure accumulates within the sealed oral cavity. Linguapalatal release occurs in the second phase of the action. The acoustic burst during stop sound production (see Figure 4–6) occurs within 20 to 30 msec after the linguapalatal release begins. Vowel onset appears later. It seems to coincide with the moment when the consonant releasing action is completed.

The anterior stop gesture is postulated to serve as a fountainhead for the remaining lingual consonant gestures. A series of specific adaptations are identifiable that can be conceived as developing directly from the basic anterior stop gesture. This tier relationship with other consonantal gestures is as follows. The articulatory posture for the [k, g] stops is viewed as the first contrastive adaptation of the front stop gesture. Velar stops are conceived as being produced by simply shifting the articulator contact location from the alveolar ridge where the [t, d] sounds are articulated to a location near the posterior edge of the hard palate for the [k, g] gesture. Again, contact against lateral margins of the alveolar ridge is a critical characteristic of the valving action. This contact extends across the palate near the hard palate/soft palate juncture with continued tongue stabilization against the lateral dental/

alveolar process. The lingual constriction release is first observed near the midline of the vocal tract. The [t, d] sounds are referred to as "front" or "tongue tip" sounds and [k, g] as "linguavelar" consonants only from the very limited viewpoint that the locus of the initial release portion of the gesture is at those sites.

Evidence of the intimate developmental relationship between the [t, d] and [k, g] gestures is found in young child sound substitutions. Preisser, Hodson, and Paden (1988) reported that the most common deviation involving the velar stop in the developmental phonology of 1½- to 2½-year-old children is stop sound fronting (e.g., *gum* → [dʌm]. This suggests that anterior lingual control is established earlier than posterior control, perhaps because of the relative visibility of the intraoral actions.

The gradual emergence of motor control over the articulators is beautifully illustrated in voice onset time[4] development during stop sound production. When children are between 1½ and 2½ years old, they gain the ability to manipulate laryngeal and oral articulation parameters independently. This is shown by refinements in voice onset time control. They first produce stops with uniformly short time lags between the acoustic onsets of the consonant and the vowel (cf. Macken, 1980). In English, these short-lag stops are heard as voiced /bdg/. In Spanish, the /bdg/ voice onset normally precedes the stop release and in /ptk/ follows it. Spanish children's short-lag stops are therefore heard as unvoiced. A gradual refinement then takes place as articulator control and timing matures. As this takes place, the child VOT moves toward adult values. The nature of adult phonetic perception clouds recognition of this transition, however. Rather than hearing the gradual transition that really occurs as the child gains independent control of the laryngeal and oral articulators, adults hear an abrupt shift to clear voice/voiceless distinctions only when the child's VOT values reach adult-like standards. Changes during the transition from child to adult VOT values are not easily discerned by adult listeners who hear speech sounds categorically.

Sibilants

The evolution of a second tier adaptation from the /t, d/consonant articulatory gesture revolves around establishing a grooved central passageway through the lingua-alveolar peripheral seal. High fre-

---

[4]Voice onset time (VOT) refers to the relative timing between an articulator constriction release and onset of vocal fold vibration. In stop sounds, the VOT is the time between the oral and laryngeal sound sources. The laryngeal tone can either precede (lead) or follow (lag) the stop release.

quency frictional noise is then generated by forcing air through this narrow channel. The amplitude of the noise as it emerges from the aperture is increased when the high velocity jet air stream strikes the teeth and is resonated in the cavity between the tongue and teeth (Fant, 1960). The resonant cavity volume is about 1 cm^3 for [s] and 4 cm^3 for [ʃ] (Perkell, 1981). The groove and small high frequency resonance cavity are thus core sibilant sound production features.

The nurturing and symbiotic relationships between anterior stop and sibilant gestures is illustrated by frequent clinical use of a stop consonant environment to develop the [s]. For example, the [s] gesture is often achieved by directing a child to repeat "ts" or "ns" then isolating and stabilizing the sibilant portion of the articulatory action. The complexity of the grooving gesture causes it to be commonly omitted during early childhood consonant cluster reduction (e.g., *spoon* → [pun]).

As the groove gesture is established, its versatility is increased by locating it at the front and back margins of the alveolar ridge to produce contrasting [s] and [ʃ] sibilants. A lip rounding gesture is also added to the [ʃ]. Wood (1986) has observed that lip rounding increases sensitivity to changes in the place of articulation in the prepalatal region of the mouth. The more posterior place and lip rounding refinements help explain the later arrival of the [ʃ] than [s] gesture in the developmental sound repertoire. Dyson (1988) reported the [s] to be present in both word-initial and word-final positions during spontaneous utterances of 2- to 3-year-old children while the [ʃ] was found only in the word-final position (but see Ingram, 1978; Ingram, Christenson, Veach, & Webster, 1980). A common origin of the sibilants is suggested by a systematic increase in [s] and [ʃ] differentiation across words spoken by 3- to 7-year-old children (Nittrouer, Studdert-Kennedy, & McGowan, 1989).

Fletcher and Newman (1991) studied the place and width of the sibilant groove during natural production of /s/ and /ʃ/ sounds by two talkers. Then they compared those results with listener perceptions as the place and width of the groove were systematically manipulated during production of sibilant-like sounds by the same two talkers and an additional one. In the natural speech experiment, one subject was found to produce [s] and [ʃ] through sibilant grooves 7 mm and 14 mm respectively from the incisor teeth. The other subject produced the same sounds 11.5 mm and 17.3 mm from the incisors. The second subject appeared to counterbalance his more posterior articulation place by reducing his sibilant groove width. In both subjects, the posterior edge of the alveolar ridge demarcated [s] and [ʃ] articulatory zones.

In the perception experiment, [s] was found to be heard when the groove was 5- to 10-mm from the incisor teeth and about 6 mm wide. Thus, consistent with Stevens' (1972) quantal theory, the anterior pala-

tal region was found to be relatively insensitive to location pertur-
bations. [ʃ] was heard when the groove was located behind the alveolar
ridge and was 10- to 12-mm wide. The physical difficulty the different
speakers experienced in achieving stipulated sibilant groove places and
dimensions also appeared to exert an important effect on the sounds
heard by the listeners. In the responses of the subject who produced
sibilant-like noise through grooves at the stipulated locations and
widths with comparatively little difficulty, a strong systematic relationship was found between linguapalatal contact place, groove width,
and the sibilant heard by the listeners. The 6-mm wide groove produced a significantly higher proportion of [s] percepts than did either
smaller or wider grooves. It was noted that this groove width was also
most common in this subject's natural [s] sound production. It is also
similar to that reported by Hixon (1966) from air pressure/flow studies
and those found in previous palatometric studies of normal speech by
Fletcher and his associates (Flege, Fletcher, & Homiedan, 1987; Fletcher,
1989a; Wolf, Fletcher, McCutcheon, & Hasegawa, 1976).

The [s] groove was typically located on the fourth row of sensors in
the responses of the second subject. This was 11.5 mm from the lingual
edge of his central incisors, suggesting that as yet undefined physical
attributes such as shape and size of the oral cavity as well as location
and size of the sibilant groove contribute to a speaker's choice of the
articulatory parameters of sounds spoken.

In the initial, natural-speech experiment, the [ʃ] was produced
through a 9- to 12-mm groove that was formed by both talkers 14 to 18
mm from the lingual surface of the upper incisors. These dimensions
are also similar to those reported previously (Fletcher, 1989a; Hixon,
1966; Shadle, 1985). It is noteworthy that in both the naturally generated [ʃ] sounds and those identified from listener classifications of
sibilants produced as groove place and width were systematically manipulated, the grooves were in close juxtaposition to the rear border of
the alveolar process. This juxtaposition would cause the jet stream to be
directed against the more vertically oriented buttress of the alveolar
process and its major rugae. These structures thus likely serve as sound
sources in [ʃ] noise generation.

In the perception experiment, noise generated through grooves
near the front border of the alveolar ridge were heard as [s]; those
formed behind the posterior margin of the ridge were heard as [ʃ]. An
interactive effect between groove place and width was evident in the
intermediate region of the alveolar ridge. In the utterances from the
subject with the most skill in linguapalatal contact placement, the noise
generated through 6 mm grooves was heard as [s] when the groove was
placed as far back as the fifth sensor row (14 mm from the incisor edge).
Noise from 10- to 12-mm grooves was perceived as [ʃ] when the groove

was as far forward as the third row of sensors (10 mm from the incisor edge). Thus, as reported in earlier studies of articulatory compensation (Fletcher, 1985; Hasegawa, Christensen, McCutcheon, & Fletcher, 19-77) groove width as well as place apparently contributed jointly in distinguishing [s] and [ʃ] sibilants. Groove place is probably easier for talkers to control in natural flowing, connected speech contexts, however.

Affricates, Spirants, and Liquids

The establishment of stop and groove articulatory gestures lays the foundation for affricate gestures. Affricates require a stop closure followed by frictional noise release of impounded air through a groove at the rear margin of the alveolar ridge (see Fletcher, 1989a; Gimson, 1972). The placement of this gesture at the posterior edge of the alveolar ridge, which is the same as that normally used during the [ʃ], distinguishes the [tʃ] onset from that of the [t]. An important observation by Gimson (1972) is that the frictional part of the [tʃ] is of shorter duration than that of the fricatives proper. This noise production property and the single location placement provide support for his contention that the affricate is a unified, monophoneme, stop-groove sound rather than a compound amalgamation of two sounds produced in close proximity. Directing the subject to produce a "tight, quick" [ʃ] is often sufficient to secure a [tʃ] acoustic output.

The linguadental slit fricative [f] and [θ] "spirant" sounds have less acoustic intensity than other consonants. The inherently reduced intensity of sounds produced at or near the incisors is attributed to the fact that noise generation is less efficient for a slit than groove-shaped channel (Lauttamus, 1984, p. 104). The [θ] posture is achieved by moving the tongue forward from its anterior stop posture. Frictional noise is then generated by directing air gently through the thin slit remaining between the forward placed tongue tip and incisor teeth. The thin slit concept may be understood by analogy with the [f] which has an articulation that may be viewed directly on a speaker's face. Vigorous practice in mimicking alternating [f, θ, f, θ] slit fricatives via direct observation and palatometric feedback can be helpful in achieving discriminant control over the linguadental and labiodental spirant gestures.

The liquid consonant [l] introduces yet another variation in the stop closure gesture. In this instance the appropriate gesture is secured by breaking the linguapalatal contact at some point behind the lateral corners of the enclosure. The [l] is thus formed with midline closure and a lateral opening, usually at both sides of the mouth. The [l] can be produced with either a front (light [l]) or back alveolar (dark [l]) tongue position. The sound may also be produced by channeling a voiced air stream through a lateral groove or around the posterior margins of one or both alveolar processes. In the latter condition the air stream travels through the buccal cavities before emerging from the mouth. Quick release of the tongue contact in repeated syllables, as in [la, la, la], helps produce a clear audible quality as the [l] is spoken. Practice in producing this sound should include a variety of vowels since the [l] quality can vary substantially in different phonetic environments.

The liquid [r] consonant is uniquely characterized by noise generated during a rapid, backward sliding movement of the tongue. The [r] is usually formed by anchoring the sides of the tongue firmly along the lateral margins of the palate then raising the tip toward the [t] posture as the contact is slid rapidly back. Instead of completing the enclosing gesture of the stop consonant, however, the outer margin of the tongue tip is simply curled *slightly* upward and sometimes backward during the combined tongue tip and body actions. The amount of backward curl varies across speakers and phonetic contexts. This led Ladefoged (1975) to suggest that the more general term *rhotic* should be used to describe the /r/ consonant rather than *retroflex*. The use of the rhotic label also deemphasizes the notion that the /r/ must have a strong backward curling component.

The /r/ gesture includes the hollowed, spoon-shaped configuration of the tongue as it is curled upward around its outer border. A posterior moving action of the tongue in this posture creates a resonant cavity between the tip and undersurface of the tongue and teeth. The [r] posture may also be approximated by producing a voiced [ð] or [z] and, while prolonging the sound, drawing the tongue tip upward toward the rear edge of the alveolar ridge. The physically demanding nature of the [l] and [r] gestures is described in a report by Preisser et al. (1988) who noted that deletion of the liquid consonant in consonant clusters (e.g., black → [bæk]) was the most frequently found deficiency in the speech of 1½- to 2½-year-old children. Vowelization by substituting a less complex gesture for the liquid (e.g., *zipper* → [zɪpʊ] and *leaf* → [wif]) was next in frequency.

Consonants in World Languages

Stops occur in the inventories of all known languages. They are therefore regarded as the *optimal* consonants (Jakobson & Halle, 1956, p. 42). The overwhelming majority of languages contrast the stops by voicing and by bilabial, dental or alveolar, and velar place of articulation. Stops are likely to be voiceless.[5] If a language has at least two stops,

---

[5]Macken (1980) pointed out that English-speaking children usually produce "voiced" stops as voiceless unaspirated sounds that are therefore more similar to Spanish and French voiceless stops.

it is likely to have a voiceless/voiced contrast. The velar and dental/alveolar places of articulation are also frequent across languages. This is indicated by Maddieson's (1984) observation that if a particular language has a /p/, it will likely have a /k/; and if it has a /k/, it will probably have a /t/. The same generalizations are true of the voiced counterparts of each of these stops.

Virtually every language has at least one nasal consonant. In general, if a consonant is a nasal, it will also be voiced. The most common place of nasal articulation is in the dental/alveolar area, but bilabials are also very frequent (Ferguson, 1963). With rare exceptions every language that has a nasal has an /n/. /m/ is the next most common. If a language has only one nasal consonant, it will be formed at the dental/alveolar place. As in English, the next most common nasal articulation place after the alveolar and labial places is velar. The presence of a velar nasal consonant implies both /m/ and /n/.

The oral obstruent/nasal consonant contrast is also important among world languages. Ferguson observed that the number of nasal consonants in a language is never greater than the number of obstruents (either a stop or affricate). In the majority of languages the nasals are a subset of the places at which obstruents occur.

The great majority of the world's languages have at least one fricative. Except for the Australian languages, the most frequent fricative is the voiceless sibilant /s/. The /s/ is not an easy sound to articulate, however. The /s/ gesture requires the articulators to be placed such that the central groove is maintained to generate a high velocity jet air stream. The requirement to achieve a near but not complete closing action rapidly during sibilant sound production helps explain the late acquisition of the groove gesture.

The next most frequent fricative in the languages of the world is the posterior palatoalveolar /ʃ/. The incidence of /ʃ/ is followed closely by the incidence of palatoalveolar voiceless affricatives (Maddieson, 1984). Voiceless sibilant fricatives and affricatives are also much more common than their voiced counterparts in languages of the world. Only about a third of the fricatives found are voiced, however. There is a general tendency for voiced fricatives to be found only when its voiceless counterpart is present. /z/ is the most common voiced fricative, but it rarely occurs without the /s/ voiceless cognate. This is also true of the other common voiced sibilant, /ʒ/, the voiced cognate of /ʃ/.

Most languages have at least one lateral liquid articulated with the blade or tip of the tongue against dental/alveolar structures. The most common liquid is the voiced lateral /l/. Maddieson (1984) suggested that the preference for tip or blade articulations during the /l/ is because it provides a free air passage behind the front closure. A lateral liquid sound may be produced by directing the air stream through a channel on either one or both sides of the tongue. No data are available on the incidence of unilateral versus bilateral emission of the air stream.

Midline articulatory actions are more common in world languages and consistently appear earlier in speech development than their lateralized counterparts. A physical maturation origin of later lateral liquid arrival than the sibilants is suggested by the fact that side to side movements are acquired later in natural development than midline tongue raising and lowering actions. The late maturation laterality principle helps explain the lower appearance of the [l] in the consonant hierarchy.

The next most common liquid is /r/. Most /r/s in world languages are produced as trilled, tap, or flap consonants. The typical language has one lateral and one /r/ sound. The vast majority of these sounds are voiced. Only about 10% of the /r/s in world languages are produced as approximants, however, and only half of the approximants are retroflex. Production of the /r/ in a retroflex manner is also less common in English. Ladefoged (1975) pointed out that the English rhoticized /r/quality can be produced either with the tip raising retroflex movement or with the more common tip down, raising of the tongue to a high bunched posture. Both moving gestures have a very similar auditory effect. The difficulty of learning to execute a moving articulatory action helps explain the late arrival of liquid [r] sounds in the consonant hierarchy.

The last sounds to appear in the English consonant hierarchy are the "slit spirants", or /θ/ sounds. As might be anticipated, the slit spirants are also uncommon among world languages and usually among the very last sounds to be acquired during English speech development. This slowness in development is attributed to the marked difficulty met in forming a wide but narrow space between the tongue tip and the teeth and generating a continuous laminar stream of air through the slit. Maddieson (1984) suggests that the low intensity spirants originate from "laxing or weakening" plosive sounds. Thus, the relatively rare appearance of these sounds in languages of the world may be explained on grounds of both physical complexity and auditory weakness. Their low intensity may help explain why, when they do occur in world languages, they are more likely to be voiced than voiceless. In fact, the existence of a voiceless spirant implies the presence of its voiced counterpart. Ferguson (1978) has noted a tendency within languages to transform /θ/ into an /s/. Such transformation is commonly observed among children during their developmental years.

The Consonant Hierarchy

The contrasts in consonant production patterns reveal a systematic increase in articulatory complexity that parallels the natural developmental order of consonant evolution. Stoel-Gammon (1985), Preisser, Hodson, and Paden (1988), and Dyson (1988) all reported that glides, stops, and nasals are among the earliest sounds acquired. Fricatives, affricates, and liquids appear later. The developmental role of front versus back contrast is indicated in observations by Templin (1957), Jakobson (1968), and Locke (1983) that nonfrontal sounds develop only after some anterior sounds have been acquired.

Dinnsen, Chin, Elbert, and Powell (1990) reviewed the phonological systems of forty, 40- to 80-month-old children with functional misarticulation and sought to extract converging principles with implied laws that governed misarticulation properties. The hierarchical order they derived is shown in Table 4–2 along with the order of the sounds following a physiologic complexity interpretation. The phonetic inventories yielded from the Dinnsen et al. study showed feature distinctions that parallel the physiologically based order, and the order of articulation development in normal children rather closely.

Dinnsen et al. (1990) also described constraints that seemed to function within phonetic categories. For example, if sounds are limited to their most general constraint, stops would be developed first in word-initial position and fricates and affricates in postvocalic positions. No apparent contextual constraints were found for glides and nasals. As shown in Table 4–2, the phonetic feature hierarchy derived fits that gleaned from developmental articulation studies and the order of sounds arranged by their order of physiological complexity rather well.

TABLE 4–2. Consonant hierarchy implied by emergence of phonetic features during speech development (Dinnsen et al., 1990), frequency of sounds in world languages, and control of articulatory gestures. Some discrepancies between the reported orders of phonetic feature and articulatory control development are evident.

Phonetic Feature	Articulatory Control
Syllabic	Semivowel glide
Consonantal	Stop
Sonorant	Nasal vs. oral
Coronal	Articulation place
Voice	Voice timing
Continuant	Groove
Delayed release	Stop-groove
Nasal	Lateral groove
Strident	Rhotic movement
Lateral	Slit groove

The consonant sound hierarchy shown in Table 4–2 may be fruitfully thought of as an extension of the basic stop gesture. In this conceptualization, the sound levels represent an order of increasingly demanding physiological complexity in articulation programming. The order derived by Dinnsen and his associates (1990) appears to reflect a natural process of motor control development. Naturalness is defined in this context by both the ease of sound production and the acquisition of the sounds in a sequential order that represents increasingly complex maneuvers. Following this definition, one articulatory action is more natural than another if it appears earlier in the development sequence *and* it occurs in a greater number of languages.

Speech clinicians have long used a developmentally derived hierarchy of consonant sounds to guide assessment of misarticulation and establish the order of sounds to be modified through speech therapy. Their hierarchy has been based on cross-sectional, broad-sample studies of children tested at specific ages. The developmental norms derived from these data reflect the age at which most children produce the phonemes of the language in an adult-like manner. They are therefore referred to as *age of sound acquisition* norms. A major criticism of these norms has been that to achieve a sufficiently broad sample of talkers at each age, the investigators limited their phoneme samples to single words, with sounds sampled a single time in initial, medial, and final positions within the word. Articulation errors were then defined in terms of deviations from the expected incidence of sound mastery in the normative studies. The magnitude and types of deviation from the norms were used to establish the degree of speech disability. Despite between-study methodological differences that led to some discrepancies in the findings from one study to another (cf. Smit, 1986) and the limited phonetic sampling methods used, the results have generally showed acceptable agreement from study to study. They have also provided very useful information for English consonant acquisition assessment and a firm treatment order rationale. The findings show nasals, stops, and glides acquired relatively early, fricatives and affricates later, followed by liquids and spirants. This order is similar to that predicated by physiological complexity and found in the review of sound frequencies in world languages. All of these data support a physiological basis for the order of sound mastery and usage.

GENERAL ARTICULATION PROPERTIES

In summary, the foregoing review of developmental, physiologic complexity, and language usage information points to the following five articulatory properties that will play a central role in the upcoming speech assessment and training considerations. Articulatory gestures are:

1. motor rule based,
2. spatially and temporally discriminable,
3. ordered by a hierarchy of articulatory complexity,
4. developed through experience across a wide action range, and
5. organized to generate maximally contrastive sound output differences that enhance meaning in speech perception.

CHAPTER 5

PROSODY:
A FRAMEWORK
FOR SPEECH

Articulatory gestures provide the physical elements in speech phonetic segments. Suprasegmental modifications in rate, amplitude, quality, and temporal organization of those elements in dynamically coupled syllables, phrases, and sentences add to, enhance, or subtly change their meaning (Studdert-Kennedy, 1979). These changes, as the phonic air stream is made audible, underlie speech melody and rhythm sensations. Collectively, they define the *prosody* of speech production.

Prosody contributes information about how a person feels about what he or she is saying, provides a general framework for the spoken message, and contributes significantly to a listener's ability to predict what will be said from what has been said. The importance of prosody as a basic property of vocal communication is indicated by experiments such as that by Darwin (1975). He asked listeners to shadow a sentence that was introduced in one ear while a competing sentence was played into the other. At some arbitrary point, the speech melody suddenly switched to the other ear while the syntactic and semantic sequences continued to be heard in the original ear. The listeners were apparently covertly tracking the intonation contour in the supposedly unattended ear. Prosody overrode syntax, semantics, and the ear of entry as it interacted with the words heard.

The major sources of prosody in speech can be grouped into four main categories: individual word stress patterns; sentence accent placement; syntactic ambiguity resolution; and pragmatic factors, such as attitudinal indicators that influence the intonation contour (Cutler & Isard, 1980).

Studies of speech with abnormal prosody can help reveal its practical importance. For example, many of the prosodic indices of meaning and emotion are missing in the slow, labored, individual-sound prolonged, rhythmically abnormal, stress disturbed utterances of deaf speakers (Hudgins, 1934; Metz, Schiavetti, Samar, & Sitler, 1990; Stevens, Nickerson, & Rawlins, 1983). They seem to deal with speech primarily on the segmental level. That is, syllables and words appear to be treated by such talkers as separate units rather than having the actions integrated across phrases and sentences. Most of the syllables are spoken as though they were stressed. Intersyllabic and coarticulatory timing is particularly disturbed. Pauses are frequently lengthened, laryngeal and oral action sequencing miscoordinated, stressed and unstressed syllables are produced with the same duration, and word duration is not adjusted to reflect the word's syntactic location or contextual significance within utterances (McGarr & Lofquist, 1982; Nickerson, 1975). These prosodic disturbances compound those from misarticulation and have a profound effect upon both the intelligibility and the naturalness of the spoken message. It may be seen that virtually every facet of prosody is influenced by hearing deficits.

Some prosody disturbances can be traced to malfunction and miscoordination at the laryngeal level. For example, malpositioned and under- or overly tensed vocal folds may result in abnormally high or low average fundamental frequency (F_0). Coupled with erratic pitch and intensity variations and harsh or breathy voice quality the speech output then takes on a bizarre quality.

Debate continues concerning the degree of deficit each prosodic disturbance contributes to the difficulties talkers experience (Maassen & Povel, 1985; Nickerson, 1975). Experiments to resolve these difficulties are limited by imprecise distinctions between speech intelligibility and naturalness and by interrelations between segmental and suprasegmental functions. Metz, Schiavetti, Samar, and Sitler (1990) made a significant contribution to our understanding of how segmental and supersegmental functions interact in deaf speech. They used regression and principal components analyses to determine the effect of 28 acoustic segmental and suprasegmental parameters on the speech intelligibility of 40 talkers who were severely to profoundly hearing impaired. Six major factors were derived that could account for 59% of the intelligibility variance. The most important single factor was temporal and spatial articulatory control of laryngeal versus oral articulations. Voice onset time (VOT), jaw opening, and tongue height represented in first formant measures, and articulator movement skill identified in speaking rate measures were included in this factor. Most of these sub-factors point to disturbances on the segmental level. The next most important factor identified suprasegmental disturbances. This factor isolated the difficulties that hearing impaired speakers experience in using falling versus rising intonation to differentiate declarative and interrogative utterances. These difficulties seemed to reflect problems in both laryngeal sequencing and in manipulating the intonation to differentiate statement versus question utterances. The third factor isolated dynamic consonant-to-vowel and vowel-to-vowel diphthongal movements and transitions, particularly in [aɪ], as a central consideration in the speech of the talkers. Higher intelligibility was associated with prominent second formant transitions in the consonants and clear fundamental frequency changes in the vowels. The next factor identified difficulties in using differences in F_0 and vowel duration to communicate emphatic word stress. Large F_0 and duration differences between the stressed and unstressed vowels, for example, led to more intelligible utterances. The investigators reported that the contribution of this factor along with Factor 1 could account for 74% of the intelligibility variance. The last two factors reflected a mixture of segmental and suprasegmental parameters that the writers were unable to interpret meaningfully. In general, this study provided clear evidence of interwoven intelligibility benefits from articulation and prosody control.

The importance of the factors identified by Metz et al. (1990) has been documented by findings from studies of experimentally altered speech. Correction of deviant phoneme durations in deaf speech has shown small intelligibility improvements (Osberger & Levitt, 1979). Substantial improvement has been demonstrated when segmental timing aspects of deaf speech were instrumentally corrected (Maasen & Povel, 1985). Improved intelligibility was also observed when 160 msec silent pauses were inserted between words in sentences spoken by profoundly hearing impaired children (Maassen, 1986). These findings again point to fundamental and complementary roles played by articulation and prosody in the speech of those with impaired hearing.

Speech prosody has also been singled out as a critical factor in the difficulties listeners experience with persons who have foreign accents. Chreist (1964) observed that abnormal rhythm and stress patterns can render English spoken by nonnative talkers both unnatural and less intelligible. The validity of these observations was attested in a study by Suzuki (1986). In a series of experiments, Suzuki examined changes in speech "naturalness" as pauses, segmental and suprasegmental durations, pitch, and vocal intensity were systematically manipulated in English spoken by native Japanese and American talkers. In one stimulus set the parameters in the Japanese sentences were systematically replaced by the corresponding parameters from American sentences.

In the other set, parameters in the American sentences were replaced by the corresponding Japanese parameters. Thus, Japanese accents were gradually introduced into the American sentences, and the Japanese sentences were given American accents. When all four prosodic parameters in the Japanese sentences were replaced by their American equivalents, the listeners found the sentences to be more natural than the Japanese accented American speech.

The contributions of prosody have also been examined in spectrally rotated speech. Blesser (1969) conducted a series of studies in which the spectra of words spoken were automatically rotated around a 1600 Hz central frequency. Low frequency components of the signals were replaced by corresponding high frequencies and vice versa. This transformation devastated segmental cues such as spectral energy concentrations and formant space relations in the sounds spoken but preserved source feature and prosodic information. Pitch sensations were maintained since the harmonic structure was intact. Suprasegmental intensity, stress, and rhythmic temporal order cues were also preserved as were segmental cues identifying consonant voicing, obstruency, and frication.

The training consisted of having adult subjects learn to converse through the frequency transformed speech. After each session, listening and comprehension tests were given to assess changes in performance and identify learning strategies. Blesser found that the participants learned to communicate through the transformed speech medium in a surprisingly short time. Even in the initial sessions they were able to use some prosodic cues remarkably well. Virtually all of their confusions were noted to be between words that were not differentiated prosodically, such as those with the same number of syllables, the same intonation patterns, and similar rhythms. Difficulties with word familiarity was also evident. Uncommon monosyllabic and bisyllabic words produced particularly low recognition scores. Sentence syntax was also helpful. In later sessions the subjects continued to confuse words in the spectrally rotated speech but recognized the syntactic structure in which they were embedded. Function words that were intimately linked with the syntactic structure of the sentence but had little semantic content were recognized more frequently than content words. Only after further exposure to the transformed speech did they begin to use segmental cues to recognize the content words in the sentences. The improvements in phonetic recognition leveled off at about 30% for vowels and 35% for consonants, however.

Contextual cues were used with increasing effectiveness by Blesser's subjects to identify words and follow the discussion. Significantly higher word recognition scores were achieved when the subjects were given semantic priming (i.e., told the semantic category, such as city names, of a word), but the use of phonetic cues, such as sound identification by place of articulation, remained difficult throughout the study. In sentence recognition, the context only helped when it provided semantic redundancy.

Interestingly, the amount of time the subjects spent in conversation through the transformed speech medium did not correlate with improvements in consonant identification, but time spent in free conversation did. During the process of learning to communicate through spectrally rotated speech, Blesser also became aware of a "breakthrough" phenomenon. He noted that after changes in phonetic recognition began to approach an asymptotic performance level, the subjects seemed to show a sudden ability to converse in transformed speech. He attributed this to their reaching an acoustic processing skill level at which the time consumed in decoding the utterance was less than the talker's speaking rate. They were apparently able to decode the information rapidly enough that they had time to "lock on" to the sentence meaning.

The major insights gleaned from this brief review are that the human central processing system will use whatever information is available to identify and interpret spoken messages. Thus, it is futile to ask whether prosodic or phonetic information is more important in speech understanding. Both domains are essential, deeply interrelated, and interdependent. All available cues appear to be accepted, integrated, and globally optimized to achieve speech understanding and intelligible output. The sudden arrival of the ability to converse through frequency transformed speech attests to the rich central interconnections used dynamically by listeners to resolve what has been said.

Attention will now be directed toward the emergence of prosody and the specific roles and functions it serves in spoken language. A child's entry into language is mediated by meaning. It is obvious that meaning cannot be conveyed by isolated features or phonemes. The earliest unit of meaning acquired by the developing child is probably the prosodic contour of speech melody. The child learns very early to use a rising pitch to indicate questions and surprise and a falling pitch for statements. Menn (1978) observed that the young child she studied discovered that high-pitched whining and squealing could gain caregiver attention and actions as babbling appeared. At other times, the child moderated his vocal pitch range toward that of the adults around him. Later, short rising-pitch utterances with a high peak were used in his babbling to obtain an object or service. Similar utterances with a moderate peak functioned to initiate or maintain social interaction. Refinement of the signaling system was thus evident as prosody was used to differentiate adults-as-instruments and adults-as-social-partners vocalizations. Menn noted that the child's free babble was also characterized by increasingly elaborate intonation contours, gestures, and actions used to convey special meaning.

A universal characteristic of human speech noted from early infancy is that the fundamental frequency and acoustic amplitude of the voice fall at the end of an utterance. Lieberman (1980) suggested that this is a natural physiologically dictated function of the phonatory system. A brief review of laryngeal structure and function is needed to clarify this facet of speech motor control.

LARYNGEAL FUNCTIONS

Four cartilages provide the structural framework of the larynx: the cricoid cartilage rests on top of the upper ring of the trachea and serves as the base of the larynx. This signet ring-shaped cartilage widens from front to back. The thyroid cartilage partially surrounds the cricoid cartilage. They are anchored together via cricothyroid joints on each posterolateral surface of the cricoid cartilage. The thyroid cartilage is shaped like two butterfly wings joined anteriorly at the thyroid notch. The angle between the wings is near 95° in men and 135° in women. The narrower angle creates the often-prominent male "Adam's apple." Toward the rear, the thyroid cartilage curves upward and downward to form long, narrow *carnua.* The upper carnua anchor the hyothyroid ligaments. The lower carnua terminate in the cricothyroid joint. Their location on the back, lateral surface of the cricoid cartilage provides leverage to rotate the thyroid cartilage up and down. This helps tense and relax the vocal folds. Two arytenoid cartilages, shaped like triangular pyramids, rest on the upper posterior rim of the cricoid plate. The cricoarytenoid joints allow the arytenoid cartilages to both rotate around their vertical axis and slide forward and back to some extent. The thyroid and arytenoid cartilages are connected by the vocal ligaments that lie along the medial edge of each fold. The final cartilage in the "laryngeal skeleton" is the epiglottis. It is attached at the inner, front surface of the thyroid cartilage just below the thyroid notch and appears to play little or no part in phonation.

Postures of the vocal folds and movements at the cricothyroid and cricoarytenoid joints are controlled by intrinsic laryngeal muscles. The cricothyroid muscles originate at the front sides of the cricoid cartilage and insert on outer surfaces of the thyroid cartilage. When they are contracted they rotate the thyroid cartilage downward. The thyroarytenoid muscles originate from the inner surface of the thyroid cartilage below the thyroid notch and insert on the vocal process of the arytenoid cartilages. They provide the bulk of the vocal folds. The cricothyroid and thyroarytenoid muscles have an agonist-antagonist relationship. When the thyroid cartilage is rotated downward by the cricothyroid muscles, the vocal folds are elongated and tensed. When the thyroarytenoid muscles are contracted, the thyroid cartilage is pulled back up and their vibrating mass is increased as the pull from the cricothyroid is counterbalanced. This separation of functions is not complete, however. The vocalis muscles are a division of the thyroarytenoid muscles. They are located beside the vocal ligaments and are attached to them along most of their length. When they are activated, they can thus help fine tune vocal fold tension and contribute to control of their mass and stiffness.

The lateral cricoarytenoid muscles originate from the upper surface of the cricoid cartilage and terminate on the outside corner of each arytenoid cartilage. When they are contracted, they cause the outer corners of the arytenoids to be rotated forward, thereby swinging the vocal folds inward and helping to adduct them. This inward movement is amplified by the interarytenoid muscles that span from arytenoid to arytenoid cartilage on their rear surface. The vocal folds are abducted (separated) by the posterior cricoarytenoid muscles which originate along the posterior surface of the cricoid and attach to the back, outer corners of the arytenoid cartilages. The contraction of these muscles causes the vocal process of the arytenoids to rotate laterally, in the opposite direction from when the lateral cricoarytenoid muscles act.

The vocalis muscle comprises the medial part of the thyroarytenoid muscle. Its fibers insert along the vocal ligament. When it is contracted, it pulls the arytenoid cartilages forward. This decreases vocal fold tension. This permits it to play a special role in fine tuning vocal fold tension.

As can be seen in Figure 5-1, the vocal fold consists of mucosal epithelium, the lamina propria, and the vocalis muscle. The superficial layer in the lamina consists of loose connective tissue which serves with the mucosal lining to provide the vocal fold "cover." The transition layer of tissue includes the intermediate and deep layers of the vocal ligament. The vocalis muscle is referred to as the "body" of the vocal folds since the thyroarytenoid is not shown.

Based on the layer structure of the vocal folds, Hirano (1975) proposed a cover-body model to explain variations in the mode of vocal fold vibration. In this model, contraction of the cricothyroid muscle elongates the vocal folds and increases stiffness of both the cover and the body to produce falsetto register phonation. Contraction of the vocalis muscle shortens the vocal fold, increases the effective mass and stiffness of the body, and decreases that of the cover. This action along with contraction of the cricothyroid is used for glottal fry and chest register phonation.[1]

---

[1]This model offers no explanation for middle vocal register. There is considerable doubt whether that register actually exists (see Hollien & Schoenhard, 1983).

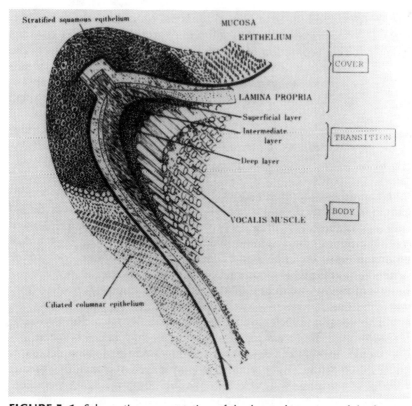

FIGURE 5-1. Schematic representation of the layered structure of the human vocal fold. From Hirano, M. (1981). Structure of the vocal fold in normal and disease states. Anatomical and physical studies. In C. L. Ludlow & M. O. Hart (Eds.), *Proceedings of the conference on the assessment of vocal pathology. ASHA Reports 11* (pp. 11–30). Rockville, MD: The American Speech-Language-Hearing Association. Reprinted by permission.

The larynx is richly supplied by sensory and motor nerve fibers. Motor innervation is via the recurrent laryngeal nerve. Sensory fibers are distributed through the internal laryngeal nerve (ILN) and, to a smaller extent, the external and recurrent laryngeal nerves. The ILN innervates both superficial and deep sensory receptors and guards the airways against entrance of foreign material. It also provides essential tactile and proprioceptive feedback for respiration and phonation. In cat and rabbit studies, for instance, Davis and Nail (1988) found that ILN fibers are capable of signaling vibratory sensations up to 400 Hz or more. They are also very sensitive to vibratory amplitude. These observations suggest that these fibers could provide a significant source of information for vocal fold vibratory amplitude, frequency, and timing control.

Since speech represents such finely integrated laryngeal, oral, and acoustic functions, one might suspect that direct linkages exist across the sensory systems. Some evidence supports this assumption. Sapir, McClean, and Larson (1983) and Udaka, Kanetake, Kihara, and Koike (1988) reported electromyographic (EMG) activity in the human cricothyroid muscle in response to auditory stimuli. Udaka et al. also found reproducible EMG detected activity in the cricothyroid and the lateral cricothyroid muscles in response to both bilateral and ipsilateral stimulation of the superior orbital branch of the trigeminal nerve. Laryngeal responses from stimulation of the maxillary and mandibular branches of the trigeminal nerve would also be likely, although this possibility has not yet been explored.

A series of electrical stimulation, lesioning, single-unit recording, and anatomical studies have been used to acquire basic information about how vocal functions are planned, adjusted, and controlled at higher nervous system levels. A major effort has been given to clarifying relationships between vocalization and neural activity in brain stem and midbrain neurons. Evidence has been found that the periaqueductal grey (PAG) area of the midbrain (Ortega, DeRosier, Park, & Larson, 1988) along with fibers in and around the nucleus ambiguous may be directly involved in vocal coordination (Larson, Derosier, & West, in press; Larson & Kistler, 1986). Some of the PAG neural units have been observed to increase their firing rate, some decrease their rate, and some become active just before vocalization. Certain units have shown activity correlated with very specific vocal functions (e.g., vocal intensity, duration, and fundamental frequency control). Electromyographic evidence indicates that sets of cells within the PAG may contribute to specific types of muscle activity. The responses from these nuclei are long lag (12 msec), however, compared with those of the nucleus ambiguous (4 to 5 msec). This indicates that their effect is probably modulated through the lower center (Larson et al., in press). Their discharge pattern indicates that the PAG neurons may be exclusively concerned with vocalization while those in the nucleus ambiguous seem to serve more as a relay for swallowing and respiration activities. In general, these findings along with those from Ortega et al. (1988) suggest that neural activity within the PAG can activate vocalization with specific acoustical properties. Elicitation of abnormal vocalizations has also been demonstrated that opens a way to determine how PAG dysfunction could lead to vocal abnormalities.

This information seems to provide a firm physical basis for control of prosody at the laryngeal, brainstem, and midbrain levels. Attention will now be directed toward more precisely defining the different facets of prosody that exist and examining roles they might play in vocal communication.

RHYTHM

Dynamic actions are intrinsically rhythmical. The rates and phases of their periodicities reflect the functions of particular subcomponents and their coupling within the system. They also reflect general bodily organization principles. For example, when subjects produce repetitive finger tapping and syllable actions at the same time, they experience difficulty if the movements are "out-of-synch." Little or no difficulty is experienced, however, if the movements are produced at identical or harmonically related times. Additionally, when one is listening to a salient rhythm, such as the cadence of a marching band, the rhythm tends to cause other actions to "fall into step." Even speaking tends to assume the beat of strongly rhythmical noise or music. These responses function as if the speech and body movements are governed by the same internal clock.

Rhythm is a central feature of infant noise making and babbling. And babbling is a widely recognized landmark on the path to articulate speech. Elbers (1982) observed that babbling progresses through four major stages with each stage representing an increment in rhythmical patterning. Babbling begins with single syllables such as [ba] produced in isolation. It progresses to rhythmic reduplicated syllables (ba, ba, ba), then acquires alternating or concatenating contrast (ba, da, ba, di, de), and culminates in jargon babbling that includes a complex rhythmical mix of syllables with real words increasingly interspersed in the utterances.

Ferguson (1986) suggests that reduplicative babbling serves several roles in phonological development. It enables the child to manipulate a unit smaller than a word as a step toward phonemic segmentation and specification, paves the way toward polysyllables with increasing phonetic complexity, and introduces syllable final consonants. These developments signal a systematic refinement of vocal rhythm and stress patterns toward those of mature speech. Beginning control of prosodic shaping thus emerges in conjunction with phonetic sound contrast.

As illustrated in Table 5-1, many *rhythmical* motor skills emerge when the infant is around 25 to 30 weeks, or six to seven months, of age (cf. Thelen, 1979). This rhythmical activity also coincides with the arrival of prosody control. Reduplicated babbling is thus part of a general developmental process in which movements become organized within dynamic cyclical gestures (cf. Kent, 1985). As reciprocal movement skills become organized, stabilized, and habitual in rhythmical actions, the child gains readiness to explore other variations in movement rates and patterns. Elbers (1982) suggested that reduplicative babbling provides a springboard for gradual progression from sound making to words, phrases, sentences, and adult speech.

TABLE 5–1. Development changes in stereotyped rhythmical movements by human infants (age in weeks).

Structure	Peak Interval	Peak Week
Legs	24–32	22
Torso, hands, and knees	24–32	28
Fingers	24–32	30
Hands	28–50	28
Arms	28–50	36
Torso,		
sitting	34–42	34
kneeling	44–52	40
standing	44–52	42

After Thelen, E. (1979). Rhythmical stereotypies in normal human infants. *Animal Behaviour, 27*, 699–515.

This discussion suggests that a major function of early sound-making activities is exploration of possible prosody parameters that can be controlled and manipulated. As these parameters are explored, movement strategies evolve to link the developing prosody with articulatory gestures. This then provides the basis for the dynamic, rhythmical, rapidly executed and integrated speech action sequences (cf. Brooks, 1983; Browman & Goldstein, 1989). Syllable rhythm and duration continuities from prespeech to speech vocalization provide one of the evidences that both periods flow together in speech and language acquisition (cf. Robb and Saxman, 1990).

INTONATION, STRESS, AND TIMING

Intonation refers to the rising and falling of the voice pitch and intensity in spoken phrases. It is described in terms of the intonation contour which summarizes time-by-frequency or time-by-intensity contrasts within an utterance. There is considerable evidence that the syntactic organization of an utterance is expressed at the prosodic intonation level. The now-classical sentences:

(a) light-house keeper
(b) light house-keeper
(c) light house keeper

where (c) refers to a "keeper of a house which is light," illustrate the role that differences in stress and intonation play in transmitting meaning.

Intonation is one of the first features of speech to develop. Even in the first months of life children employ intonation to give "meaning" to vocalizations. Two types of cry are differentiated at birth. The normal cry lasts one to two seconds. It typically has an initial rise in its contour then remains steady or falls gradually to a more rapid drop-off at the end (Ostwald, 1963). The "scream" of the excited infant demands immediate attention. It is louder than the usual cry and becomes atonal as vocalization rises to its peak. The use of intonation to transmit the attitudinal and emotional feelings of the person continues throughout life. Mature talkers use voice quality, F_0 range, and the pitch contour type to indicate their emotional state (Ladd, Silverman, Tolkmitt, Bergmann, & Sherer, 1985). The slow, flat, hopeless tones and rhythm of defeat; the lilting qualities of sadness; the vibrant, staccato tempo of excitement all provide prosodic indices that tell as much about a speaker's message as the words spoken.

The physical bases of prosody are found in both laryngeal and respiratory support system functions. In a neutral emphasis utterance (one with no explicitly stressed word) the intonation curve rises briefly to a peak at the onset of a phrase then falls gradually throughout the remainder of the utterance (Lehiste, 1970). This pattern reflects subglottal pressure buildup at the onset of the breath-group. This is followed by a declining air supply as the utterance continues (Lieberman, 1967). If the tension of the laryngeal muscles is not increased to counterbalance subglottal air-pressure fall, the fundamental frequency of the voice will drop systematically. The expiratory muscles are normally not brought into play until the volume of air in the lungs falls below the point where their elastic recoil is insufficient to maintain the subglottal pressure for natural voice production. In the newborn, cry vocalization often continues into inspiration. This simply indicates that coordination between laryngeal and respiratory vocal support has not developed fully although coordination of the cry act is essentially mature at birth. Postnatal vocal expression may thus be described as "the addition of upper pharyngeal and oral modulations to an already well-developed laryngeal vocal coordination" (Bosma, Truby, & Lind, 1965, p. 91).

One of the earliest ways that children learn to communicate specific meaning is through rising versus falling intonation contours in declarative and interrogative utterances. The final falling tone in vocalization is present from infancy. In mature speech the early rise, gradually falling intonation curve is used semantically to signify finality. The end of the utterance is denoted by a final drop in the intonation contour. A high fall in the same part of the utterance may convey surprise or indignation, a low fall indifference or disgust. A contrasting rising intonation is used to indicate uncertainty, as in a question.

The contour of the intonational curve in connected speech helps determine how prosody is used by talkers to transmit meaning. A repeated observation is that a spoken phrase will have a brief rising then falling intonation unless there is some specific reason why it should not. Crystal (1980) reported that in "any sample of data" (p. 61) from normal talkers between 50% and 60% of the phrases will have the neutral intonation contour, and this contour is typically associated with statements. He suggested further that the vast majority of these contours will be low falling in type. Rondo (1980) indicates that a falling intonation is associated with assertiveness, new information, and finality. Half of the remaining contours will be low, mid-rising, or level "whose use is wholly conditioned by the accompanying syntax" (Crystal, 1980, p. 61).

Lieberman, Katz, Jongman, Zimmerman, & Miller (1985) examined spontaneous speech and found evidence that challenged the syntactical declination model described previously. First, they noted that one of the most striking aspects of the F_0 contour is its extreme variability in both read and spontaneous speech. Given this variability it seemed unlikely that listeners would track a sentence declination slope to derive putative linguistic distinctives from the subtle F_0 variations. Additionally, the spontaneous sentences fit the breath group model better than a syntactically based declination model. Recall that the breath group model predicts that subglottal air pressure will be adjusted to maintain an essentially constant air flow and level intonation curve until a strong rise or declination is instituted to signal the speaker's intent at the termination of the phrase. Finally, they demonstrated that an "all points" line with a generally falling slope, calculated from a least-squares analysis, provided the best general description for both spontaneous and read sentences. The most common means of illustrating the intonation of an utterance is a straightforward frequency-by-time or intensity-by-time plot. This type of plot produces an almost infinite number of possible variations that are difficult to categorize and explicitly differentiate. Some generalizations are possible. A rising intonation is most frequently associated with questions or with statements associated with an expected positive answer. The tag question, "It's a beautiful day, isn't it?" is an example of a part-statement and part-question which may or may not have a concluding rising intonation curve. In some questions, such as "Did John tell that to you?", the tone rises early and remains high until the end of the phrase where there might be a further rise. For detailed discussions of variations in question intonations and contrasting use of question and statement intonation, the reader is referred to Chafe (1968) and Rondo (1980), respectively.

Stress is defined physiologically as the degree of effort exerted to produce an accented syllable (Lehiste & Peterson, 1959). It is identified perceptually by the prominance of a particular syllable relative to other syllables in the phrase (Folkins, Miller, & Minifie, 1975) and acoustically by in the voice fundamental frequency and intensity. Timing is defined by durational phenomena within segments and temporal relations across segments.

Emphatic stress is one of the most robust measures of speech and the amplitude integral over the duration of a syllable is one of the most robust means of distinguishing stressed from unstressed syllables. Lieberman (1960) compared the amplitude integral, peak envelope amplitude, syllable duration, and fundamental frequency in 25 noun/verb contrasting syllable stress pairs (CONtract/conTRACT, REbel/reBEL, and so on) spoken by 16 talkers. Within the words 92% had a greater amplitude integral, 90% greater fundamental frequency, 87% greater peak envelope amplitude, and 66% greater syllable duration for the stressed than the unstressed syllable. When comparing the word pairs, correct identification of the stressed syllable in one word with its unstressed counterpart showed 90% accuracy using the peak envelope amplitude, 72% using F_0, and 70% using syllable duration. Medress, Skinner, and Anderson (1971) corroborated Lieberman's findings in a study of syllable stress in isolated polysyllabic words and words embedded in short sentences. They found the amplitude energy integral to be the best predictor of stress in 97% of the sentence test words. It was followed by duration with 91% prediction and fundamental frequency with only 52%. These findings counter the previously held belief (Bolinger, 1958) that vocal pitch serves as the primary word *prominence* cue in an utterance.

As children mature, many of the rhythmical and timing characteristics of childhood physical actions, including speech, may be found in refined form and with identifiable subcomponents. For example, rhythmical walking still includes lift, stride, heel contact, and support phases. An important sign of maturation is that the proportion of time spent in each phase is maintained at different walking speeds (Shapiro, Zernicke, Gregory, & Diestal, 1981). For example, if the lift requires 20% of the stepping time cycle duration at a slow speed, it consumes about 20% of the time at a faster rate. This constancy holds only within a rather limited walking range, however.

Similar relative constancy has been claimed as a function of timing in stressed and unstressed sound production. Mackay and Bowman (1969) described an experiment in which they had a group of subjects produce a sentence as rapidly as possible over 12 practice trials. Maximum speech rate increased systematically with practice. More importantly, they reported that the relative duration of the words and syllables remained essentially constant at the faster speeds. These observations dovetail with the belief that stressed syllables within an utterance are timed to occur at equal intervals. Much early research on syllable rhythm revolved around this "isochrony" concept (rf. Coleman, 1974).

More recent experiments by Carlson, Erikson, Granstrom, Lindblom, and Rapp (1975), Folkins, Miller, and Minifie (1975), Fugimura (1981, 1986), and Weismer and Ingrisano (1979) have challenged important claims in the *relative time constancy* hypothesis alluded to earlier. Carlson and colleagues studied the effect of phrase level timing as the location of emphatic stress was systematically manipulated during production of an eight-syllable Swedish phrase by a single talker. They found large increases in the durations of the syllables receiving emphatic stress but little change in the unemphasized syllables compared with their duration in a "neutral emphasis" utterance.

Folkins and his colleagues examined syllable timing differences when the phrase *Bob bought a big box* was produced with primary stress on *Bob, bought, big,* or *box* at normal and fast speaking rates. The three judges who scored the perceived stress also tapped the rhythm of the utterances on a transient generating device. Analysis of the data indicated that the rhythmic tapping patterns produced similar data to those from the acoustic measures. Syllable duration was significantly longer when the stress was on *Bob, bought,* and *big* or *box*. In other words, duration changes across the five talkers were similar for the last two words but different from each of the first two. They also found systematic differences in the intervals between syllables and highly significant differences in both the manner and amount of syllable variation across talkers. The variability was smaller but still present at the fast speaking rate. They concluded that isochrony was not present except perhaps between the two or three most prominently stressed syllables in the phrase.

Weismer and Ingrisano essentially replicated the Carlson et al. (1975) experiment except they used the English phrase *Bob hit the big dog,* spoken by three talkers. The subjects produced the phrase at conversational and fast speaking rates with a nonemphasized stress pattern and with emphatic stress on each of the four content words. Their data again showed each word to differ significantly between emphasized and nonemphasized conditions. They also observed a spreading effect from the stressed to nonstressed words. The duration of a particular word was generally longer when it was adjacent to an emphasized segment than when it was displaced from the emphasis location. In other words, the influence of emphatic stress was not confined to the stressed segment.

In contrast with the data reported by Folkins et al. (1975), Weismer and Ingrisano (1979) observed that for the most part the data from the individual subjects were consistent with group trends. In agreement with reports from the other investigators, they reported that the nature of the duration change varied with the segment. In other words, the changes were not isochronic. The *hit* segment, for example, was associated with the greatest mean percentage duration change at both speaking rates. They wondered if the difference in *hit* might be because it was closest to the "optimal accentual realization" location since the intonation curve in a neutral emphasis utterance normally rises briefly to a peak nearing the beginning of the utterance then falls thereafter (Lehiste, 1970). To test this hypothesis, they conducted a post hoc analysis of *Bob caught a bad cold* spoken by one of the original subjects. These data showed the percentage change from nonstressed to the emphatic stress condition to be 13%, 40%, 18%, and 11% for *Bob, caught, bad,* and *cold,* respectively. This finding supported the posited interaction between phrase timing and normal intonation of the utterance.

Fugimura (1981, 1986) studied temporal adjustments within the articulatory constituents of phrasal units. His data indicated that rate changes did not always give rise to uniform compression or expansion of all elements. Rather, portions of the movements were found to be particularly susceptible to temporal compression and/or gesture reduction. Other portions, referred to as "solid icebergs," were relatively incompressible. The "rigid" elements were noted to be distributed more or less independently across different articulatory dimensions. Fugimura suggested that this allowed them to overlap if they were not in the same dimension. Thus, the phrasal unit was posited to include compliant linkages between articulatory and prosodic variables that allowed sensitivity to physical and physiological constraints of specific gestures. Phrase boundaries were identified by temporal deceleration or real pauses during the final part of the phrase.

Faure, Hirst, and Chafcouloff (1980) also challenged the commonly held belief among phoneticians that intervals separating stressed syllable onsets in the English language are roughly equal. To test this hypothesis explicitly, they submitted a set of recorded sentences from two British speakers to three separate English phonetician judges who marked the stressed syllables and pauses. Pauses were defined as "any break in the rhythm of the utterance, including any type of segmentation with or without an accompanying silence." Their findings showed the judges to differ widely in the between-stressed-syllable intervals they identified as "approximately equal." This confirmed the now common observations that stressed syllables have longer durations than unstressed ones and that speed and length of unstressed syllables varies with the number of syllables between the "strong beats." The investigators speculated that the difference between the judged impressions of equal stressed syllable intervals and the actual length of the intervals could have arisen from the *rhythmical* occurrence of the stressed syllables with respect to the unstressed syllables. This may have caused the intervals to *seem* equal despite considerable variation.

TRAINING

Crystal (1980, pp. 62–63) proposed a simplified shorthand procedure that summarizes six widely identified "nuclear tones" or accent locations within connected speech contexts.[2] This system provides a means of documenting both intonation patterns and changes sought in intonation training.

- or ′   Nonfinal accent in sentence: *syntactic dependence,* for example,
[what he SAID/was are you CÒMING]
[he won't go HÒME/until she comes BÀCK]

′   Final accent in sentence: *continuity,* for example, in an incomplete listing:
[would you like MÌLK/or WÀTER] (cf. . . . MÍLK/or WÀTER])

Final accent in sentence: *expectation of response,* as in a tag question,
[he's CÒMING/ÍSN'T he]) (cf. . . . ÌSN'T he], and a question vs. an exclamation:
[how WÈLL she sings/DÓESN'T she]

↑′   *Contrastive question* in an echo utterance, as in,
a: [John's going to the ÒFFICE]
b: [to the ↑WHÉRE]

This marking is also used in certain rhetorical questions and to indicate the next to the last word in a list, as in,
[we want ÉGGS/BÚTTER/ ↑BRÉAD and MÌLK]

↑   *Contrastive focus* in rising-type emphatic stress accent, as in,
[he's HÀPPY/in fact he's ↑VÈRY happy]

v   *Contingency,* especially with a negative implication, where the polar contrast is clear, as in,

---

[2]This notational system is introduced and justified theoretically in Crystal (1973). The example phrases listed were drawn by Crystal from published English grammar.

[I didn't give her ÁNYTHING] (cf. ... ÀNYTHING])
[I SHǑULD go/(but I won't) cf. ... SHÒULD ...]
[we do admit STǓDENTS/(but not ÀNY STÚDENTS])
[its GǑOD/(but not THÀT GÓOD])
[John won't sit still until the TÁXI comes
(cf. ... STÍLL/... TÀXI ...]

↓`   Final accent in sentence: *unmarked*
Nonfinal falling-type accent in sentence

In prosody training particular attention must be given to tying gestures together in dynamically coupled syllables, phrases, and sentences made audible by the phonic air stream. Rhythm in the suprasegmental patterns of stress, intonation, phrasing, and rate control must also be used to allow listeners to predict what will be from what has been said (Martin, 1972). Much of the information that suggests how this might work has been summarized in the earlier discussions. Segmental information, such as interarticulatory delay and phonetic production rate, may also be added to help predict syllable functions. For example, syllable midportion durations predict the overall speech rate (Keller, 1989). Normal hearing but not low intelligibility deaf speakers are also known to adjust timing within the syllables to enhance the overall rhythm as well as rate (Metz, 1980). As some functions are changed others are also affected. For instance, unstressed vowel nuclei may decrease in length as syllables within an utterance become more complex (Crystal & House, 1988; but see Farnetani & Kori, 1986). Emphatic stress effects may also be expected to overflow from prominent words to the surrounding segments (Weismer & Ingrisano, 1979). An important goal in suprasegmental training is to help talkers develop skill in using both the prosody and syntax to help define the meaning that reveals the emotional intent of an utterance. These many considerations that influence prosody would seem to make the task of building new prosody skills through training inordinately complex. However, since many of the skills are acquired as natural extensions of normal speech skill development, the task may be seen as less overwhelming. For example, changes in stress are known to modify the duration of vowels in spoken utterances rather naturally (Harris, 1974).

Particular attention seems to be needed on how to produce and time syllable stress. Misleading syllable stress timing cues inserted into normal speech have been shown to cause large reductions in talker intelligibility (Huggins, 1978). This effect is also shown by substantial improvement when segmental aspects of speech are instrumentally corrected (Maassen & Povel, 1985). Improved intelligibility has also been observed when 160 msec silent pauses were inserted between words in sentences spoken by 10 children who were profoundly hearing impaired to provide a more rhythmical output (Maassen, 1986). Temporal differentiation and rhythm thus appear to be among the most important components of speech intelligibility. Contrastive stress follows closely (Metz et al., 1990). Normal rhythm within intonation is therefore considered to be a prime target for intonation training.

A way to expose speech prosody so it can be developed more readily is to imitate the perceived beats of the syllables in an utterance. Syllable rhythm reflects phrase level stress patterning rather directly (Allen, 1972; Folkins, Miller, & Minifie, 1975; Martin, 1970). During normal speech the basic temporal regularity is clouded by many simultaneous and near simultaneous events. This makes it difficult to learn timing and rhythmical patterns. A solution to this problem is to strip away, as much as possible, the influence of segmental articulatory variation. Teaching prosody through "reiterant" speech was strongly advocated by Kelso, Vatikiotis-Bateson, Saltzman, and Kay (1985). In this speaking mode a consonant-vowel syllable, such as [ba] or [ta], is substituted for each real syllable in an utterance. In principle, this procedure exposes the utterance's prosodic structure and affords analysis of its patterns in a simple, accessible form. Although the absolute duration values in repeated syllables are very different from those in contextual speech (Liberman & Streeter, 1978), reiterant speech can serve both as a training and an analysis tool. Care must be taken, however, to maintain a close association between the syllable pattern mimicked and those in the modeled phrase. In essence, this involves introducing a standard phrase and its simplified substitute reiterant pattern at the same time. The learner is then taught to maintain the standard word pattern in memory as a constant mental reference during reiterant syllable practice. This close linkage paves the way later for transferring new prosodic skills to natural speech contexts.

Testing Materials

Ultimately, success in speech training will be defined by the extent to which the prosodic patterns of the person who is speech handicapped duplicate those of normal talkers. Testing materials for this purpose are becoming available. The Revised Prosodic-Reception Test (Rpros$_2$), described by McGarr (1987) is an example of a test developed to document perception of speech prosody in children who are younger or markedly handicapped, such as those with impaired hearing. It and its counterpart, the Prosodic-Feature Production Test (Ppros), also described by McGarr (1987), can be used to help describe the current prosody status of children with impaired speech and document changes as it is altered in training.

The Rpros test (Table 5–2) uses nine sentences with four variations of each to examine listeners' ability to detect speech stress, pause, and rising or falling intonation. The subject is required to render "same or different" judgments when the sentences are presented following practice trials with nontest sentence pairs. Practice stimuli are used first to verify or establish the subject's understanding of the same-different concept.

The Ppros test was devised to assess stress (indicated by italicized words), pausal juncture (indicated by ellipses), and intonation (indicated by question marks or periods) in speech production. It uses six of the nine sentences from the Rpros test. Practice trials with nontest sentence pairs are again used to establish the subject's understanding of the expected prosodic contrasts. Normally the sentences would be elicited and audiotape recorded. The recorded responses could then be replayed later to listeners who label the prosody type and judge its "naturalness." Speech naturalness has been found to be more highly correlated with intelligibility ratings than simple word stress scores (Gordon, 1987).

Consistent use of normal talker modeling and shaping routines is suggested in developing prosody through pitch and duration contrasts. Specific procedures to do that are detailed in later chapters of this book. Careful attention to setting an appropriate training framework is also time well invested. The training should begin with an objective description and demonstration of the key differences between how the client now manipulates prosody and changes that are planned to help him or her improve. The major goal is to improve the ability to transmit meaning through use of the explicitly defined prosodic cues described previously. Another important function of prosody training is to help the client develop strategies for resolving contextual ambiguity through stress and intonation cues. That these changes will be of personal benefit to the client must be clear to ensure motivation to change. If possible, the client should be directly involved in planning the training program and selecting materials.

For maximum benefit, the plan formulated should also include provision for brief out-of-clinic practice sessions in carefully structured settings at stipulated intervals each day. Direct personal involvement in the training routines can both motivate the desire for out-of-clinic practice and prepare him or her to be successful in doing so.

In the reiterant speech training, segmental phonological variation is stripped away and the prosodic structure is exposed in simple consonant-vowel (CV) syllables such as in the following sentences.

These sentences illustrate how Crystal's (1980) shorthand method may be used for identifying the prominent stress and intonation pat-

TABLE 5–2. Revised prosodic-reception test (McGarr, 1987).

Sequence Number	Test Number	Set Number	Stimulus	Number of Syllables	Prosodic Feature
5	1	1	Oh boy.	2	Early stress
16	2	1	Oh boy.	2	Late stress
32	3	1	Oh . . . boy.	2	Pause
35	4	1	Oh boy?	2	Question
33	5	2	Thank you.	2	Early stress
36	6	2	Thank you.	2	Late stress
24	7	2	Thank . . . you	2	Pause
18	8	2	Thank you?	2	Question
1	9	3	Come here	2	Early stress
11	10	3	Come here	2	Late stress
30	11	3	Come . . . here	2	Pause
4	12	3	Come here?	2	Question
22	13	4	I can run.	3	Early stress
6	14	4	I can run.	3	Late stress
14	15	4	I . . . can run.	3	Early pause
9	16	4	I can . . . run.	3	Late pause
15	17	5	John drinks milk.	3	Early stress
28	18	5	John drinks milk.	3	Late stress
31	19	5	John . . . drinks milk.	3	Early pause
29	20	5	John drinks . . . milk.	3	Late pause
20	21	6	Bob eats cake.	3	Early stress
17	22	6	Bob eats cake.	3	Late stress
10	23	6	Bob . . . eats cake.	3	Early pause
7	24	6	Bob eats . . . cake.	3	Late pause
25	25	7	My new hat is blue.	5	Early stress
27	26	7	My new hat is blue.	5	Late stress
19	27	7	My . . . new hat is blue.	5	Early pause
13	28	7	My new hat . . . is blue.	5	Late pause
3	29	8	I want to see it.	5	Early stress
26	30	8	I want to see it.	5	Late stress
23	31	8	I . . . want to see it.	5	Early pause
2	32	8	I want . . . to see it.	5	Late pause
12	33	9	He has one big dog.	5	Early stress
8	34	9	He has one big dog.	5	Late stress
21	35	9	He has . . . one big dog.	5	Early pause
34	36	9	He has one . . . big dog.	5	Late pause

Summary

2-syllable sentences	**3-syllable sentences**	**5-syllable sentences**
3 questions		
6 stress (3 early) (3 late)	6 stress (3 early) (3 late)	6 stress (3 early) (3 late)

(continued)

TABLE 5-2 (continued)

2-syllable sentences	3-syllable sentences	5-syllable sentences
3 pause	6 pause (3 early)	6 pause (3 early)
	(3 late)	(3 late)

Adapted from McGarr, N. S. (1987). Communication skills of hearing-impaired children in schools for the deaf. In H. Levitt, N. S. McGarr, & D. Geffner (Eds.), *Development of language and communication skills in hearing-impaired children* (pp. 91 107). ASHA Monograph No. 26. Rockville, MD: American Speech-Language-Hearing Association. Reprinted by permission.

She was a light housekeeper.

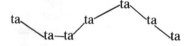   which contrasts with

She was a lighthouse keeper.

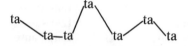

It was yellow ice cream.

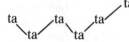   which contrasts with

It was yellow; I screamed.

terns in both normal text and reiterant syllable contexts. The ellipses identify breaks in the natural rhythmical flow of the syllables. In developing prosody through pitch and duration contrasts, certain syllables, such as "house" and "light" in the sentences shown below, can then be made *prominent* by pitch or intensity changes within the outlined stress pattern. They may be made *dominant* by pauses such as that before "I screamed," which would focus attention acutely on a particular syllable within an action sequence. Such manipulations of rhythm and stress would be expected to help both the client gain control of stress within the syllable set and listeners discern meaning (see Martin, 1972).

CHAPTER 6

ESSENTIALS OF MOTOR SKILL LEARNING

In this chapter, our goal will be first to uncover heuristics and meta-strategies that govern motor skill development. This discovery will lay a foundation for efficient and effective speech instructional practice. The ultimate goal of this approach is to increase the likelihood that an individual will acquire desired speech motor skills more rapidly and predictably than heretofore and that the skills attained will transfer to natural speaking conditions.

A field matures scientifically as its practitioners learn more about what information to seek as evidence, how to formulate its problems, and how to gain access to specific information needed to solve problems and evolve general solutions that are successful, essentially doubt-free, and relevant to the central issues facing its members (Shapere, 1987). In a real sense, developing speech motor skills is an individually creative process governed by basic principles which dictate success.

The mathematician and science philosopher Poincaré identified four processes that seem to underlie creativity: preparation, incubation, illumination, and verification (cf. Boden, 1990). In *preparation*, the individual becomes motivated to solve a challenging and perplexing problem and begins to focus intensive efforts on discovering a solution. When a reasonable solution is not found despite an intense desire to do so, the person may consciously shift foreground attention to some other topic. But the brain continues to combine and recombine ideas through unconscious background rehearsal. In this state, new and old possibilities can be freely intermixed. This period of *incubation* leads to *illumination* in the form of a flash of conscious insight. But the task is not over. The apparent solution must still be tested. *Verification* arrives as the solution is considered in the crucible of evidence. Some possible solutions fall by the wayside, victims of an inability to fulfill their own promises. Others fail because there is no way to verify their truth. Others survive because they make it possible to derive more precise, detailed accounts of experience. Evidence of each of these creative processes was found in our earlier discussion of early speech development. As in other scientific discovery endeavors, new understanding was "created" by building on prior concepts but altering them profoundly.

The opportunity to observe others who have already solved certain aspects of the challenging and perplexing problems of motor skill development opens a new avenue for creative problem solving. These studies suggest that solving problems in this type of task encompasses the following subprocesses:

1. having an action plan;
2. presetting responses by focusing attention on a relevant feature within a targeted action;
3. using modeling, imaging, and rehearsal strategies to organize and activate acquisition of key properties, gestures, and intergesture movement patterns in goal directed responses;
4. setting specific, difficult goals that lead to high task performance levels;
5. executing sequences smoothly without consciously thinking about physical details of the actions;
6. using internal and external feedback and short and long term transfer procedures to verify, guide, and stabilize response patterns;
7. applying principles of massed, spaced, and variable practice to maximize improvement, enhance training effectiveness, and foster skill transfer into daily life activities.[1]

In this conceptualization, preparation consists of focusing intensive attention on some aspect of the modeled articulatory behavior that is to be learned. The person who serves as the model may be doing so intentionally or unintentionally. During observational learning, incubation becomes a process of gaining a specific mental image of what the model is doing and mentally rehearsing actions perceived. Illumination

---

[1] A similar set of subprocesses has been described for sports skill development by Singer (1986, 1988).

comes through trial execution. Verification is then required to quantify and evaluate the degree of error or success in achieving the modeled pattern. Thus, parallel processes or strategies appear to be used in solving problems whether understanding is sought through creative internal analysis or external observation. Each of these activities involves principles, rules, and strategies related to the tasks and situations involved. These aspects of creative learning will now be expanded and discussed within a framework of speech articulation concept development and motor skill building procedures.

In this chapter you will be systematically introduced to basic and applied research pertinent to attending, focusing, imaging, rehearsing, executing, and verifying motor skill learning. Specific examples will be used to illustrate the potential use and utility of such procedures in the speech articulation teaching-learning process. You will also be introduced to metastrategies individuals may use in task-specific ways to help change speech articulatory behaviors through palatometric modeling and shaping routines. The application and use of these principles will then be expanded and applied in a deeper and broader discussion of specific articulation tasks in later chapters. The general goal of the articulation motor skill approach is to provide a rational and scientific basis for establishing and modifying speech articulation.

ESTABLISHING AN ACTION PLAN

One of the speech clinician's major tasks in articulatory skill development is to arouse the client's intent to develop or improve articulatory gestures and movements. The more often a task is repeated, the more likely it is to be learned, but unless the subject intends to remember the various activities within the task, mere repetition is not enough (Tulving, 1966).

The central importance of planning in learning motor skills has been examined by Dickinson (1978). He compared learning and recalling four arm positioning movements by subjects given instructions with no particular reason for learning the positions and subjects given instructions designed to promote intentional learning. Greater skill retention was found in the second group, and their superiority increased with time.

The term *attention* has been used to describe a person's fluctuating level of arousal or alertness to changes during efforts to increase skilled performance. Attention is a key factor in planning to learn. Moray and Fitter (1973) stress that attention is an intensely dynamic process which changes from moment to moment. Landers (1980) reported a direct relationship between arousal level and attention. The inverted-U hypothesis, proposed by Fitts (1964), posits that performance is progressively enhanced with increased arousal until an optimal arousal level is attained. Maximum performance occurs at that level. Beyond the arousal plateau, performance deteriorates with increased arousal. The so-called *optimal arousal level* is thought not to be the same for all activities. Rather it seems to vary within a range that depends upon a number of variables including task complexity, individual sensitivity to arousal and stimulus conditions, and experience with various kinds of arousal stimuli. For best performance, gross motor skills that emphasize strength, endurance, and speed seem to be performed optimally at relatively high levels of arousal. Tasks such as speech articulation that emphasize fine muscle movements, accuracy, and coordination may be impeded by excessively high arousal levels. Perceptual selectivity increases when arousal shifts from low to moderate levels (Oxendine, 1979).

It is helpful to consider attention from a central neural processing standpoint. Attention has long been identified with electroencephalographically (EEG) recorded "α-wave" changes. Reductions in α-wave activity are associated with drowsiness. A gradual drop in α-wave prominence as a person "drifts off " into sleep has been identified since early human EEG recording studies. The α-wave disappearance is also associated with drops in heart rate and short lapses of attention — described as "microsleep" — during monotonous visual and auditory tasks (Bjerner, 1949; Groll, 1966).

Kety (1970) suggested that arousal for learning may originate from neurosecretions of biogenic amines in the brain and cerebrospinal fluids. Neurones using catecholamines as neurotransmitters have many branched axons that are induced to secrete the amines by biologically significant events, just as they do in the peripheral autonomic nervous system. The amines then induce changes at synapses that are active at the time. Whether such activation of biogenic amines takes place in associative conditioning is not yet known, but such concepts point to an emerging belief that a close biological relationship exists between motivation to learn and acquiring new motor skills.

All motivated behaviors have the property of expectancy that facilitates performance through associated reward and reinforcement. Most theorists believe that goal-directed behavior is dependent upon specific arousal of the organism. A series of studies have shown that alertness in a motor task may be heightened by signals that prepare the organism to respond. These signals have been found to be registered centrally by a cortical CNS "wave of expectation" starting in the frontal lobes of the brain. Studies of "vigilance" have indicated that this wave is directly related to the subject's intent to react to an alerting signal (Walter, 1966) and to the intensity, size, vividness, and novelty of the stimulus itself (Bandura, 1969; Thompson & Bettinger, 1970). Observed evidence of active attention should thus be sought by the clinician as a means of verifying the focus or unification of a learner's vigilance. Vigilance will multiply the likelihood of success in training routines. Once learning takes place, the changes themselves become incentives either through secondary reinforcement or natural rewards and arouse motivated behavior (Bindra, 1968).

The action plan — which includes structured representation of goals, subgoals, choice points, and action operations — activates *attention* and *motivation* and rouses an internal state of expectancy. That state then primes or potentiates a response mechanism so *sensory stimulation* can direct and shape resulting behavior, and *experience* can be used to integrate and generate new strategies and behaviors. Inattention, or lapses of attention, reduces productivity.

Attention is not an all or nothing phenomenon. It can be partitioned across a series of different activities. For example, 4- to 5-year-old children have been found to attend to as many task-irrelevant as task-relevant cues when the child's attention is not focused on particular features of a modeled activity (Yando, Seitz, & Zigler, 1978). To a 4-year-old child the act of simply imitating a modeled event is satisfying. The older child is spontaneously more selective in determining the specific facets of a modeled action they choose to mimic. Thus, both the level of alertness at the moment and general sensitivity to stimulation must be considered to arrive at a level of attention that will activate an action plan with subjects of different ages.

Attention also has a social side. Bandura (1969) has noted that:

> Simply exposing a person to distinctive sequences of a modeled stimuli does not in itself guarantee that they will attend closely to the cues, that they will necessarily select from the total stimulus complex the most relevant events, or that they will even perceive accurately the cues to which their attention has been directed. An observer will fail to acquire matching behavior at the sensory registration level if he does not attend to, recognize, or differentiate the distinctive features of the model's responses. To produce learning, therefore, stimulus contiguity must be accompanied by discriminative observation. (p. 136)

In a situation such as articulatory skill learning, an incentive value is attached to success or failure. That is, the consequence of improving or not improving has potential outcomes such as material reward (tokens redeemable for toys, clinician compliments, cash), internal satisfaction (joy, exhilaration), deprivation, and embarrassment or punishment of some sort. The use of such incentives is based on the presumption that the client makes a "what's in it for me?" assessment prior to participating or performing an activity. The clinician's task is to answer that usually unspoken query in terms of expectancies that may follow success or achievement. This information along with the individual personality traits of the subject that influence the level of involvement and goal achievement aspirations can help us understand why some persons gravitate toward achievement while others do not (McClelland, 1965). Some individuals have a strong tendency to avoid situations that might cause them to fail.[2]

A number of formal strategies have been used in an effort to increase a subject's personal attention in a motor skill learning task. Among these strategies are contracting to learn a specific task or set of tasks, establishing intermediate goals and pathways to desired goals, organizing learning tasks into modules that may be achieved in step-like fashion with intermediate successes reinforced along the route, and applying firm, goal directed guidelines that enhance successful performance. Use of such procedures has been shown to produce substantially higher performance in goal-relevant efforts.

GOAL SETTING

Actions are motivated, undertaken, and controlled by goals that have their origins in past experiences. A *goal* represents the transformation of *wishes* to *wants* to *intentions.* In Lewinian terms (Lewin, 1935), *wishes* are not yet endowed with critical potency to motivate a transition from fantasy to reality. When the probability of attaining a goal exceeds a critical magnitude, the wish is transformed into a *want.* As opportunity, time availability, personal importance, and urgency arise, and the means become available for achieving desired goals, wants are transformed into *intention,* commitment, and finally action. Goals are the endstate whose attainment requires actions and anticipated outcomes (Heckhausen & Kuhl, 1985). Goals themselves have a hierarchy. For instance, an individual may enjoy a particular action and also perceive the action to be a step toward a higher-order goal state. An important part of a goal is a specific standard of proficiency on a task, usually specified as a targeted achievement within a limited time period. During the past two decades, goal setting has come to the forefront as one of the most predictable ways of enhancing human performance and productivity. Goals provide a sense of purpose and direction as well as stimulate effort by letting individuals know when performance falls below an acceptable threshold. Attainment of short-term goals gives the person a sense of task mastery and bolsters efficacy which, in turn,

---

[2]For a more detailed discussion of motivational factors in motor achievement, the reader is referred to Carron (1980).

increases subsequent aspirations and perseverance in the face of discrepant feedback.

Most of the current research on the goal setting topic can be traced to Locke's (1968) model of motivation, based on intentions and consciously established goals. He hypothesized that specific, difficult goals lead to higher levels of task performance than easy goals, no goals, or do-your-best goals. The story of *Alice in Wonderland* by Lewis Carroll provides cogent insight into the role of planning to reach a particular goal:

> Alice was wandering through the forest in Wonderland when she was startled by the sudden appearance of the Cheshire Cat sitting on a tree bough. She was concerned about being lost, so she said:
> "Would you tell me, please, which way I ought to go from here?"
> "That depends a good deal on where you want to get to," said the Cat.
> "I don't much care where ... " said Alice.
> "Then it doesn't matter which way you go," said the Cat.
> " ... so long as I get somewhere," Alice added as an explanation.
> "Oh, you're sure to do that," said the Cat, "if you only walk long enough." (p. 51)

Goals establish the direction of progress as well as define conditions that signify our arrival. The challenge of the goal itself becomes motivating as we experience success in working toward it. Individuals learn throughout life that easily achieved goals are less satisfying than those that are more difficult to achieve. The surge of joy on solving a difficult problem rewards the person for perseverance. Garland (1985) suggested that those who set high goals for themselves develop effective task strategies that bolster their feelings of efficacy. This hypothesis has been supported in a variety of rapidly multiplying laboratory and field studies.

In a thorough review of the literature Locke, Shaw, Saari, and Latham (1981) reported that 99 out of 110 studies they surveyed found support for the difficult goal hypothesis. They noted further that most of these studies were well designed with control groups, random subject assignment, negligible attrition, and a wide variety of tasks and situations. Thus, considerable confidence can be placed on both the internal and external validity of the findings. Miner (1984) analyzed 32 theories in organizational science and concluded that Locke's goal-setting theory was one of only four that were both useful and valid. Finally, Mento, Steel, and Karren (1987) conducted a meta-analysis of goal setting and task performance studies conducted between 1968 and 1984. Their analysis also supported the hypothesis that hard goals enhance motor skill performance.

Goal Attributes

Some confusion has existed between *task difficulty* and *goal difficulty* in specifying the level of expected achievement in a training task. A task may be difficult because it requires a high level of skill and knowledge, because it is physically demanding, or because it requires both greater knowledge and physical effort (Locke, Shaw, Saari, & Latham, 1981). Task difficulty thus refers to the nature of the activity and the work to be accomplished.

Goal difficulty refers to the relative ease of attaining a specific level of task proficiency, usually measured against a time-limited standard. Presumably, harder goals demand greater effort and time to achieve them. But if the harder tasks require more ability and knowledge, initial efforts to achieve a goal may be less successful even if the subjects try harder. More complex goals require time to develop strategies for their accomplishment. Locke and Latham (1985) suggested that for greatest progress goals should be difficult and challenging but attainable. This is consistent with the belief that goals that expose participants to repeated failure will undermine both motivation and performance.

Garland (1983) questioned the goal attainability assumption. He noted that many laboratory experiments have shown improved performance despite the assignment of goals that were seemingly beyond the reach of the participants. Some subjects experience repeated failure with no evidence of a decline in either motivation or performance. The expected inverted-U relationship between goal difficulty and performance is not found in experimental studies. For example, Locke (1982) himself examined the effects of 14 difficulty levels on performance with the top 9 beyond the reach of the participants. The predicted performance decrement did not occur. In fact, subjects with unrealistic goals set for them performed slightly better than those assigned more realistic performance standards. This finding has since been replicated in a variety of studies. Participants do not necessarily lower their efforts nor drop in their performance despite repeated failure to reach assigned goals.

Several possible explanations have been suggested to account for the apparent lack of performance decrement despite repeated failure to achieve targeted goal standards. The most important of these seems to be the individual's belief in her- or himself. A person needs a healthy self-respect to continue pursuing a novel learning experience despite mistakes, failure, and criticism from others. Most people seem to have developed a sufficient reservoir of success that they can endure such situations for a surprisingly lengthy period of time when eventual success, or at least satisfying improvements in performance, is anticipated.

Motives and the goals they generate are the origin of specific actions. Bandura (1986) argued that as individuals succeed in increasingly diverse tasks and settings, they develop a general sense of efficacy that is positively related to subsequent trials and challenges. Once established, self-efficacy generalizes to other situations, particularly those similar to ones performed well. Bandura and Cervone (1986) observed that many people remain unshaken in their self-efficacy despite failure to achieve lofty goals. They noted that individuals with high efficacy are stimulated to greater efforts when their efforts meet with performance below their goal aspirations. Others, however, become less sure of themselves when faced with failure. If an activity is painful or has been punished in the past, the stimulus situation produces an inhibitory force that serves to block expression of the activity (Atkinson, 1977). These individuals seem to lose faith in their capabilities as an outgrowth of the past negative experiences. Those with subnormal self-efficacy lower their efforts in the face of subgoal performance. In essence, lofty goals seem to be motivating for most individuals but not for everyone.

Solomon (1982) suggested an opponent process theory that could help explain the motivational states of different individuals to aversive learning conditions. He posited that powerful new motivational states are induced by arousal of opposite sign reactions. For example, an electric shock initially induces pain and fear in a dog through avoidance conditioning. In the process of developing the avoidance reaction, a *countering arousal* of excitement and euphoria is also evident, however, after the dog is released from the apparatus. Both fear and joy become associated with the conditioning training. A similar analogy may be drawn with regard to the effects of defective speech. Defective speech has been shown to be associated with fear, risks, and failure in previous speech experiences. Trepidations in articulation training with lofty goals may be counteracted by pleasure that accompanies success in performance when progress is made, whether or not targeted goals are fully met. Aroused motivation may be expected to lower the level of fear or aversiveness as a high performance action plan is successfully introduced and followed.

The importance of attitude in striving to reach goals has been documented by Weinberg, Bruya, Garland, and Jackson (1990). They found a correlation of .87 between a subject's expectancies and subsequent performance. Reaction to lofty, unattainable goals again seemed to be conditioned by the personality of the individual. Nevertheless, the presence of a specific, challenging goal appears to be the single most important factor in achievement. "Do your best" is no better than no goal at all.

Goals must not only be high, but they must be specific. Locke et al. (1981) cited 24 studies which showed that individuals given *specific,* challenging goals either outperformed those trying to do their best or surpassed their own previous performance when they were not channeled toward specific goals.

Some claim has been made that personal involvement in goal setting is an important ingredient in progress toward its fulfillment. Mento and his associates (1987) included six studies in their meta-analysis in which results from assigned versus participative goals could be compared. Four studies yielded data favoring participative goals while two favored assigned goals. This difference is not very impressive. Findings by Earley and Lituchy (1991) suggested, however, that the indeterminateness of the differences Mento and colleagues found between assigned and participatory derived goals may have been because of the intimate connections between different types of involvement in the goal-setting task. They conducted a series of three interlocking studies to examine interrelationships between goal setting and the estimates of their capacity to perform. From the findings, Earley and Lituchy concluded that assigned goals influence both self-efficacy and personal goals. Self-efficacy and personal goals, in turn, have direct effects on task performance. They also noted that the participants' personal abilities influenced their performance and motivation as well as their self-efficacy.

On an individual basis, successful progress toward a goal, care given to delineating goals and setting specific performance standards, the relevancy of the tasks assigned to the goal, total time allocated to the effort, personal feedback and evaluations, and the personality of the participant all appear to influence achievement. Early and Lituchy (1991) noted that their experimental findings on goal setting and results attained indicated that helping a person develop self-assessment skills may be of particular benefit in guiding him or her to expectations that are consistent with abilities. Such guidance should bring congruity between goals and optimal performance.

ATTENTION FOCUSING

A fundamental requirement for motor skill learning is directing attention to the location where key operations are taking place then focusing on actions that are transpiring there. The process of *selective attention* or achieving attentional focus has been studied empirically, both psychophysically and physiologically. These diverse studies still do not provide a complete picture of the shifting operations of attention and their use in the analysis of perceptual information. They do provide, however, strong support for the notion that selective attention plays an important role in sensory information processing. Landers (1980), for instance, reported a direct relationship between arousal level and perceptual selectivity.

The notion of selective attention often implies that the processing of sensory information is restricted to avoid "overloading" the system with excessive information. Attempts to process additional information would then cause interference and deterioration of performance. The notion of focused attention does not necessarily imply such generally unproven notions as general capacity or overload, however. The main purpose of focusing is to enhance an expected response, rather than to avoid excessive capacity demands. The process is structured, but not necessarily in a simple manner. In the course of learning a motor skill routine, both the locations and operations performed must be controlled and coordinated according to the requirements of the routine in question.

Researchers in motor skill development have learned that efficient motor skill acquisition requires control of sensory or motor interference sources once considered to be peripheral to the task at hand. Kahneman (1973) used the term "structural interference" to identify negative effects that competing events taking place at the same time have on each other and on the outcome of desired action sequences. Navon (1985) has isolated four potential sources of selective attention conflict that arise when events occur in parallel: cross talk between targeted and nontargeted events, difficulty in perceiving transitions between unfamiliar targets, failure to match subordinated modules, and disablement from introducing competition for a single processing mechanism too early in the training regimen.

Functional interference is also a factor that influences an individual's preparation to participate in a motor learning activity. Weiss, Bredemeier, and Shewchuk (1985) observed that children may be grouped on the basis of those who act primarily on internal feedback from their own actions and outcomes and those who prefer external guidance in judging performance in motor skill learning tasks. Little and McCullagh (1989) found supporting evidence that differential results can be obtained when children are primed for a motor learning task through instructional strategies that fit the individual's intrinsic versus extrinsic motivational makeup.

The skill with which the environment is searched or scanned for information changes with age. From infancy through the early grade school years, scanning behavior is neither extensive nor systematic. The young child's gaze is concentrated on visual field areas that contain only the most salient stimulus elements. This results in "piecemeal intake of information" with figure parts rather than whole figures perceived (Elkind, Koegler, & Go, 1964). At about age nine, scanning and response patterns become more systematic and broadly oriented. Judgments of similarities and differences then begin to approximate those of adults (Tanaka, 1964).

In a typical palatometric training session, subjects are given verbal instructions to focus attention on modeled actions that will occur at specific locations on the video screen. Other movements are to be ignored as they fix their gaze. The subject's task is to discriminate "target patterns" within the moving actions of speech production. The goal of these efforts is to prime the subject to perceive a particular articulation target or set of targets. Considerable evidence exists that spatially focused information is attended to and processed differently than more peripheral, nontargeted inputs. Hillyard, Munte, and Neville (1985) reported for instance that, in vision, inputs from the central foveal field are gated preferentially into the more posterior portions of the occipital cortex while the peripheral events are routed to the parietal cortex to be processed. Posner (1978) has shown that when subjects expect an event, such as a light illumination in a particular location within the visual field, they detect it more quickly. On the other hand, when a stimulus such as light is directed toward a location on the retina that is different from that which is expected, greater processing time is required, and the response is slower. The response facilitation is referred to as attentional *benefit*. The inhibition for stimuli at unexpected locations is called attentional *cost*. Lateralized right hemisphere attention effects have also been described, but they seem to be limited to reactions to stimuli in peripheral visual fields (Hillyard, Munte, & Neville, 1985). Asymmetries are not observed in foveal attention.

When stimuli are selected on the basis of sensory features such as place, shape, or size, the evoked cortical response pattern indicates a hierarchical preference for location. This preference, which is of particular interest in structuring a motor task sequence, is lost, however, when the stimulus locations are so close that they are difficult to discriminate spatially. In the latter situation, selection of other features such as shape or size then proceeds without regard to stimulus location. Each of these observations supports the generalization by Treisman and Gelade (1980) that "features come first in perception." They also suggest that spatially focused attention is a prerequisite for combining feature information into a unified percept. From such observations, Hillyard et al. (1985) concluded that:

> Focal attention, then, seems to enable a further processing of events falling within its spotlight, which includes a more detailed examination of the relevant features and their integration into perceptual objects. (p. 74)

Perceptual observations may be subdivided into *defining* attributes and *reported* attributes. Defining attributes distinguish targets from nontargets; reported attributes describe the subject's attentional focus during a goal directed activity. For example, if a subject's task were to name a red letter in a display with five green letters and one red one, the defining attribute would be color. Shape would be the reported attribute. Similarly, in a task to identify a sibilant in a palatometrically displayed sentence with words having stop and sibilant sounds, the defining attribute would be the central linguapalatal contact groove. The reported attribute would be /s/ or /ʃ/, determined by the groove location. In a situation where *targeted* stimuli are to be detected and *nontargeted* stimuli rejected or ignored, defining attributes must therefore be distinguished from targeted attributes (Duncan, 1985).

One of the major changes in attention research has been a shift to response output modulation. For example, Wurtz, Goldberg, and Robinson (1980) found that in vision, neurons in the superior colliculus respond more strongly when a target is presented in a saccadic eye movement context than when the gaze is focused on a fixed point. And the enhancement is directly associated with the eye movement as a response is anticipated. A similar effect has been described by Johnston and Hale (1984) who found word identification to be facilitated by its prior context. In these situations, a *preparatory set* is developed as a means of improving efficiency of operations that take place during central processing (Requin, 1985). The preparatory set can thus be interpreted as an optional process that is similar to attention focusing in mediating the effect of an experience.

Experimental evidence increasingly indicates that providing advance information about features such as the place, direction, or extent of movement reduces the time required to initiate an action and enhances the response. There is some evidence that in speech, comprehension is also improved by drawing the listener's attention to other features such as contrastive stress in an utterance (Pechmann, 1984).

A number of studies have identified "filtering costs" when focused attention is required to select a visually guided response from multiple alternative targets in a display (e.g., Kahnéman, Triesman, & Burkell, 1983). Navon (1985) postulated that visual search is conducted in two successive perceptual stages. An initial parallel, preselective search is executed that involves coding perceived information covertly by targeted attributes or features and excluding nontarget data. Interfering nontarget effects — such as disturbance from nontargets too close to or partially overlapping the target — seem to influence the search process at this covert stage. The second stage involves a serial, limited capacity search linked with the subject's overt awareness of the action.

The two-stage process may be illustrated by a competing message listening task where messages are presented by a man or woman talker to either ear. In the first stage, the listener would be expected to code physical characteristics such as location of the talker and voice qualities that differentiate talkers. In the second stage the message content would be extracted. If the assigned task required two messages to be derived, the second stage would be very difficult since its capacity is limited. But if only one of the messages were targeted, the nontarget message could be excluded at the first stage. Performance would then improve. Preparation for selective attention might thus include guidance to attend to the defining attribute (e.g., left side of palatometric screen or woman talker) first then focus on a targeted attribute, the tongue placement. Attentional conflict could presumably be reduced or prevented by assigning a sequential order for processing the arriving information thereby spacing the events in time. Using the computer metaphor, preselecting subroutines readies the program to be loaded. It can then be executed accurately.

Three kinds of neurons have been identified in the motor cortex that support the outlined separate preparatory and motor execution concept of action sequences. As described by Requin, Lucas, and Bonnet (1984), the activity of the first neuron in the three-step motor preparation model is not movement related. Its discharge is activated shortly after a "Ready" warning signal is presented. The response is then sustained during a variable duration foreperiod and ends with onset of the intended movement. This type of neuron thus plays a specific role in the presetting process. The second kind of neuron is successively preparatory set then movement related. Its resting discharge changes shortly after the ready signal is presented and increases progressively until the movement actually occurs. It then continues until the action subsides. The third kind of neuron is a true motor unit. Its activity is related only to movement and is unaffected by a warning signal. These motor neurons remain completely inactive until just before (200 msec or less) the peripheral EMG activity appears during a movement. They then exhibit a strong movement-related response. Their function thus appears to convey program instruction commands to the peripheral effectors.

The first two kinds of neurons are labeled permissive, because they preset the motor system for a response. The second and third kinds are labeled as executive, because they receive program instructions and convey orders to the peripheral structures for movement execution.

MODELING, IMAGING, AND REHEARSING

A natural tendency to imitate is a long recognized trait of the animal kingdom. Imitative behavior studies indicate that even in the first hours of life human infants are capable of copying simple oral motor and vocal acts performed by adults. Wyrwicka (1988) cites experimental evidence from electrophysiological, surgical lesion, and conditioning studies that indicate that adult gestures provide powerful visual stimuli which activate representations in the infant's brain and motor systems. The fact that these acts are imitated without training or reward helps confirm the assumption that the imitative behavior is initially based on *innate unconditioned reflexes.*

Studies have suggested that imitation of complex acts may result from earlier associations between reflexive imitation and instrumental reward (cf. Wyrwicka, 1981). Innately determined reflexes prime the motor system to respond in certain ways and trigger cognitive and motor processes that lead to action pattern refinement. Basic response mechanisms emerge first and are gradually transformed into larger cognitive-motor response units under the organizing and integrating influence of maturation and rewards experience. The motor subsystems that develop in this process are thus more complex than reflexes, but simpler than the later motivated behaviors. Motor development may thus be interpreted as a hierarchical process with mature movements emerging as an expression of a succession of motor and cognitive refinements built upon innate tendencies.

The most natural form of imitation is for a learner to attend a patterned performance by a person skilled in a task then extract and imitate the essential elements of the actions. The person imitated thus becomes a *model* whose actions and expressions serve as cues in behaviors of the observer. In the process of observing and imitating models in their environment, children are thought to form goals for their own actions and, through rehearsal and action channeling, to discover complex sensorimotor repertoires that underpin many of the physical and social competencies of the culture they experience.

Skills also develop as a consequence of the child's increasing capacity for perceiving, symbolically coding, and rehearsing actions that are translated into goal driven performance (Kuczynski, Zahn-Waxler, & Radke-Yarrow, 1987). Special, age-related sensorimotor capacities exert a systematic effect on motor skill development. For example, Weiss and Bredemeier (1983) cited a study by Williams who compared the ability of 6- through 11-year-old children to judge the speed and direction of ball flight. He found that the 6-, 7-, and 8-year-olds responded quickly, but were unable to use the visual information to make accurate judgments about ball flight. The 9-year-olds were very precise but slow in their ball direction predictions. By ages 10 and 11, both speed and accuracy were integrated into a smooth, skilled performance by the children. The psychomotor developmental process seems to take place with little intervention by socializing agents. From such observations, theories of imitation have developed in parallel with those of learning (Kymissis & Poulson, 1990).

Modeling may be intentionally employed to elicit imitation. In modeling, a performer uses demonstrations as stimuli to induce images of desired actions, increase understanding of action sequences, and shape changes in an observer's performance skills. Sequential modeling, or scaled demonstration, builds skills through a progressive series of modeling, imitation, and response-shaping procedures.

Bandura (1969) defines observational learning as that which occurs through modeling when an individual displays new behavioral patterns that had no probability of occurring prior to modeling despite motivational inducements. Through goal directed social prompts, modeling can also strengthen or weaken inhibitions to perform previously learned activities.

Although modeling is a pervasive form of instruction, questions persist about the most effective person to serve as a model, how to use modeling most effectively, and what specific strategies should be employed to enable goal setting and modeling procedures to be used jointly to establish action and movement patterns most efficiently. Such questions have been the fountainhead for scientific investigation of learning through mimicry. Efforts to answer these questions during the last decade have stimulated a major forward surge in understanding the basic principles governing modeling, mimicry, rehearsal, and response shaping. In the following paragraphs, current understanding of those principles will be reviewed then applied to speech articulatory skill development through palatometry. The goal will be to outline a set of theory-oriented demonstration, modeling, rehearsing, and shaping procedures that when applied systematically will lead to efficient development of new or improved articulatory gestures and movement patterns and eventually to intelligible, socially acceptable speech.

The Model

From a theoretical standpoint, modeling is a form of social comparison influenced by perceived similarity between a model and an observer (Berger, 1977). The model's social status, attributes, and skills have been found to predict the functional value an observer assigns to behavior to be imitated. A model's social attributes may be particularly influential in situations where individuals are uncertain about their capabilities, lack task familiarity, or have self-doubts from difficulties in previous tasks they have tried to perform well (Bandura, 1986).

An experiment by Landers and Landers (1973) illustrates that a model's social status and skills both play important roles in motor skill learning. They compared the effects of observing a highly skilled teacher, an unskilled teacher, and unskilled peer models on grade school children learning to climb a Bachman ladder. In this task the individual balances a freestanding ladder and climbs as many rungs as possible before losing balance. The children who observed the skilled teacher model were found to outperform those who viewed either the unskilled teacher or skilled peer models. Interestingly, failure on the part of a model had a greater detrimental effect than failure on the part of a peer. For example, those who observe an unskilled peer generally outperform those who watch an unskilled teacher, but the precise age of the model is an important factor. Children seem to judge the preferences of children younger than themselves as inappropriate for their own actions.

Schunk (1987) reviewed a series of adult versus peer model studies in motor skill learning and concluded that model competence overrides any effect of model age. Individuals are simply likely to be aided by performing modeled behavior they judge to be successful. Given equal competence, learners seem to pay closer attention to a higher status adult teacher model and gain more benefit from a skilled adult demonstration, however. Peers appear to be more influential in improving feelings about self-efficacy, particularly among low-achieving children and others who are uncertain about their own capabilities. Schunk speculated that observing a skilled adult model may lead some children to wonder whether they are capable of becoming as competent as the model. Because of this possibility, he suggests that teachers may wish to supplement instruction of low-achieving children with peer model demonstrations to enhance their feelings of self-efficacy to learn a challenging task.

When to Model

The timing when a model is used to demonstrate a motor task also influences the learning process. Landers (1975) shed light on when modeling should be introduced into the training program in a study comparing motor performance of 180 adult female subjects in a Bachman ladder balance learning task. One subgroup observed the task modeled four times prior to performing 30 trials on the task. The task was modeled twice prior to having the second group start their performance and twice again midway through their trials. For the third group the task was modeled all four times at a point midway through the trials. The final group simply performed the task four times without ever observing a model. The before-model and interspaced-model groups achieved higher scores on the initial block in the five-block training program than those who had no modeling exposure. The interspaced group also performed better than the middle-model group on the fourth block. In other words, seeing the model before they began the task helped the subjects "get the idea of the movement," but seeing it again after they had had an opportunity to practice was even more beneficial.

Thomas, Pierce, and Ridsdale (1977) examined the effects of age on the time when modeling should be introduced into a training program. They examined stabilometer[3] performance by 7- and 9-year-old girls when modeling was introduced before trying the task and halfway through the training. The modeling was found to facilitate performance by both age groups, but its effect differed by age of the subjects when the modeling was reintroduced halfway through the trials. It lowered performance by the 7-year-olds and raised performance by the 9-year-olds. In seeking to explain this unexpected finding, the investigators suggested that the older subjects may have been able to adapt their strategies to take advantage of the new information presented midway through the trials whereas the younger group became locked into their own strategy and were unable to change it once the training was started. It seems likely that the modeling provided clues to new response patterns that both groups wished to incorporate into their strategy but, perhaps because the original strategy of the younger subjects was rather hazy and thus more tenuous, they were simply unable to expand their strategy to include the newly discovered possibilities midway through the training program.

Allen (1985) described a series of studies that provide enlightening examples of the problems children face in developing strategies for new learning. They were interested in how children and adults differ in visualizing space during a walk through an urban neighborhood. They specifically questioned how child and adult subjects might use the same landmarks along a travel route. To address this question, 7-year-olds, 10-year-olds and college adults first walked through a selected neighborhood. They were then shown photographs and asked to select those which could best serve as reference points along the route traveled. The scenes selected most frequently by the adults depicted either actual points or intersections for possible turns. Conversely, less than half of the scenes selected most often by the 10-year-olds and less than one fourth of those selected by the 7-year-olds coincided with those selected by the adults. Instead, they often chose scenes from the middle of blocks which portrayed attention-getting scenes such as colorful window displays and bright awnings that were not distinctive in a spatial sense. A second study was then conducted to investigate the utility of the scenes selected by the original group of child and adult

---

[3]The stabilometer consists of a platform centered on a fulcrum, much like a seesaw. The subject stands with both feet on the platform (one on either side of the fulcrum) and attempts to maintain the platform in a level, balanced position. Performance is scored by the number of times the platform touches the base on either side or the time the platform is kept in balance.

subjects for judging distances along the same walk. Performance of the 7-year-olds was found to be poor whether they used the adult-selected or child-selected scenes. Performance of the 10-year-olds was also poor with the scenes selected by the other 10-year-olds, but comparable to that of the adults when they used the adult-selected scenes to judge the distances.

Younger children also have difficulty attending to modeled events and distinguishing relevant from irrelevant cues (Bandura, 1986). In other words, skills in "knowing" or developing metastrategies that can be applied in solving new tasks mature very slowly. This slow maturation is likely a major source of their lower performance in using modeled performance midway in the stream of motor skill learning. Younger children may need a longer, more repetitive series of trials to foster metastrategy development.

In general, these findings suggest that introducing a model pattern both before practice begins and later in the training program will enhance performance of a motor task by both child and adult subjects. Younger subjects may need both more opportunities to witness demonstrations and more carefully modeled patterns than older subjects to develop fully integrated action strategies once they have begun to practice.

Mental Imagery

Mental imagery is based on the principle that *all things are created twice:* a mental concept is created first followed by a physical creation. People use this two-fold creation principle in varying degrees and in many different ways. A traveler usually plans the destination and routing before starting on a trip. A gardener envisions the arrangement and appearance of vegetables in a garden before the seeds are planted. A seamstress lays out the pattern for clothing before starting to cut the cloth. A builder selects a plan before the first nail is driven.

A period of mental incubation is often required during the initial stage of idea creation and activation. Friedrich von Kekulé, for example, developed a new account of molecular structure by discerning the key structural component in the following reverie (Findlay, 1965):

> One fine summer evening, I was returning by the last omnibus through the deserted streets of the metropolis, which are at other times so full of life. I fell into a reverie, and lo! the atoms were gamboling before my eyes. Whenever, hitherto, these diminutive beings had appeared to me, they had always been in motion; but up to that time, I had never been able to discern the nature of their motion. Now, however, I saw how, fre-

quently, two smaller atoms united to form a pair; how a larger one embraced two smaller ones; how still larger ones kept hold of three or even four of the smaller; whilst the whole kept whirling in a giddy dance. I saw how the larger ones formed a chain. . . . I spent part of the night putting on paper at least sketches of these dream forms. (p. 39)

From his sudden insight, Kukelé was able to develop a new account of molecular structure in which individual atoms could be located in organic molecules based on strings of carbon atoms. Visual imagery provided a powerful source of the new sight obtained by Kekulé who had been an architecture student before turning to chemistry.

To a large extent, success in the physical creation is a result of careful mental creation followed by diligent application of the concept formed. The immediate goal of articulatory modeling is to create a clear mental percept of postures and movements that generate intelligible phonetic outputs. This use of mentally formulated spatial images to guide concept development is commonly referred to as "mental imaging" or "visual motor behavior rehearsal" (Suinn, 1980).

Rehearsing

After a mental image is formed, it can be rehearsed as a central construct in a more complex and dynamic context, still without overt movement. This stage has been called "cognitive rehearsal" (Sage, 1984) or simply "mental practice." Examples of this behavior include a ball player imagining how to "meet the ball" in batting practice, a basketball player mentally rehearsing how to release the ball in a jump shot, and a talker mentally reviewing tongue placement and movement sensations that will accompany correct production of a particular sound or series of sounds in a word or sentence.

The literature on mental practice that includes imagery and rehearsal is voluminous. After an extensive review of this topic, Weinberg (1981) summarized the findings as follows:

> What are "the proper conditions?" A major factor seems to be that the mental practice include rehearsal of movement sequences as symbolic components of the task. According to this notion mental practice enhances motor performance to the extent that cognitive factors are inherent in the activities. When the cognitive and motor components of a mental practice task have been studied separately, the findings indicate the major source of benefit is from the cognitive rather than the motor component of the tasks. (p. 211)

This interpretation was firmly supported by Feltz and Landers' (1983) meta-analysis review across 60 studies having 146 different effect sizes.

They observed that:

> In spite of different populations, designs, and methodologies employed in the mental practice studies, the distinction between symbolic and motor aspects of motor skill learning are very robust and provide very strong support for the symbolic learning explanation. (p. 45)

Considerable controversy exists about whether mental practice is more effective for novice or highly proficient learners. Most of the research has been done with beginners, and their learning rate has been found rather consistently to be facilitated when they have been taught how to image, rehearse, and accomplish a task. More proficient subjects have also been shown to benefit from mental practice. The findings with these subjects indicate that in the early stages of learning a new task, the experienced performer seems to use mental rehearsal to gain a rough idea of how a particular task *might* be performed. Feedback from actual practice is then used to refine both the rehearsal and the motor skill in executing the desired response patterns. Feltz and Landers (1983) noted that nearly all of the studies they reviewed in their meta-analysis of the literature on this topic found greater mental practice effects for experienced than novice subjects. They concluded that for tasks high in symbolic or cognitive elements, mental practice is most effective when subjects have had some prior experience with the task. In other words rehearsal became an increasingly effective tool in aiding motor skill learning as experience accumulates. This conclusion is consistent with the effects found in the modeling literature where observational learning during as well as preceding performance trials enhances motor performance.

In certain tasks, mental rehearsal may contribute comparatively little to the physical aspects of the performance. Minas (1978) had subjects throw balls into bins in particular sequences under different mental and physical practice conditions. In this task, mental practice was found to facilitate learning the sequence (cognitive component) but had little effect on the throwing (motor component). This difference was corroborated in later studies by Ryan and Simons (1981). Sage (1984) noted, however, that mental practice generally appears to help correct execution errors, increase concentration, and develop improved motor strategies.

Studies of imagery in motor skill development have traditionally treated it as a form of cognitive rehearsal that may be applied as an adjunct to, or replacement for, actual practice. Even within this limited framework a beneficial effect on skill learning has been consistently shown. For example, Johnson (1982) observed that imaging of a movement appeared to bias later motor performance in the same way as an actual movement biased motor reproduction.

Paivio (1985) suggested that the beneficial effects of imagery arise from a combination of increased desire to achieve specific goals and cognitive insight gained through covert practice of imagined actions and strategies. Following this line of reasoning Van Gyn, Wenger, and Gaul (1990) hypothesized that a key factor in gaining benefits from mental practice is that learners image the specific task they intend to perform. If that hypothesis were correct, they reasoned that mentally rehearsing an intended task even while engaged in nonspecific physical training could enhance later performance. To test this hypothesis, they studied changes in peak power and 40-meter (m) sprint time under four training conditions. In one, the subjects simply pedaled an ergometer-controlled cycle set to simulate the energy output demands of the 40-m sprint. Another group was instructed to image or rehearse actual involvement in the sprint while they were involved in the same cycle pedaling activity. The third group was guided through an imagined sequence of activities during a timed 40-m sprint. They were specifically instructed to visualize warming up, responding to the "go" signal, running the sprint, and jogging back to the start line. During this rehearsal activity, the subjects actually maintained a sitting, relaxed posture in the classroom. The fourth group, which served as a control, received no specific training.

The results from the Van Gyn, Wenger, and Gaul (1990) study showed the post-training "peak power" scores[4] of both groups trained on the cycle to be greater than those of the others. Those who exercised increased their physical power. The others did not. The more interesting finding was that the cycle trained group who also explicitly imaged the sprinting task was superior to all others both in physical power and in sprint times. No sprint time differences were found between the cycle-only, imaging-only, and control groups. The apparent absence of benefit for the cycle-only group in the sprint is consistent with findings in prior physiological studies, which have shown poor transfer from practice to performance when the practice and task conditions are divorced from each other even though similar energy may be expended in the training and performance sessions.

To ascertain the reason for the superior performance of the group with imaging plus cycle power training, Van Gyn, Wenger, and Gaul (1990) queried the subjects about their imaging process. The participants reported that they "put a great amount of effort" into creating and sustaining clear images of the actual sprinting action throughout the sprint phase of the ergometer cycle training. In other words, during their exertion they focused their attention keenly on imaging and rehearsing the actual task they were being trained to perform.

---

[4]Determined by the pedaling rate and resistance to a 90 g/kg body weight during the 30-sec interval of peak power output.

Image focusing in motor skill training emphasizes the need to isolate and rehearse the specific task the training routine is intended to improve. A common tactic in speech training is to have a subject mentally review an erroneous response before trying it again. A critical consideration in this situation would seem to be to determine whether the error was because the individual had not acquired the essential gestures and movements of the targeted articulation pattern or because of difficulties in transferring the gestures into the highly constrained phonological contexts of speech production. In the first condition, the specific context hypothesis would suggest that rehearsal should focus on imaging the specific spatial and temporal properties of the sound to be produced whether the sound was practiced in isolation to remove possible conflicting motor actions and simplify the motor requirements of the task, or placed in real words to simulate a more natural speech context. When the basic articulatory actions *are mastered,* the training sessions could then shift to imaging, rehearsing, and executing the articulatory actions in contextual speech with emphasis given to contrastive changes in the articulatory sequences. The reader should be cautioned that although such extensions from motor skill learning studies appear to be very logical, their effectiveness for speech motor skill learning has not yet been fully tested in speech research. Imaging and rehearsal strategies appear to offer fruitful avenues to explore in our efforts to increase the power and efficiency of speech articulatory training.

One of the major benefits from mental practice may be that it primes the system for maximum proficiency in the motor activities that follow. It may also enable the performer to concentrate more attention on the task at hand while blocking disrupting thoughts. The aroused attention set could be particularly helpful for younger children as they are striving to focus their efforts on the task at hand. Imaging and rehearsal would be expected to help more experienced learners sort through different aspects of complicated routines as they refine their response strategies.

Finally, it is worth noting that it is not necessary to devote a large amount of time to any single mental imaging task. Shick (1970) reported that three to five minutes spent in mental practice at one time seemed to produce the best results. It is likely that in most speech articulation applications even shorter periods of mental practice would contribute beneficial results.

EXECUTING

All skills are grounded in tacit knowledge. The motor-program concept stipulates that movement is a natural extension of instructions and movement parameters. Commands from the motor-program are translated into directions that are relayed to the motor system where biomechanical features of targeted movements are added (e.g., Requin, Semjen, & Bonnet, 1984). In speech, recurrent spatiotemporally coordinated articulatory postures and gestures become encapsulated into respiratory driven action series. The spoken word is thus a lawful consequence of the articulatory gestural planning and action patterns. Under pressure from an expanding repertoire of increasingly lengthy and complex utterances, the central articulatory program is presumed to organize and activate different combinations of recurrent postures and gestures to achieve specific phonetic goals. The program must contain rules that govern the patterns and range of motion by individual structures, resolve potential movement interference, and enhance coordination across articulatory actions.

Thoroughly practiced actions tend to become "automatic" in the sense that they are performed without conscious control. This is an essential part of the process of developing complex actions and movement series. Consider the centipede as a homely example. The centipede would be immobilized if it were required to specify the temporal order and action patterns involved in walking. By the same token, it seems apparent that if talkers were required to continuously monitor and control the highly complex postures, gestures, and action sequences involved in speech production, man would be much less vocal. The speech motor system must have some means of relegating action sequences to routines that can be activated and executed in an essentially automatic fashion.

That highly repetitive human tasks are carried out in an automatic manner has been well demonstrated in multitask activities. For example, certain women carry on a continuous stream of conversation while knitting, provided the knitting includes only simple patterns or highly repeated action sequences. Beyond a certain level of complexity or non-repetitiveness, however, the knitter must devote an increasing share of attention to the knitting task, after which conversation is again resumed. Some evidence is found that even complex tasks can be performed at an essentially unconscious level. Leonard (1953) described an experiment in which signals were used to activate overlapping actions. He used a signal to activate a second response before a previously signaled response had been initiated. Contrary to what might have been expected, performance of the second task under this condition was much faster than in a previous experiment in which the second response was signaled after completion of the previously signaled one. A further interesting and important observation was that in the second experiment the subjects seemed to be unaware of their actions. In fact, they reported the sensation that the actions were being executed without conscious control. This situation created an uncanny feeling that they were spectators in their own actions.

The task imposed in Leonard's second experiment required the subjects to initiate one response and at the same time prepare to initiate a second set of signaled responses before the currently demanded one was underway. These complex, seemingly conflicting requirements were apparently solved by a physiological time-sharing strategy. The "out of control" sensation could perhaps be explained by positing that both the current and preparatory responses were executed as background physiological actions. The feedback may thus not have been relayed to the subject as the actions were transpiring. This explanation presumes that conscious monitoring was bypassed to permit the motor control program to devote full attention on executing the two concurrent, intricately interwoven action sequences. The fact that performance improved under these conditions suggests that efficiency in executing required motor commands is a direct by-product of the physiological activate-monitor-feedback-modify control system which in this circumstance was freed from parallel reporting to the conscious sensing system.

Processing information without conscious awareness is not unusual. It is a common experience in recalling something from memory. Often a person realizes that some desired information, such as a person's name, is known but not available through central recall at the moment. So, attention is switched to another task. The mental search does not stop at this point, however. In a few moments the name suddenly appears in the person's consciousness. In a similar way, well learned but seemingly forgotten motor sequences such as the combination of a lock can often be retrieved by simply activating the physical actions associated with them. For example, beginning to turn the tumbler on a lock and allowing motor memory to lead the hand movements through a previously well learned sequence of number locations on the dial may be successful in opening the lock. Interestingly, when this type of action is completed, the memory of the number sequence may also be restored. The movement information thus refreshes the conscious awareness of stored knowledge. Such activities demonstrate the intimate, reciprocal relationship that exists between cognitive and motor systems involved in foreground-background information processing functions.

A benefit of an automatic response is that it permits attention to be focused on the outcomes rather than the mechanics of a response. Faster and smoother task performance is an apparent consequence of achieving automatic, unconsciously controlled movements. Welford and Bourne (1976) cited a study by Klein and Posner (1974) that showed that when visual and kinesthetic signals are relayed to the nervous system, the externally referenced visual information is likely to take precedence in attention. From this, they posited that when a higher priority system such as vision provides sensory information sufficient for accurate outcome prediction, automaticity is a natural consequence. If this is so, a major goal of any skill training program must be to establish and foster a dependable set of automatic responses. The ultimate aim would be to integrate multiple action sequences and enhance execution of concurrent, overlapping tasks such as those required in speech production.

The strategy of freeing the motor system during the execution of intricate motor commands can be applied rather directly in motor skill training routines. After the elemental postures and gestures have been established and the action sequences have been accurately conceived and rehearsed, execution should be emphasized without conscious monitoring. In the speech context, this would be expected to free the speaker to attend to more global information such as verifying the content of the utterance and visually confirming the transmission of the message by observing the listener's reaction. At the same time, execution of the motor response without conscious oversight would enable confirmation of the articulatory action sequences as the motor commands are carried out. In palatometric training, this perceptual freedom can provide an opportunity to impose an intermediate step in the speaking process: visually confirming the general integrity of articulatory sequences displayed on the video screen.

The capability of monitoring the flow of activities as a speaker seeks to transmit a given message seems to be used on a periodic schedule throughout life. Mature talkers appear to refer to auditory sensations now and then during the natural flow of speech to confirm that the motor sequences being executed are accurate. It seems likely that continuous oral sensory monitoring is applied as a background phenomenon. The presence of continuous physiological monitoring of the articulatory actions is indicated by speaker reports describing their sensations when oral structures are still anesthetized following dental treatment. Anesthetization of the speech articulators typically rouses sensations of speech disturbance that far exceed the actual degree of change in the output. The discrepancy between the speech sensations and the actual output suggests that mature talkers usually rely primarily on the continuous oral physiological feedback to monitor and control integrity of the articulatory actions. The automatic nature of this monitoring in natural speaking situations is suggested by the difficulty that even phonetically trained talkers have in describing the disturbances they sense when the sensory system is temporarily disabled.

Increasingly consistent, precise actions with their elements tightly integrated into unified whole patterns are symptomatic of developing motor skill expertise (Chi & Glaser, 1980). In the process of development, there is also a general trend for action sequences to become longer and longer. For example, utterance length increases from early childhood onward and is longer with familiar than unfamiliar material. Welford and Bourne (1976) stressed that when a task is encountered repeatedly, routines are developed that merge the actions together as a single order "unit." The building of such units depends upon establishing the ability to execute the individual movements and gestures accurately without being interrupted to make corrections. Changes due to factors such as fatigue or momentary distractions that impair accuracy tend to break up the emerging routines and necessitate a return to dealing with the task in a piecemeal fashion.

It follows from that line of reasoning that a major goal of training in speech production skills is to enable articulatory execution to proceed automatically. Known derivatives of automaticity are faster performance, greater efficiency, and a sense that each action can be initiated without being required to wait to observe the outcome of a previous one. Accurate, habitualized performance also engenders a feeling of being unhurried since the performer's entire attention and effort can be devoted to global information processing without attending to the details of action monitoring. Bartlett (1947) and many others have emphasized that speed and accuracy are the prominent characteristics of highly skilled performance.

In a modular system such as speech, errors may still be expected when words with new sound combinations are attempted and when nonhabitualized patterns are incorporated into longer phrase and sentence sequences "on the fly." These errors are likely to be resolved as subordinate articulation modules become more fully coordinated, habitualized, and tagged to distinguish their roles in sequential actions. In a training program, arousal of conscious monitoring should be limited to establishing and rehearsing basic postures and gestures needed to underpin speech actions. The achievement of relatively rapid change may be enhanced through the use of the previously described focusing, modeling, imaging, rehearsing, and the following verification procedures.

VERIFYING AND EVALUATING MOTOR SKILL LEARNING

Verification is the process of determining the degree to which an intended action has been executed correctly. The process of verification includes obtaining, delineating, and evaluating information about differences between targeted and actual actions after a motor command has been executed. It plays a central role in the repeated try-assess-revise cycles that are part of motor skill learning. Verification provides opportunity to analyze progress toward established standards of performance and to evaluate the extent to which objectives and goals have been reached.

The "matching law" (Herrnstein, 1970) states that organisms will distribute their activities between behavioral options in proportion to the rewards offered by the options. In other words, motor skill learning is predicted by the extent to which actual responses match modeled, imaged, and rehearsed patterns. Verification of "successful" pattern matching may in turn be expected to activate increased attention focus and effort, particularly in the early stages of learning. Accurate modeling, valid imitation, appropriate rehearsal, and authentic response execution strategies are thus all verified by the output accuracy. Successful actions are likely to be repeated.

Evidence of success in a speech skill learning task includes minimizing variability in the motor control process and maximizing the likelihood that the skills gained will transfer automatically and naturally to social speaking conditions outside the laboratory. The information derived in the process of response verification can also be used to establish the costs and benefits from training which is the essence of accountability.

Feedback is the springboard for skill assessment and verification, and response contingent feedback is a central issue in motor skill verification. Performance theory predicts that *accurate* feedback will increase interest in a task, enhance skill in performing the behaviors, accelerate the rate of change in response patterns, and reduce fatigue during the learning process. The importance of feedback is undisputed. Bilodeau and Bilodeau (1961) flatly state:

> Studies of feedback . . . . show it to be the strongest, most important variable controlling performance and learning. It has been shown repeatedly, that there is no improvement without [feedback], progressive improvement with it, and deterioration after its withdrawal (p. 250).

Verification includes reviewing feedback information to document the validity and accuracy of responses, implement possible corrective changes, and confirm benefits from changes made. Feedback is thus an integral part of controlling the functioning unit. It enables an organism to be both self-acting and self-regulating. The use of feedback presumes a detection device, standards against which performance can be measured, and sufficiently rapid analysis that the feedback is available when it is needed to regulate the output. When feedback is prevented, the output differs radically from that observed under normal conditions.

Actions are controlled by sensing differences between the present state of the system and *intended* goal states. In cybernetic and action theory, the try-observe-revise cycles that are part of motor skill learning continue until differences are eliminated. The *combined spatial* and *tactile-kinesthetic image* of the goal supplies the sensory criteria that must be met before the test is passed. Feedback is used to assess the goal directed actions, optimize strategies conceived to achieve them, assess and guide actions as the strategies are put into play, and verify and adjust the degree of coincidence between targeted and executed action patterns.

As currently applied, the term "feedback" has a variety of meanings. In its historical sense, feedback refers to automatic furnishing of data concerning the output of a machine for the purpose of control and error correction. When the term is used behaviorally, it refers to using data as a consequence of actions by an organism to influence or modify further performance. Biofeedback combines these basic functions. It is defined as the use of instrumentation (usually electronic) to reveal normal and abnormal internal physiological events through visual and/or auditory signals which enable an organism to control otherwise involuntary, unfelt, or unperceived events by manipulating actions identified in, and controlled through, a displayed output (adapted from Basmajian, 1979, p. 1). As indicated, a critical aspect of feedback is that the information is presented in a format designed to *facilitate* monitoring and changing selected physical performance attributes the subject is normally unable to sense accurately.

Events that take place within the body are normally sensed through *tactile* (touch) or *kinesthetic* (position and movement in space) interoreceptors within the various organs. For example, you know where your tongue is within the oral cavity by kinesthetic feedback generated as the tongue moves through oral space and tactile sensations as it touches structures such as the palate within the oral cavity. Events that take place at a distance are sensed through auditory (hearing) and visual (sight) *teloreceptors*. *Feedback* from the interoreceptor and exteroreceptor sensory systems *is normally combined, reviewed, and compared with* information from previous experiences stored in memory. Through such comparisons, we can assess skills already attained in tasks that are performed and judge success during current performances in terms of changes with respect to specific goals and standards. The standards themselves are developed as current and previous abilities and capacities are explored. They are also derived from actions modeled intentionally or unintentionally by others in similar circumstances and from instructions by teachers or clinician instructors as they guide subjects toward skilled achievements. Thus, feedback can have a series of different referents, each of which is important in the teaching/learning process.

Information provided by another person or by an instrumental device such as the palatometer that measures and displays response patterns is called *augmented feedback*. Augmented feedback can be used in different ways. Biofeedback is a form of augmented feedback that is provided continuously during the activity being monitored. If the feedback information is stored during the activity and the level of accuracy in achieving a specifically targeted goal is reported only after a response has been completed, it is termed *knowledge-of-results* or, in abbreviated form, simply KR. KR provides a numerical score or verification rating of motor response accuracy. It may be from either instrumental measurements or instructor rendered judgments. The data summarized graphically in Figure 6–1 illustrate the clear value that KR provides in such motor skill learning.

Finally, if the information being fed back is used to extract an evaluation of an action after it has been carried out, the feedback is termed *knowledge-of-performance,* or simply KP. KP provides *kinematic* or movement-related response assessments or evaluations that help identify how well actions explicitly involved in a response are performed with respect to a set goal or standard (Newell & Walter, 1981). For example, the accuracy of producing a targeted articulation pattern would be indicated by either an instrumentally or clinician derived KR score and a KP description "Your tongue was too far forward."

The three sources of augmented feedback play supplementary and complementary roles in speech treatment regimens. Biofeedback provides information to the motor control system about moment by moment changes in response patterns related directly to planned actions and performance goals. KR supplies a measured evaluation of the goal-driven performance after the response has been completed. The resulting KR data can be used to assess, compare, and establish consequence-based changes in performance and document the rate of change and learning trend patterns. KP adds a means of guiding motor skill change toward established goals through specific temporospatial interpretation of the pictorial feedback displays. KR and KP combined provide opportunity to channel the subject's actions toward explicitly defined goal postures and movement patterns and to evaluate progress and reward successes attained as the subject moves toward targeted temporospatial action patterns. Each form of augmented feedback can thus be used to pinpoint aspects of the training program that need revision and enhance the utility of internal tactile/kinesthetic feedback and self reports as skills are transferred to everyday life.

Documented changes in motor skills also provide a reference mechanism for examining performance and assessing changes in performance patterns as training conditions are manipulated experimentally. Used in this way the resulting data can be used to appraise investigators of effectiveness of different sensory systems in processing specific types of information. Rubow (1984), for example, compared differences in breath pressure control through visual and auditory biofeedback and visually based KR. Breath exhalation was controlled at 66, 100, and 133 cc per second under each condition. In the visual tracking condition, targeted and actual respiratory rates were demon-

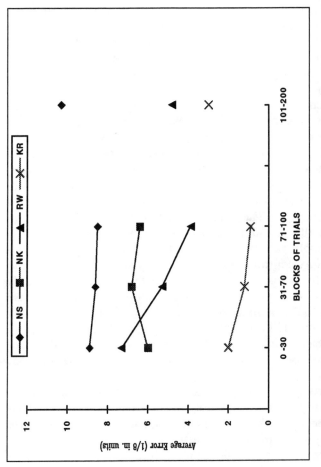

FIGURE 6–1. Differences in the average line drawing error as a function of the type of feedback (NS=Nonsense, NK=No Knowledge, RW=Right-Wrong, KR=Knowledge of Results) provided during acquisition (TRIALS 0–100) and retention (TRIALS 101–200) of motor skill learning. From data in Trowbridge, M. H. & Cason, H. (1932). An experimental study of Thorndike's theory of learning. *Journal of General Psychology, 7,* 245–258.

strated by rises and falls of light spots crossing a CRT screen. The storage scope used retained the light spot traces until each 5-sec trial period was completed. In the auditory pursuit task, respiratory pressure was represented by a 250 Hz tone with acoustic intensity proportional to the air pressure. The resulting pattern was routed to the subject's right ear. Targeted exhalation rates were represented by constant tones in the left ear. In both the visual and auditory conditions, feedback was relayed to the subject within 1 msec of the response. The KR feedback consisted of the stored, static traces from the targeted and actual respiratory rates. The display was presented with an average time lag after the response of 2.5 sec.

The subjects in Rubrow's study consisted of normal 21- to 35-year-old individuals and two mid 40-year-old, cerebral-palsied dysarthric individuals. One five-member normal group was assigned to each of the three experimental conditions and one to a no-feedback control condition. The subjects were familiarized with the respiratory tasks, pretested under the 3 feedback conditions and a nonfeedback condition, then trained during 3 sets of 6 feedback trials under each of 3 respiratory rate conditions. They were then retested without feedback immediately after the 54 training trials and 10 min later.

Despite highly variable results, Rubrow's data showed that although respiratory control errors were initially smaller in response to the KR and auditory conditions, the visual feedback group was the only one to retain improved performance in the training transfer test. These results support findings from previous studies indicating that visually based biofeedback is likely to produce greater temporospatial control than auditory-based biofeedback. The findings also indicate that continuous, dynamic feedback is likely to be superior to static KR in motor control tasks.

The importance of dynamic information in motor skill development is increasingly apparent. Action theory conceives human behavior as goal directed with hierarchically arranged plans that utilize feedback from the environment to articulate and guide actions. The central construct of the goal-oriented action theory is that understanding is fostered by feedback from objects acted upon. The theory stresses that in the process of motor skill learning specific plans are created in specific environments to reach specific goals. Situations that do not permit the perceiver to act upon objects perceived truncate the processes by which we normally come to know the world (Frese & Sabini, 1985).

It is self-evident that the feedback is in vain if it is insufficient or, worse, erroneous (Schönpflug, 1985). A general presupposition is that individuals strive toward efficiency and economy of effort through minimizing problems which restrict actions. There is no activity that does not consume resources. Failure consumes resources, including time, and risks unintended negative effects.

Actions often fail to produce intended results or produce unintended ones because the action space is not well represented in the actor's model. This situation poses a salient problem in traditional speech therapy where learners must depend on auditory sensation to infer what is happening in another person's mouth during speech sound production. Incorrect inferences in this matching process would create unrealistic images with missing, nonessential, or irrelevant details in the representational model. Each of these conditions would heighten the risk of error (see Schönpflug, 1985). Thus, knowledge of conditions and functional relations concerning the articulation action space becomes a potent factor in seeking accurate data for efficient and effective motor skill training.

In palatometric work, biofeedback evolves from linguapalatal contact detection and signal transduction into representative video displays that can guide movement patterns as the action is underway. Modeling and shaping routines are then applied with KR and KP used systematically to guide change in articulatory behaviors. An immediate question is what role might hard, specific speech articulation goals play in achieving the modeled articulation patterns?

Mento, Steel, and Karren (1987) conducted a meta-analysis which compared experimental results when subjects received feedback with respect to goal driven performance versus those with no goals. The data analysis provided clear support for the efficacy of coupling feedback with hard, specific goals for enhanced performance. In fact, the more varied and complex the goal task, the more the person apparently needs higher level structures such as personal aspirations, rules, and accurate feedback to organize response behaviors and develop successful integrated strategies.

As described in the previous section, conscious monitoring and simultaneous use of internal feedback is likely to be detrimental to performance of an intricate skill. For actions to be executed rapidly, accurately, and smoothly in continuously integrated movements, the motor program must be free to carry out the coordinated gestures without the process being consciously sensed, modified, or reported during the stream of ongoing activities. The key muscle contraction sequences and forces involved in a skilled motor act must be monitored physiologically and the information stored in memory from where it can be accessed, retrieved, and used later to verify accurate functions and movements. Such stored information is also needed to provide KR and KP auxiliary feedback and to update the central motor schema.

An important consideration in providing feedback to guide actions is how and how often it should be provided. Salmoni, Schmidt, and Walter (1984) reviewed a number of studies that showed that decreasing the relative frequency of KR during acquisition led to better performance during no-KR retention tests. They suggested that when KR is overly abundant, the subject may not engage in the information processing needed to maintain performance without KR. Lavery (1962, 1964) also observed improved retention when KR was presented in a summary fashion rather than immediately after each trial. Schmidt, Young, Swinnen, and Shapiro (1989) also found that performance improved with the number of trials summarized during acquisition.

Sidaway, Moore, and Schoenfelder-Zohdi (1991) suspected that it was differences in the KR frequency rather than the number of trials summarized that led to differences in the amount learned. To test this possibility, they examined the effects of providing KR on only the last of 1, 3, 7, and 15 trials during acquisition scores and on no-KR scores obtained 10 min and 2 days after the training. They found learning to be unaffected by the number of trials summarized. The group that was given KR on each trial exhibited the best performance on both acquisition and retention. From this they concluded that "it is the frequency of KR presentation during acquisition rather than the number of trials [summarized] that determines retention performance." Sidaway and colleagues suggested that perhaps a major reason for the difference between their findings and those of Schmidt and his associates was that the apparatus they [Sidaway & colleagues] used permitted the subjects to execute their movements at a rather leisurely pace. In the Schmidt and associates study, the subjects were required to execute the movements at close to their maximum speed. All studies show that the frequency of KR presentations, and perhaps the temporal delay of KR, is important in motor skill learning. Evidence is still lacking concerning the most effective variations in KR to provide the greatest long-term effect on retention and generalization. The data provide convincing evidence that both KR and KP provide important information for motor skill learning. Trials followed by both KR and KP lead to better performance.

PRACTICING AND DIVERSIFYING

Among other things, learning usually means acquiring skills through practice. The gauge of motor skill practice is how well a targeted action is performed. Thus, practice and performance are inextricably intertwined. In motor skill performance, retention is a vital dimension. A person who learns lines of a play, may not be expected to recall the words beyond the final performance. However, in the motor skill domain retention is usually required. A talker is forever obliged to retain and recall the correct actions involved in speech articulation, for example. Although the vocabulary may change, the mechanics of speech production remain fixed. They must not be forgotten.

Specificity Versus Variability

Active, goal-directed practice is essential for acquiring and retaining complex motor skills. The question specifically raised at this point is what should be practiced to facilitate motor skill learning and retention? Two opposing viewpoints have been posited in answer to this question. One is called the *specificity of learning principle* (Adams, 1971, 1987; Hull, 1943), the other the *variability of practice hypothesis* (Schmidt, 1975). A central assumption of the specificity of learning principle is that practice should focus on one and only one task. Under this assumption changing the motor task even slightly would mean implementing a new motor program. Application of the specificity of learning principle to speech articulatory skill building would indicate that practice in training should focus on one and only one task.

An apparent application of the specificity of learning principle is in speech articulation training routines where clinician efforts are focused exclusively on a specifically missing or defective articulatory skill. This approach may be needed with children such as those described by McReynolds (1989) who are rather quiet, rarely practice sounds orally, seldom imitate the sounds of the environment, and miss key phonetic learning experiences due to shifts in their attention. McReynolds contends that these children may need highly structured, specifically targeted speech training routines. She comments that in speech articulation training the usual procedure is to:

> . . . . reinforce responses in the presence of a specific stimulus until responding has stabilized. Then stimuli similar and dissimilar *in a particular dimension* [italics added] to the training stimulus are presented in the presence of extinction, to determine which stimuli will function to evoke the trained response. (pp. 1–2)

In this type of training, expansion of the new skills through variable practice would be delayed until later stages of training when the aim becomes transference of new skills to conversational speech.

The variable practice hypothesis emphasizes the use of contrastive sensory consequences in task learning. Hypotheses are presumed to be formed, tested, and rejected as conditions are varied until an action pattern is found that consistently produces acceptable responses across a range of possible actions. In essence, the subject makes the choice where effort will be allocated in the face of alternatives. The heart of the variable practice method is thus seen to be the tradeoff between possible choices. Variations around a central task are thought to form the basis of flexible skills within a broad scope of possible actions. Breadth of experience is used to test and refine emerging rules. For example, a lifelong immersion in music lay behind Mozart's ability to abstract subtle musical structures and develop powerful exploratory strategies for finely integrated compositions. A person needs time and effort to amass the mental structures for other complicated acts such as speaking and to explore and refine the rules or meta-strategies that utilize them to their potential. These rules may then be applied and extended as the basis for new patterns and experiences. This means that the greater the variety of speech experiences, the more flexible will be the set of articulatory responses that could produce potentially intelligible outputs in a variety of speaking contexts.

Errors also play an important role in variable practice theory. During the concept development stage of motor skill development, learners appear to enter a search mode for a brief time after errors are made (Trabasso, Rollins, & Shaughnessy, 1971). At that time they are thought to make decisions about which specific dimensions to vary in a motor task and set values on these dimensions. Certain dimensions are presumed to be more noticeable (more *salient*) than others. These dimensions are likely to be tested first in the process of developing viable hypotheses for guiding action patterns. When a response is correct (receives positive feedback during a trial), the hypothesis that dictated that response is confirmed and the action retained. Through such hypothesis testing, learners are thought to narrow the action possibilities until only correct responses remain. Those patterns are then stabilized and automatized. The responses are still not unchangeable, however. If an error is made on a subsequent trial, the search mode may be reactivated and the testing operation re-entered to refine and recheck the program. The development of skill is thus postulated to be directly related to the variations practiced as a subject works within a particular class of responses.

A number of motor skill studies have shown that variable practice during early learning activities enhances later transfer of learning to a novel task (cf. Lee, Magill, & Weeks, 1985; Newell & Shapiro, 1976; Wrisberg & Ragsdale, 1979). Shapiro and Schmidt (1982) noted that the advantage of training variability is especially evident during childhood. In their review of motor skill learning, they found that performance on a novel task was more effective "in nearly every study" when earlier practice was variable as opposed to constant.

One of the most cited studies of the relation between variability during practice and motor skill learning was conducted by McCracken and Stelmach (1977). They examined skill in moving the hand across

15, 35, 60, and 65 cm distances, each in 200 msec. The subjects were assigned to constant and variable practice groups. The constant practice group was subdivided into four subgroups each of which was given 300 trials at one of the distances. The remaining variable-practice group was given the same number of trials but with 75 trials at each distance. The results showed average timing errors by the group that received training at variable distances to be considerably larger than for those who had practiced 300 times on the same distance. At the end of the training period, all subjects were given a series of trials at a novel 50 cm distance. The results were switched under this novel condition. As would be predicted by the variable practice hypothesis, the average timing error for the subjects who had learned constant distance movements was now substantially *larger* than for those who had practiced movements at different distances. These results, along with a series of others cited by Sage (1984), indicate rather clearly that practicing a variety of maneuvers within a movement class is likely to facilitate skilled movements when they are needed in new situations.

An interesting twist on the role of variable practice in motor skill learning was reported in a study by Shea and Kohl (1990). They compared the outcome of predictions by the specificity of learning principle and the variability of practice hypothesis in a motor learning task. The task consisted of developing controlled handgripping force. One group of subjects practiced solely on a targeted value. The other group practiced achieving the targeted value plus others that clustered around it. As might be expected, the results from the study showed variable practice produced significantly better accuracy during both motor skill acquisition and retention. Of particular interest was the additional observation that when the number of specific target trials was increased by subjects who practiced solely on a targeted value, they did even worse than when a smaller number of spaced trials was given. This raises the spaced versus massed practice issue in motor skill learning.

Language and associated articulation skills are normally acquired in an unstructured, highly flexible environment. In the normal environment, children master a wide variety of vocal skills with surprising ease and relatively little direct attention. Variable practice thus characterizes the usual life patterns of speech development.

One trend in speech articulation training is to aim at generalization from the start of treatment (Baer, 1981; Costello, 1983). This shift is consistent with the central assumption of the variable practice hypothesis, namely that natural and intentional variations are used by talkers to test and confirm or reject hypotheses about the role specific vocal parameters play in speech. This also supports the assumption that trial variability should be an integral part of any training routine.

The concept that speech development should be enhanced by variable practice is founded on the belief that an individual does not store specific sensory consequences from each action in a learning task. Rather, a talker is assumed to compare his or her own speech output with that from other talkers in order to determine the contributions specific parameters make to speech intelligibility as they are varied in vocal communication. The variable practice itself is thought to lead to the discovery of explicit actions that consistently produce acceptable matches between targeted and actual listener reactions across a range of possible variations. At the same time, the variations are thought to help localize sources of acoustic contrast arising from different movements within articulatory gestures. Variations within a set of responses may also permit a talker to use the consequences of actions to help isolate movements that are physiologically easiest to produce as they contribute to a highly contrastive phonetic repertoire. Variable practice is thus treated as a means of screening response patterns, weeding out those that are unsuccessful, and stabilizing those linked with successful performance in a wide variety of phonetic contexts and speaking situations.

Sounds produced by a single talker are remarkably consistent both acoustically (Hughes & Halle, 1956) and physiologically (Fletcher, 1989b; Fletcher & Newman, 1991). But when articulation details are compared across talkers, important differences emerge. As noted earlier, Fletcher and Newman (1991) described one subject who produced [s] and [ʃ] through sibilant grooves 7 mm and 14 mm respectively from the incisor teeth. Another subject produced the same sounds 11.5 mm and 17.3 mm from the incisors. The second subject counterbalanced his more posterior articulation place by reducing his sibilant groove width. In both subjects, the posterior edge of the alveolar ridge demarcated [s] and [ʃ] articulatory contact regions, however. Thus, substantial individual variation may exist in basic articulation parameters across talkers who differ structurally while still yielding normal sounding speech.

Stevens (1972) posited that articulatory configurations or states that allow a range of articulatory parameter values with little change in the acoustic output should be favored in speech production. Those that precipitate an abrupt acoustic change with small articulatory modifications should be avoided. For example, the combined results from a series of studies, including the two experiments described by Fletcher and Newman (1991), suggest that a groove width of about 6 mm for the [s] and 10 to 12 mm for the [ʃ] may be near optimum for these sounds. The data in the perception study conducted by Fletcher and Newman suggested moreover that articulatory targets that are unusually difficult for a particular individual to reach may have a detrimental effect on the output. Unusual effort required to achieve certain specified articulatory goal postures appeared to disrupt the listeners' perceptions of spoken sounds. This observation raises interesting questions about possible roles that such factors as muscular tension, special compensatory articulatory postures, air pressure-flow dynamics, and articulatory strategies introduced by talkers to achieve difficult-to-reach articulation postures may play as they seek optimal articulatory posture and movement patterns during speech development. Such information could bear directly on speech sound acquisition principles and misarticulation interpretations. Additional research will be needed to define more precisely the conditions, attributes, and possible aberrations in sound production and perception from structural and functional differences.

It may be evident that a key element in gaining full benefits from practice is providing opportunity for the subject to participate creatively in solving the puzzle of the place, shape, and timing of articulation gestures. Varied involvement can be fostered through use of multiple models producing a pool of meaningful, intelligible words that is expanded systematically during clinical intervention.

Leonard (1981) has suggested that procedures used to guide speech skill development should be intentionally "loosely structured." In other words, the client needs to be given considerable flexibility in how he or she achieves particular gestures and uses feedback such as palatometric displays to improve speech production patterns.

Traditionally, speech stimuli are introduced initially in training routines through isolated sounds, simple syllables, or single citation form words. The phonetic repertoire is later expanded by locating the stimuli in phrases and connected speech contexts where stress, rhythm, and intonation can be used to give global meaning to the utterance and highlight key words. Gaining skill in producing sounds in words spoken in citation form or other severely restricted phonetic environments is relatively simple compared with their production in conversation where the talker must store and retrieve correct sounds while attending to both contextual demands and pragmatic, syntactic, and morphological aspects of verbal communication. Caregivers help in the use of the usual speech context by articulating carefully, simplifying the utterance complexity, and using high lexical redundancy in their speech model (Snow & Ferguson, 1977). On practical grounds, it would seem important to provide a learner with as much experience as possible about what could possibly happen during speech articulation where words spoken and speaking conditions are constantly changing. This would prepare the individual to develop effective meta-strategies that enable the talker to cope with a wide variety of speaking situations.

To illustrate, suppose that one subject practices only on isolated sound production, another on bisyllabic nonsense syllables, a third on citation form words, and a fourth practices on isolated sounds, nonsense syllables, citation form words, and words in phrases and sentences. If the results of training under all four of these conditions are then tested in a novel connected speech discourse, the variable practice principle would predict that subjects provided with a variety of articulatory experience will produce the best performance. The variations would enable those speakers to learn more naturally what variations in the sound can be tolerated within a category and what variations critically differentiate the sound category from others in the language.

Spaced Versus Massed Practicing

Considerable evidence has been found that when a particular task is overpracticed, beneficial changes may be countered by arousal of inhibiting forces within the system. This leads us to question how the distribution of practice may affect speech articulatory learning. Specifically, should the practice follow a *distributed schedule* with rest periods between trials or blocks of trials across spaced periods of time (distributed practice training)? Or should the schedule call for repetitions one after another within a short time span (*massed* practice training)?

Researchers have produced conflicting data about whether distributed or massed practice training produces better learning. A consensus has gradually emerged, however, favoring distributed over massed practice training. Lee and Genovese (1988) documented this agreement through an in-depth, meta-analysis review of 47 published papers on this topic. The results of their analysis showed surprisingly consistent performance benefits during both acquisition and retention motor skill tests in favor of distributed practice schedules. They noted further, however, that all except one of the over 100 studies they had initially considered in their survey had used "continuous" motor tasks in their research. A *continuous* task is one like cycling or swimming that is repeated over and over with no obvious beginnings, endings, or pauses between parts of the action. The whole movement pattern is repeatedly "replayed." Once learned, this type of skill is known to be highly resistant to forgetting — even across periods encompassing many years. This type of skill maintenance can therefore probably be explained by the large number of times the actions are repeated in an almost identical manner.

Dart throwing is an example of a discrete skill. Discrete skills have specifically defined beginning and ending points with loosely connected movements that are not critically dependent upon one another. The dart thrower, for instance, raises the arm, moves it forward rapidly, releases the dart, and allows the arm to follow through. The action sequence is completed quickly with readily identifiable and isolatable phases. Performing a single, isolated articulatory gesture is also an example of a discrete skill. The speaker moves the articulators to a particular position, activates a stream of air, then molds the ensuing air stream in certain ways to generate specific sound patterns.

Skills that entail a series of movements in a highly prescribed sequence are also known as *serial skills.* Speaking a sentence is an example of a serial action. If the movements are executed in an improper sequence, the utterance will be incorrect. Each part is more critically related to antecedent or subsequent events than in a strictly discrete action. Another way of viewing a serial skill is to interpret it as a number of connected discrete skills.

Lee and Genovese (1988) noted that the one study they found which had studied motor skill learning in a discrete task was conducted by Carron (1969) and described by Schmidt (1988). In Carron's study, the subjects pulled a small dowel out of a hole, reversed it end for end, and replaced it in the hole as rapidly as possible. Unlike in continuous motor tasks, massed practice in this task produced slightly better skill retention than distributed practice.[5] To test the possibility that massed trials may be generally superior in discrete motor skill tasks, Lee and Genovese constructed a task that could be performed in both modes. It consisted of moving a probe stylus between targeted points on two metal plates in a time that was as close to 500 msec as possible. In the discrete version of this task, the subjects were required to move the stylus from the neutral position, tap one of six metal plates then another in a specified but variable order within 500 ± 10 msec. The subjects were then given a 0.5 sec intertrial rest interval during which they were informed by high- or low-pitched tones whether the response was above or below the targeted time span. The continuous version of the task was similar in every way to the discrete one except a "trial" consisted of repeating the tapping cycle 20 times in succession. After this set of responses, the subjects were given a 25 sec intertrial rest period before the next set. Each group of subjects performed 50 trials during task acquisition.[6] Skill retention was tested 10 min following the acquisition training and 6 to 9 days later. Half of each group was tested under an opposite condition from that in training. Auditory feedback was also withheld during the retention tests. The findings from the distributed practice trials were consistent with that generally reported in the literature. Better retention was found in the randomized trial condition. Under the discrete ver-

---

[5]On the average, the dowel rotation consumed about 1300 msec at the end of 120 practice trials.

[6]Note that the definition of a "trial" differed between the groups in this experiment.

sion of the task, however, both performance and retention were superior following massed practice. These findings suggest that the dictum that randomized practice always produces greater learning than massed practice may not be true for all training tasks. Rather, when the task consists of single short-term discrete actions, massed practice may produce both the most rapid learning and the greatest retention of skills gained.

An obvious extension of spaced versus massed practice concepts to speech production would be the prediction that concentrated massed practice will yield superior results in isolated articulatory skill training, such as moving the articulators into a particular posture to establish a particular gesture. Conversely, if a series of gestures are demanded in a continuously executed response set, as in the naturally repeating articulatory movements during connected speech, then spaced practice will likely yield better and longer lasting results than massed practice. The reader should be aware that these predictions are still untested for speech.

It should be pointed out that "rest" periods between spaced trials need not be periods of total inactivity. Rather, a rest interval could be filled by simply switching activities. For instance, an articulatory learning task could be switched back and forth from connected speech to isolated sound drill as production of a particular gesture is perfected. "Rest" in this context would simply mean "diversion" achieved by introducing a different task.

Whole Versus Part Practicing

Another question is whether to practice a skill broken down into its component parts or to practice it in its entirety. The answer to this question depends upon the nature of the task. In tasks with less complex but highly organized actions and with critically related parts but comparatively little information processing required, the *whole model* may be the better choice. An example of this "whole" method would be to use the following instructions to teach an articulatory gesture:

> Notice that the display on the right side of the screen shows that none of the sensors on my pseudopalate are now contacted. Now watch as I show you what happens when I make a [t] sound. Watch closely so you can make the [t] in the same way after I model it.

The "part" method may produce better results when the skill demanded in motor task performance is high in complexity and low in organization. For example, a series of words in a sentence may be best taught by using part method drills to solidify achievement of targeted postures in stipulated gestures. The actions may then be combined and taught as a whole. Carnahan and Lee (1989) demonstrated a distinct advantage in skill transfer when a task was practiced within three unique phases identified in an action response. They attributed the benefit to developing higher order timing skills within the response hierarchy.

UNCERTAINTY

In a motor skill paradigm, the probability of successful action depends at least partly on expectations and *experience* as a task is approached. Unpredictability creates uncertainty. As in information theory (Pierce, 1980; Shannon & Weaver, 1949), uncertainty is defined as a joint function of the number of possible outcomes and the probability that each outcome will occur. This relationship is expressed in the formula:

$$H = \Sigma(i) \, log_2 \, p \, (i)$$

where H represents a weighted average of the uncertainty, in bits, across n outcomes; $p\,(i)$ represents the probability of event i occurring; the sum is over n. As the equation indicates, the average uncertainty changes when either the number of competing alternatives or the occurrence probabilities change. Thus, unpredictability increases as competing expectations equalize (Wentworth & Witryol, 1990). That is, uncertainty is greater when a variety of concurrent expectations produce future unpredictability.

Successful experience plays an important role in uncertainty. It allows us to discount the probability of certain outcomes and increase the probability of success when other actions are followed. Nelson (personal communication, February 6, 1968) described a study in which he and his associates attempted to discover how olympic-caliber athletes differed from those who were simply good athletes. A series of tests revealed no significant physical skill or intellectual differences between the different subject classes. Attitudinal differences were found, however. The olympic-caliber athletes approached essentially all motor skill tasks with supreme confidence of success. In other words, based on valid evidence, or *knowledge,* from past experience (Shope, 1983) they were able to devise logical strategies of performance that enable them to approach new physical tasks with a high degree of assumed success. Success added to success. This highlights the important difference between learning in the sense of simply acquiring experience as a function of information gleaned from experience consequences used by the actor to extract fundamental action principles and apply them strategically. Past rewards and punishments experienced enter into the learning process as stored information to modify later choices among alternative actions. Different aftereffects can thus lead to different rehearsal strategies which directly influence how actions are executed (Estes, 1971). The empirical law of effect can thus be used to drive performance principles that influence both motivation and success during execution of an action plan.

Uncertainty may be further defined in terms of indecision stemming from inadequate knowledge about alternative actions (Goldman, 1986). Under this definition uncertainty is derived directly from, and accountable to, objective standards of evidence (Hawkins, 1977). It expresses the degree of belief held by an individual with respect to an assumed knowledge standard. In action theory it covers a continuum of dimensions that past evidence has suggested will condition success. Uncertainty is thus a product of memory, reasoning from experiences that foster beliefs, and judgments against a truth standard (Smith, Benson, & Curley, 1991). At its core, it is the consolidation of results that inhibit or otherwise influence the intent to act.

A fundamental component of uncertainty is the probability of success. It is driven by experiences that represent the proportion of successes and failures, each with related stimulus-response dimensions. Lacking adequate data, an actor is likely to qualify predictions of success. Past failure causes prudent actors to be tense and unsure as they "feel their way" rather cautiously toward a stipulated challenging goal.

The evaluation of successful experience is also directly related to the quality of feedback we receive, and judgments of success are based at least in part on the perceived reactions of other persons who serve as judges. As knowledge becomes increasingly tenuous, outside feedback is likely to be less questioned. Behaviors also become coupled with irrelevant actions and superstitious behaviors linking events that are more tenuously associated with the demanded responses. The performance of complex activities thus involves a combination of existing knowledge, action strategies, and trial data that may or may not be related to the degree of accomplishment achieved. Relevance may become more tenuous as task difficulty increases and mistakes occur. When direct cause and effect relationships are unclear, uncertainty and hesitancy tend to increase rather than decrease with experience.

Anticipated social consequences also provide reference standards that regulate behavior. People continually observe the behavior of others and the occasions on which actions are rewarded, ignored, or punished. When a stimulus is paired with aversive consequences, it becomes a source of cognitively induced arousal and/or withdrawal with negative performance effects whether experienced directed or simply observed (Bandura, 1971). Individuals with speech disorders, for instance, experience failure in speech production and often exhibit aversive and uncertainty symptoms in self-evaluations and reactions to listeners. These effects change both the determination to perform and the performance itself. The speech of the deaf is a classical example of uncertainty stemming from lack of knowledge which leads to abnormal speech articulation patterns and negative listener reactions. Inadequate data about key articulation dimensions limits the hearing-impaired talker's ability to learn by experience how to stabilize the articulatory system and execute needed articulatory maneuvers. Uncertainty is thus high. Their lack of information and resultant unsureness is evidenced by slow, choppy speech production with predictable sound distortions, omissions, and consonant cluster errors. Information upon which the responses should be predicated is critically incomplete. Accurate auditory feedback has simply not been available to help resolve discrepancies between possible and actual results from the energy devoted to changing the speech output. For instance, effort involved in striving to move the tongue into desired articulatory postures may generate excessive tension which overflows to the larynx. This may then trigger the high pitched, falsetto-like voice often habitualized in deaf talker responses. Inadequate feedback compromises the ability to set appropriate standards of performance and self-administer rewarding or punishing consequences based on firm evidence. When performance falls short of social comparison standards, it is easy for the actor to enter a cycle of trials and failures. Physiologically efficient solutions then become less and less likely. In fact, speech may become increasingly divergent from normal response patterns as efforts are exerted to search for alternative articulatory actions, institute needed changes, and eliminate errors.

In articulatory training, an obvious goal is to reduce uncertainty through exposure to the actual physiology of normal speech production. Experience-based success must also be sought through accurate sensory feedback and clinician verification as articulation patterns are modeled and mimicked. Improved responses may also be fostered through systematic motor-skill-theory based procedures. With the procedures geared to the person's own experiences, performance becomes a self-reinforcing event rather than an externally managed system. The goal of replacing hesitant, unrhythmical, inaccurate responses with smoothly connected, rapid, accurate actions based on an "I can do it" pool of success then becomes realistic.

It has been repeatedly shown that performance standards are a major determinant of productivity. When performance falls short of one's evaluative standards, the actor experiences negative reactions. When responses are punished, the power of modeled stimuli to increase the likelihood of achieving acceptable matching behavior is compromised by the suppressive effects of adverse consequences. Under these conditions, whether experienced directly or observed in the punished responses of others, the facilitative effects of modeling are at least partially nullified. On the other hand, confirmation of attainment beyond past performance standards would tend to activate positive self-reinforcement and accelerate improvement. Marlatt (1968) reported that positive vicarious reinforcement of success can also facilitate change. In fact, he noted that observed improvement may produce greater and more enduring changes in behavior than direct positive reinforcement of an individual's own responses. This may be explained by the fact that persons involved in responding may be slower to discern response contingent reinforcements than an observer whose vantage point allows him to evaluate the situation of another performer more objectively than his own responses in the midst of action (Kanfer, 1965). For these reasons the participation of more than one peer user is advantageous in articulatory motor skill training.

FATIGUE

Fatigue is one of the consequences of continuous physical effort or attention. It is defined as reversible impairment that takes the form of lowered sensitivity, responsiveness, or capacity to continue a particular task. Physical fatigue is attributed to a drop in oxygen available to support muscular contraction and an increase in accumulated waste products in the muscle. As contraction begins to fail in one muscle, others nearby become more active, suggesting the use of unconscious *recruitment* to reduce the muscle load and reduce fatigue. Recruitment gradually spreads to more remote muscles. Approaching fatigue is signalled by sensations of tiredness, then pain, as an individual's fatigue tolerance level is exceeded. Evidence of fatigue includes a slowing in performance and reduction in the mental or motor output across time.

In developing intricate physical skills such as speech production where attentional focus is a central concern, "mental fatigue" is a primary consideration. In their review on this topic Welford and Bourne (1976) described a number of changes in performance that have been attributed to mental fatigue: reductions in the attention span with loss of perceptual acuity and the ability to discriminate small changes in stimuli, slowing of sensory-motor reactions combined with increased variability, slower rate of execution, timing irregularities with an associated rise in the error rate, and impaired short term memory. They noted a surprising performance improvement that is often the first sign of oncoming fatigue. This was attributed to the subject's increased effort that may, for a time, more than offset fatigue losses. Performance deterioration follows if the action continues.

An alternative explanation of mental fatigue is that it arises as a blurring effect from neural noise when mental activity exceeds some optimum level (Crawford, 1961; Woodworth & Schlosberg, 1954). Especially intense neural activity rouses increased neural noise. This noise then masks desired signals and causes distractions. Welford and Bourne (1976) note that the data support each of these viewpoints to explain fatigue in certain circumstances.

C H A P T E R 7

DESIGNING A
TRAINING APPROACH

In our discussions of early motor development certain basic reflexes were identified that were retained, refined, and used to foster new action patterns. For example, a grooved lingual posture was noted to be part of the human infant cry. A refined form of this posture was found to be the key gesture in later sibilant sound production. We will now explore more deeply how such skills might be developed under controlled conditions.

Because of the intricacy and plasticity of human behaviors, scientists have turned to animals with simpler communication systems to identify and clarify variables that may influence vocal and gesture skill development. Although there is little or no evidence that any species other than humans possesses a flexible, syntax-based language system, a wide variety of animals communicate with one another using auditory, visual, tactile, or olfactory cues. Many species, such as chimpanzees, convey quite complex information to one another through manual gestures and vocal patterns without an integrated language system (e.g., see Menzel & Halperin, 1975; Van Lawick-Goodall, 1968). One of the most influential animal communication research lines has been developed through ethological studies of instincts. Pacesetting ways to examine the role instincts play in communication have been convincingly followed in animal studies by Lorenz (1935) and Tinbergen (1951) and in avian studies by Marler (e.g., see 1970, 1984, 1991) and his associates. This research has shown that even the most creative aspects of communication development are imbued with instinctive influences attributable to the organism's genetic constitution. These influences pervade all aspects of ontogeny (Johnson, 1988). Despite this common genetic element, each species also fosters the development of actions that are uniquely compatible with the individual organism's environment and personal nature.

Marler has repeatedly shown that instinctive responses that influence vocal behaviors are not immutable. Rather, the messages are susceptible to environmental forces and individual endowments influencing both the senders and receivers. Development of communication skills is clearly a joint function of instinct *and* environment. This conclusion led Marler (1991) and others following ethological lines of investigation to change the questions they asked from "Do instincts exist which directly influence vocal development?" to "What is the nature of vocal instincts and by what behavioral and physiological mechanisms do they operate?"

INNATE DEVELOPMENTAL MECHANISMS

Many skilled behaviors have their origin in innate, primitive responses that are shaped into more complex, voluntarily controlled functions by the environment and personal attributes of the animals involved. Skilled movements may, in fact, be defined as the combined outcome from genetically endowed, environmentally shaped, self-regulated actions. These fundamental forces permeate the developmental process: *Innate* mechanisms cause organisms to be responsive to identifiable *sign stimuli* which function as *releasers* to activate change. *Sensitive* periods exist during which organisms have unusual potential for change. In the following paragraphs, each of these forces will be examined in greater detail as possible sources of information that can contribute to our understanding of how to activate and control changes in communication functions.

Instinctive Behavior Hierarchies

Tinbergen's (1951) definition of instinct provides a starting point for launching a deeper discussion of contemporary concepts of instinctive behavior and its causation:

> Instinct is a hierarchically organized nervous mechanism which is susceptible to certain priming, releasing and directing impulses of internal

as well as of external origin, and which responds to these impulses by coordinated movements that contribute to the maintenance of the individual and the species. (p. 112)

The word *hierarchy* in the above definition identifies instincts as a system with subassociations or subassemblies bound by coordinating relations at higher and higher levels (Colgan, 1989, p. 16). The definition of an instinct as a hierarchy is useful. It implies the presence of basic acts which combine to form assemblies that in turn lead to more elaborate patterns. Functionally, hierarchies with independently administered subassemblies permit quick and efficient responses and decrease redundancy in nervous system controlled actions. This definition of instinct allows a clear distinction to be made between reflexes, defined as fairly rigid response patterns elicited by specific stimuli, and instincts which are more complex processes motivated by internal and external factors. At higher levels, the hierarchical arrangement results in a patterned output array such as that found in many aspects of speech production.

Genetic endowment plays a major role in the hierarchy of behavior. It has been shown to influence how animals map their environmental niches and solve environmental pressures. For most learning to occur there must be a specific mechanism that makes this possible (Gallistel, Brown, Carey, Gelman, & Keil, 1991). For example, rats have an innate preference for sweet foods and an aversion to those that are bitter (Rozin & Schull, 1988). Sweet foods tend to be high energy compounds that are readily absorbed and used in the nutritional system. Bitter foods tend to be toxic alkaloid poisons. Since food biases alone do not guarantee protection against poisons, rats follow distinctive, largely innately dictated feeding habits. They eat familiar foods and avoid novel foods; eat only small amounts of novel foods when such foods are first tried; and wait a long time between novel food meals for illness to develop if the food is poisonous.

Animals also use species-specific, or *conspecific,* communication behaviors innately to guide their functional habits. For example, Galef, McQuoid, and Whiskin (1990) described an experiment in which an "observer" rat was exposed to the smell of one of two novel foods on the breath of a "demonstrator" rat. Seven or eight days later the observer rat ate both novel diets and became ill. When next tested with the two novel foods, the rat rejected the food it did *not* smell on the breath of the demonstrator a week earlier. This was true regardless of the health of the demonstrator at the time of the original exposure to the food smell. The rat thus appeared to operate on the implicit assumption that other rats know what they are eating. The smell gave the one food a seal of safety no matter what the health was of the demonstrator rat. The universality of this modeling principle is seen in the inherent trust human learners give teacher and peer modeled behaviors, as described in Chapter 6. These observations highlight the importance of using normal talker models to develop natural postures and movement patterns as new speech production skills are sought.

Attentional Predispositions and Environmental Influences

Innate self-regulatory forces also play a central role in attentional predispositions that guide learners to focus on certain stimuli and exclude others in the environment. Selective responses to particularly salient stimuli lead learners to isolate specific stimulus classes from others in the environment. One of the outgrowths of this tendency is development of special vocal dialects within restricted geographic regions. This principle is nicely illustrated in avian song learning. For instance, each male white-crowned sparrow has a single song type which is about 2 seconds in duration. Embedded within the song features are special characteristics that identify the bird's local dialect (Figure 7–1). The dialect is so marked that a blindfolded listener with a cultivated ear can identify where a bird lives within a surprisingly constricted geographic region, such as that roughly bounded by the state of California (Baptista, 1975).

Striking differences between song dialects may also be the source of spurious communication disturbances. Chiff-chaff dialects differ so greatly that one bird from Germany does not recognize the song of a conspecific from Spain or Portugal (Burton, 1985). Similar dialectical extremes are found in the many human languages.

The combined impact of the environment and an individual organism's special sensory endowment also influences the development of specific vocal communication skills. Male birds reared without hearing males of their own kind develop simpler songs with no local accent. Environmental influences interact with these genetically dictated instincts. Closely related swamp and song sparrows hatched and reared in the laboratory and exposed to tape-recorded songs under essentially identical conditions still show preference for songs from their own species and develop very different songs. Song sparrows acquire about three times as many song types.

Special gender, tuning, and developmental effects also influence vocal skills. Both male and female bullfinches sing, but young males learn only the song of the conspecific male that helps raise them. *Selective tuning* thus fosters special communicative functions. Selective tun-

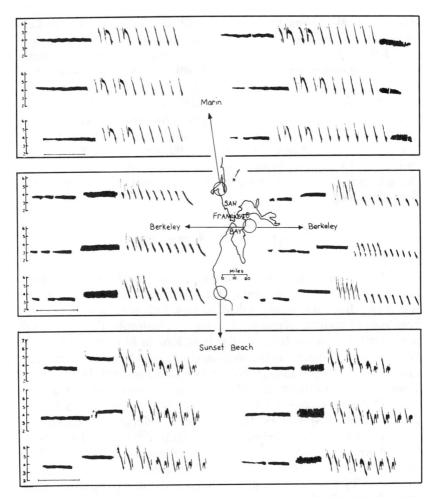

FIGURE 7-1. Song dialects of the white-crown sparrow in the San Francisco Bay area of California. The patterns represent six male birds from Marin County, six from Berkeley, and six from Sunset Beach. Local dialects are clearest in the second, trilled part of the song. (From Marler, 1970. Reprinted by permission.)

ing refers to the tendency for animals to be sensitive to certain types of stimuli and to block out or reject other stimuli. For instance, mature velvet monkeys respond selectively to certain vocal patterns. Different alarm calls signal specific sources of danger from other animals, such as pythons, leopards, and eagles (Seyforth, Cheney, & Marler, 1980). Snake calls lead other monkeys to look down. Leopard calls cause listeners to run up into or remain in trees. Eagle calls stimulate them to run under bushes and/or look up. Similar signals are found in infant monkey vocalizations, but they are not used so discriminantly. Leopard calls are used by the infants to signal danger from walking animals but not birds or snakes. Eagle calls are used to signal the presence of perceived danger from a variety of birds, not just eagles. Snake calls are used to signal danger from long thin things that move along the ground. Accuracy in signal calling develops as the monkey's perceptual skills and experience increase. Changes in the vocal patterns they acquire parallel their growing ability to identify and code critical predator features. Signal stratification built upon inborn response sets and the influence of the environment thus function in tandem as the animal matures in its ability to manipulate the basic elements of communicative utterances.

Shape and Movement

The observations concerning monkey innate vocal patterns suggest that shape and movement play special roles in activating central representations that guide communication signal choices. Speech relevant behaviors of human infants provide an apt illustration that these environmental derivatives have similar functions in human communication. Human neonates are intensely and tenaciously attracted by forms that move and shapes that have sharp contours and light-dark contrast. They innately discriminate and imitate lip protrusion, mouth widening, and visible tongue actions (Field, Woodson, Greenberg, & Cohen, 1982; Melzoff & Moore, 1977). Early speech-relevant movements appear to be built upon this foundation of natural perceptual awareness and inborn oral motor skills. The newborn infant stares intensively at the mother's face and is particularly attracted to those parts of the face — the eyes and the mouth — that are visible as the young child expands its ability to mimic the actions of the mobile facial and oral structures. These skills will serve important roles in the child's future speech. In the mimicry process, the infant appears to develop an internal representation of facial features that is systematically expanded and refined. For instance, the 4-month-old infant prefers faces with regular facial features over those with scrambled features (Fantz, 1965).

Maturation of spatial awareness and manipulation skills expands rapidly during the first years of life. Piaget's widely substantiated research (Fischer & Hogan, 1989; Piaget, 1936/1952) has demonstrated that before children are 2 years old their fundamental interest in spatial features leads them to construct internalized sensorimotor models that enable them to manipulate both external and internal spatial percepts. The models of external space then empower them to retrace routes they have followed and invent novel routes to positions in space that are blocked by obstacles. During this same time infants appear to form an oral sensory map that allows them to begin the process of accurately controlling tongue placement and movements within the oral cavity. This map then appears to be used to refine innate articulatory postures and movements and use them as basic building blocks in later dynamic rhythmical speech sequences.

The above discussion and examples point to the fundamental principle that for most kinds of learning to occur there is a specific mechanism that makes that kind possible. An organism's innate sensitivity to conspecific modeling and use of mimicry play central roles in the ensuing skill development and refinement. The environment within which the organism matures and the sensory capacity of the organism then interact to foster special skills required in dynamic communication activities. In the human, this includes speech production. Each of these factors may thus be used in planning efficient and effective instructional programs to meet the special needs of individuals who are speech impaired.

ENVIRONMENTAL RELEASERS

Animals react to only a small part of the changes in the environment that they are capable of sensing. Many of their reactions reflect biological needs for information that help them adapt to the natural environment (Seligman & Hager, 1972). The proclivity of animals to be more sensitive to certain stimulus complexes must be carefully considered in planning training routines since those stimuli may be expected to influence the learning process rather directly.

Some associations are formed easily, others with some difficulty, and others not at all (Gallistel et al., 1991). Stimuli which arouse instinctive, ontogenetically moderated responses without requiring any specific experience are defined to be *sign stimuli* (Lorenz, 1935/1970). When such stimuli are used to elicit genetically determined, stereotyped actions in normal members of a species, they are identified as *releasers*. Releasers enable organisms to achieve biologically important goals such as eating, mating, surviving dangers, and perhaps talking through behavior patterns coded in their genes. The responses are said to be *primed* when the arousal effects outlast the presence of the stimulus. For example, the sight of food primes a pecking response in pigeons. In a learning experiment pigeons can be taught readily to peck a key to obtain food, but they have difficulty learning to peck to avoid shock. The natural response of a bird to the threat of shock or similar aversive stimuli directed toward its foot is to fly, not peck. Danger signals release running in rat responses. In learning experiments, rats learn rapidly to run to avoid shock but slowly, if at all, to rear up on their back feet. Running is a natural component of a rat's fleeing from danger. Rearing is not (Bolles, 1970). Hamsters learn quickly to dig or rear for food, but slowly or not at all to wash their face and scent mark to obtain food. The latter two behaviors are not natural in exploratory activities. It is not surprising that nonhunger-related behaviors are unlikely to be established easily in a feeding context. Training must thus be tailored to the natural functions an organism may be expected to meet as it copes with life. Humans are prone to vocalize.

Vocal Motor-Control Functions

As human vocalizations mature into speech, they take on a new role. Words are used to help control actions. For example, Luria (1961) demonstrated that when a ball is placed in the hands of a 3- to 3½-year-old child with the instructions "When you see the light, squeeze the ball," the child's response is erratic. When the ball is in the child's hands, the child may or may not be able to resist the contact stimulus and wait until the signal is given before acting. Luria observed, however, that when the child was told to say "Go" *and* press the ball when the light was lit, the child was able to control the motor response. In his words, the speech "fully eliminates the diffuseness of the motor processes, strictly coordinates the movements with signals and imparts to them a distinct and organized character" (p. 46).

The use of speech to help organize and facilitate movements is further refined during maturation. For example, Fletcher (1962) studied the role played by the word "Go" in facilitating hand movements by 8-year-olds. In the experiment, two groups of children were first carefully matched for reaction times in removing their hands from a response key. They were then given a choice reaction test. Both groups were told to do nothing when a left light on a stimulus box was lit. One group was then told simply to lift their hands from the key "as quickly as possible" when they saw the right light come on. The other group was told to both lift their hands and say "Go" when the right light came on. In each of the latter instances the children had to make a decision then react as rapidly as possible. Those who were to say "Go" had an additional task. They were to perceive which light was lit, lift their hand from the key, *and* say "Go." This extra act would be expected to slow them down if speech were simply an independent physical requirement. Fletcher found, however, that although the groups were previously equally matched, the slowest child in the "Go" group was now faster than the fastest of those who simply lifted their hand. This finding supports

Luria's contention that speech mediation may significantly facilitate related motor actions. Transferring new articulatory motor skills to speech contexts as quickly as possible in training routines appears to be a practical extension of this principle.

Conspecific Stimuli

Birds and animals have a special proclivity to attend to and learn conspecific vocal stimuli. Marler (1991) reported that when conspecific songs are heard, birds become suddenly attentive, as though a brief time window is being opened. The stimulus "becomes more salient, more likely to be memorized, and probably destined to be used later for guiding song development" (p. 48). Birds are not completely bound by their innate preferences, however. If conspecific songs are withheld, they can learn nonpreferred songs when the songs are introduced using strong stimulation, as with a live tutor of another species (Baptista & Petrinovich, 1984). It is important to note that although there is ample evidence that birds can discriminate songs of other species, even at the level of individual differences (Dooling, 1989), they do not learn them in the normal environment. Or if they do, they forget them again unless the exposure is massive, continuing day after day, and associated with strong arousal. Care must thus be exercised to distinguish natural from forced learning contexts to maximize the learning rate and ensure retention of vocal skills gained.

By using computer-synthesized stimuli with independently varied acoustic features, Marler and Peters (1988) were able to isolate which aspects of the vocal signal were naturally influential and noninfluential in bird song development. Figure 7–2 shows examples of natural songs and songs of birds isolated from their own species during vocal development. Innate "release" mechanisms are evident as each species is shown to favor its own species-specific songs. Swamp sparrows copied syllables more readily than whole songs. Song sparrows included the number of segments, the internal trilled or unrepeated phrase structure, and attributes such as tempo along with the syllabic structure in the songs they learned (Marler, 1991).

Sensory Priming

Sensory priming may also be expected to play a central role in speech articulatory learning. From our earlier discussion, we would anticipate that the innate focal interest of human infants would lead them to form

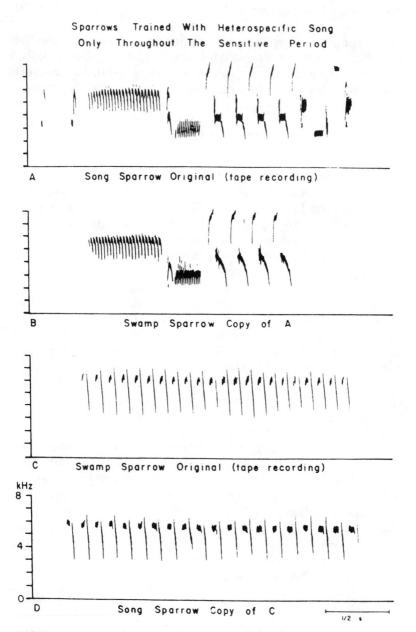

Sparrows Trained With Heterospecific Song
Only Throughout The Sensitive Period

A   Song Sparrow Original (tape recording)

B   Swamp Sparrow Copy of A

C   Swamp Sparrow Original (tape recording)

kHz

8

4

0

D   Song Sparrow Copy of C   1/2 s

FIGURE 7–2. Sound spectrographic song patterns from swamp and song sparrows reared in the laboratory and exposed only to tape recorded songs of the other species. The examples show a swamp sparrow copy (B) from a song sparrow model (A) and a song sparrow copy (D) of a swamp sparrow model (C). Song sparrows copy swamp sparrow patterns more often than vice versa, but when they do, they usually recast the syllables into song sparrow-like syntax. (From Marler, 1991. Reprinted by permission.)

concepts that define locations as well as functions of the articulatory organs. This interest should then prime the system for specific vocal skill and vocabulary development. Since auditory, visual, and motor sensations are linked together centrally, mimicry of intraoral articulatory patterns would normally be primed by both auditory and visual stimuli. Support for this supposition is shown by the axiom that sounds with viewable articulatory movements are likely to arrive in spoken words before those with unseen movements. This principle may be illustrated by the order of stop sound acquisition. In general, labial stops (e.g., /m/ in "mama") are mastered in the child's developing vocabulary first. They are followed by the partially seen anterior lingua-alveolar stops (e.g., /k/ → /t/ in "tat" for "cat") and finally by the nonviewable /k, g/ posterior linguavelar stops as the sensory field for articulatory learning shifts more and more to the audible aspects of the speech signal.

With the close integration that exists between visible and audible priming during articulatory learning, it might be anticipated that a reduction in either sensory avenue would be directly compensated by a shift to the other one. This assumption is supported by speech of the blind. It is also supported by the recent studies of the present author and his associates (e.g., Fletcher, 1983; Fletcher, 1989c; Fletcher, Dagenais, & Critz-Crosby, 1991a, b; Fletcher & Hasegawa, 1983; Fletcher, Hasegawa, McCutcheon, & Gilliom, 1980) who showed that visual patterns could be used in articulatory modeling routines to establish basic articulatory skills rapidly and accurately by talkers who are deaf (Fletcher, 1983, 1989c; Fletcher, Hasegawa, McCutcheon, & Gilliom, 1980). Additional data are needed to uncover the special roles played by command centers, feedback loops, and specific phonetic components in priming and executing speech patterns in these and other handicapped population groups.

SENSITIVE PERIODS

The widespread occurrence of age-specific learning has provoked consideration of possible biological factors that may foster learning during different periods of life. Many studies have claimed superior performance in speech learning by child subjects compared with adults. One of the most persistent beliefs concerning human vocal development is that a limited period exists during a person's lifetime when vocal skills may be acquired. This has lead to the *critical period* hypothesis which claims that definable limits are placed on speech learning capacities and capabilities, particularly those that contribute to phonetic skills.

These differences in the speech learning capability have, for example, been cited as the source of dialects that accompany learning a second language. Walsh and Diller (1981) noted that, although a second language may be acquired at any age, the rate of learning is not uniform. They claimed that complete success in mastering pronunciation beyond the childhood years is "impossible," because articulation is a "lower order" linguistic function and such functions are genetically specified and consolidated in early development.

The popular belief that language learning aptitude is confined essentially to the youthful years of life, as expressed in the *critical period* hypothesis, makes two important predictions concerning speech articulatory skill development. The first prediction stems from the observation that articulation is a complex motor pattern that integrates respiratory, vocal fold, and oral posture and movement components. The motor neurons involved in activating and controlling this composite system are widely dispersed anatomically (Jürgens & Ploog, 1988). At birth, vocalization is physiologically controllable only during the genetically dictated separation cry which is the most primitive and basic mammalian vocalization. Time is required for this system to develop the capacity for the precisely integrated, coordinated, and rapidly executed series of postures and movements required in speech production. This physical capacity places a time limit on the acquisition of articulate speech.

The second prediction of the critical period hypothesis is that a speech learning window will be open only during a sensitive period which fosters fairly durable articulatory skills. Thereafter, the system will become increasingly resistant to change. New articulation learning should thus slow dramatically as neural plasticity which presumably nurtures the sensitive period drops. These changes in laryngeal control and neural plasticity thus presumably place constraints on what age and for how long articulatory development will occur. At the end of the sensitive period particular brain centers are thought to become effectively inert.

The critical period hypothesis has received some support from lower animal studies. Distinctive learning phases have been identified within the developmental period. In these situations, however, the concentration of learning in the early stages of development is usually closely related to the age at which the offspring leaves its parents or their breeding ground. Separate stages of change have also been identified within the general developmental pattern that apparently have separate control mechanisms. Bird song, for instance, often shows a sensitive period, a gap, the beginning of subsong, then song crystallization with little or no further vocal change thereafter. The process of change ends near the end of the bird's first year of life. Birds, such as canaries and mockingbirds with larger song repertoires, however, continue adding to their song skills throughout life.

Sensory input and feedback each play key roles in fostering the process of birdsong development within each song learning phase. Figure 7–3 shows examples of song learning by birds with normal hearing in their natural habitat, those with normal hearing but isolated from other birds, isolated birds exposed to tape recordings of normal songs from their species, and birds that were isolated and deafened. These patterns illustrate that some basic normal song features develop irrespective of song stimulation. Deafness disrupts singing the known repertoire and blocks new song learning. Sparrows deafened prior to any singing develop highly abnormal, extremely variable songs that are almost amorphous in structure (Konishi, 1965). How less dramatic disturbances in sensory endowment might influence song progress during the song learning period remains to be explored.

Oyama (1979) and Flege (1987) each reviewed the concept that a critical period exists in human vocal development which places a limit on the ability to learn sounds in a new language and specifically imposes a temporal boundary on articulation skill development. They found little experimentally tested support for this belief. Much of the apparent child superiority cited in earlier studies of second language (L2) phonetic development could be explained by the simple observation that children are more deeply immersed in the language learning process than adults (Cochran, 1977). Child talkers tend to speak with a greater number of people outside the home than adults and are obliged to use the new language they are learning in a greater variety of social contexts. Moreover, adults are apt to discuss abstract concepts without tangible references; whereas language used with and by children tends to be simplified. They are exposed to shorter sentences, names assigned to things, and more carefully articulated words. These adaptations would presumably help them in the processes of learning to map their perceptual world onto an abstract speech sound system.

In certain circumstances adult phonetic learning has been shown to be superior to that of children. Winitz (1981), for example, reported that English-speaking adults discriminate Chinese tones and obstruent consonants better than English-speaking 8-year-olds, and Snow and Hoefnagel-Höhle (1978) found that after a small amount of L2 experience, English-speaking adults produce Dutch sounds more authentically than 8- to 10-year-old children. Despite these counter arguments regarding speech learning competency, in many kinds of learning a *sensitive period* has been identified. These periods consist of a biological time interval when an organism is particularly susceptible to learning specific new behaviors. Young children, for example, who differ widely in mental and motor skills acquire about seven new words a

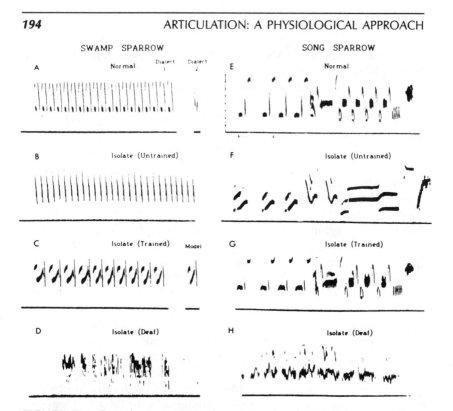

FIGURE 7–3. Sound spectrograms from typical songs of swamp and song sparrows reared under four conditions: learning in the wild (A and E), reared in acoustic isolation but with normal hearing (B and F), reared in isolation but trained with tape recorded normal conspecific songs (C and G), and isolated and deafened (D and H). The acoustic frequency markers indicate 1 kHz intervals, and the time marker = 0.5 sec. (From Marler, 1991. Reprinted by permission.)

day, day after day, week after week during the period from about 18 months to 6 years of age (Marshall et al., 1984). The evidence that adults cannot match this performance is firm. Perhaps, as suggested by Oyama (1979), the apparent superiority of early versus late speech learning may be indicative of little more than a broadly defined "sensitive" period during which responsiveness is heightened then gradually fades. Flege (1987) hypothesized that heightened speech sound sensitivity by children may be largely a product of their still-evolving sound category central representations. He suggested that less firmly established, or less thoroughly elaborated, first language (L1) categories may make children less likely than adults to identify the phones of a new language as belonging to already familiar categories in the old one. In other words, phonetic differences may be more salient to L1 learners. This would make them less likely to simply merge new phonetic classes into their speech output as acceptable variants of their current articulation patterns.

The issue of time-based articulatory sensitivity in the learning process remains unresolved. The arguments presented, and the fact that evidence supporting an age limitation on speech articulatory learning is weak, would seemingly allow us to at least conclude that there is little justification for limiting training opportunities to any age group. This conclusion would appear to be particularly appropriate for articulatory training routines such as palatometry where the principal exposure is shifted from auditory to visual sensory avenues.

VOCAL DEVELOPMENTAL STAGES

We now turn to considering what roles are played by the different stages of vocal development and how they contribute in the process of vocal skill maturation and change. The three stages of bird song development appear to have at least roughly analogous time periods within human infant vocal development. The first of these is subsong. As in human infant prebabbling vocalizations, bird subsong is thought to be important for development of vocal motor skills and for strengthening the linkage between sounds heard and imitated (Nottebohm, 1972). The subsong of a bird usually has a rather amorphous structure with a noisy spectral organization. The combination of innate and environmental influence is evident even in this initial stage of development, however. Differences in sound duration are present in infant vocalizations and in the subsongs of both hearing song and swamp sparrows. They are lacking in those of deaf birds (Marler & Sherman, 1985) and deaf human infants (Mavilya, 1969; Oller, Eilers, Bull, & Carney, 1985).

Mature structure begins to appear in the second stage of vocal development. In humans, this period spans the very important time during which a succession of vowels and consonants appear in what is called marginal babbling. Marginal babbling is identified at around 6 months. True consonant babbling with reduplicated and nonreduplicated syllables arrives at about 9 months of age. Bird vocalizations during the somewhat comparable stage are called *plastic song*. The first rehearsal of previously memorized song patterns appears at this developmental stage. But what is first heard has little in common with adult speech or bird song patterns. Innate processes bias the response selection during the plastic period but do not usurp the need for learning. As with human infant babbling, the plastic song period of birds is characterized by practice and experimenting with many more vocalization types than will be found later when the mature, *crystallized* song appears. During this time period both birds and humans apparently discover the kinds of actions that nurture the structure of vocalizations, then practice applying and elaborating those sequences as they move toward crystallized mature songs or toward human speech. In other words, a central schema, or template, seems to be formed which is used to monitor response patterns and guide vocal practice. As indicated by the wider set of responses during plastic song and human babbling than in mature vocalizations, more is memorized than is manifest in the final crystallized product. One cannot, however, conclude that during this period the young members of any species are locked into the utterances of their parentage. Not only do birds, for example, recognize exemplars of songs sung by other species, they learn songs outside the range of their species if such "novel" songs are the only ones heard during their sensitive period. But they tend to learn these patterns in species-specific ways.

MODELING AND GOAL SEEKING IN NATURAL VOCAL LEARNING

In the previous discussion the importance of modeling is clear. Only rarely is normal song developed in complete absence of a model (Gallistel et al., 1991). Sometimes the model is imitated faithfully. In other cases syllables are copied faithfully then recombined into novel patterns, or phrases are gradually modified as the song is elaborated. The mockingbird combines both processes. Syllables are copied from other species then incorporated into a specific pattern, sometimes modified and sometimes not. There is no single process that predicts bird song learning in different species. The differences highlight the variety of roles played by genetic and environmental factors in selective attention and learning. Factors such as the strength of stimulation, recorded or live tutor modeling, and access to conspecific models are all important. Innate processes seem to set the species-specific context within which experience operates (Marler, 1991). Experience builds upon that platform.

One of the basic principles that emerges in the consideration of vocal learning is that organisms will distribute their activities according to success attained in achieving targeted goals. Vocal responses, particularly speech, were noted to be a powerful tool in human goal achievement. During the first few months of life both vision and audition play significant roles in fostering vocal production skills. In human vocal development the pool of sounds used by infants expands during sound play then contracts to fit the phoneme repertoire of the environmental language. Hearing occupies an increasingly dominant role in this process as the articulatory postures and movements of sounds learned are executed farther back within the oral cavity and are thus not visually perceptible. This limitation can now be largely removed through computer-controlled instrumentation, such as the palatometer which exposes the user to precisely where and how articulation occurs within the oral cavity. A new opportunity for assessing and changing speech functions and dysfunctions is thus provided. Specifically, through such information it is now possible to recapture and extend the use and power of vision for articulation-relevant detection of spatial and movement patterns within the oral cavity during ongoing speech production. Exploring the full ramifications of that capability awaits more basic and applied research.

THE PHYSIOLOGICAL APPROACH

The premise followed in the physiological approach to articulation is straightforward: Parallel definition of articulatory actions and their acoustic derivatives opens a rather direct avenue to isolating, describing, and defining normal articulation and to changing abnormal articulation. It makes the goal of reducing uncertainty by exposing learners to natural processes of normal speech production through all available sensory avenues and applying experimentally proven, physiologically based training procedures to modify articulation abnormalities realistic. Reaching these goals includes using insight from developmental maturation, sensorimotor capacity, understanding sounds inherent in speech production, and applying emerging understanding of the roles played by genetic endowment and innate mechanisms. Inborn articulatory postures and movements and responses to sign stimuli thus become key considerations in efforts to develop self-regulated, environmentally shaped oral spatial awareness and articulatory manipulation skills in natural and normal speech production. That is a tall order! An obvious step toward filling that order is the design and development of instrumentation and procedures that enable clinicians to use the basic physiologic and acoustic principles outlined for efficient and effective articulation assessment and training. Some additional detail will now be provided to help the reader understand the working parts and functions of the Fletcher and associates' palatometric instrumental system.

The Palatometer

One of the most promising tools recently added to the clinician's armamentarium is the palatometer. The palatometer was originally designed by Fletcher and his associates to register the place and pattern of lin-guapalatal contact against the palate, alveolar ridge, and inner margins of the teeth and to generate spatially accurate measures of the postures and actions identified. Use of the palatometer rests on the common-folk premise that a picture is worth a thousand words. It portrays articu-latory events in a spatial fashion easily assimilated by the relatively untrained human eye. By constructing a geometric representation of tongue actions in three-dimensional Euclidean space, the instrumenta-tion provides an opportunity to approach speech disability from a mo-tor skill framework. Thus, no longer need the speech clinician or the handicapped person be limited to auditory and phonetic *impressions* to discover and change articulatory deficiencies. The clinician can now help clients gain physiologically based percepts and concepts of speech production as speech skills are modified.

The palatometer was developed to help define normal and abnor-mal articulation functions more accurately and to discover natural ways to overcome speech abnormalities at the physiological level. It should be pointed out, however, that the palatometer is simply a tool. Nothing more, nothing less. The usual way of thinking about tools is that they are invented to solve problems, but tools also shape the way we come to see the problems we meet. The value of a tool thus depends on both the special characteristics of the tool and the understanding and skills a user can bring to bear in its operation.

Pseudopalates

Several technical questions must be considered with respect to using palatometry for speech diagnosis and training purposes. First, pala-tometry requires the use of pseudopalates in the mouth to accommo-date the presence of tongue contact sensors. Since any intrusion into the oral cavity is a potential source of articulatory irregularities, the pseudopalate must be very thin and carefully constructed to fit snugly against the user's palate and maxillary teeth. Fortunately, the articula-tory system, at least in normal talkers, is remarkably resilient. Our pre-vious research has indicated that little or no disturbance is found in lingual postures and movements when a pseudopalate is less than 0.5 mm thick and fits the contours of the teeth and palatal surface closely.[1]

---

[1]The primary source of pseudopalate retention in the mouth is from salivary bonding developed between it and the dental/oral surfaces. Occasionally denture paste or powder may be needed to increase the saliva bonding power. Pseudopalate retention can be tested by having the subject count or produce a series of words after the bonding agent has been added. Additional material can be added if necessary to increase retention.

If the pseudopalate is still not retained, it may be necessary to use soft lining material to hold it in place. A number of soft lining materials are available. Ramitec[R] material

An accurate, custom fit pseudopalate may be obtained by taking an impression of the teeth and palate, casting a stone model from that impression, then heat-molding an acrylic base plate onto the model. The pseudopalate sensors are then mounted on that baseplate.

The distance between the sensors is another important consideration in using the palatometer as an articulatory measuring device. When an alternating current is used to sense linguapalatal contact, Fletcher and his associates found that the sensors could be located on a pseudopalate as close as 1 mm apart without serious salivary bridging between them. A rather large number of sensors can thus be mounted on a pseudopalate to define linguapalatal contact sites and patterns.

Other important measurement considerations in palatometry include establishing the precise locations of the sensors across the pseudopalate surface. Our experience suggests that 96 sensors distributed at 3- to 5-mm intervals is adequate for most articulation measurement purposes (Fletcher 1982; Fletcher, 1985; Fletcher, 1989a; Fletcher, Mc-Cutcheon, & Wolf, 1975). Precise measures of the place and pattern of linguapalatal contact are also fostered by locating the sensors a standard distance apart within an X-Y grid format. Dimensions within the oral cavity can then be gauged by establishing distances from the centerpoints of each sensor to surrounding landmarks, such as the lower edge of the central incisor teeth. The ease of using such measurements may be increased by using an *origin electrode* reference system (McCutcheon, Hasegawa, Smith, & Fletcher, 1981). For instance in the palatometric system developed by Fletcher and his associates, an origin electrode was located at the intersection of an *intercuspid line* that crossed the palate at the rear edge of the cuspid teeth and a *midsagittal line* that bisected the pseudopalate from front to back (see Figure 7–4). In edentulous subjects the location of this origin point was approximated by using the midpoint of the maxillary foramen which is usually very close to the intercuspid-midsagittal (IM) intersection. Other dimensions within the oral cavity could then be ascertained by establishing distances between the origin sensor and points on the teeth or other landmarks such as the

---

from Premier (Norristown, PA 19401) works well for this purpose. To use it, simply squeeze equal lengths of base paste and catalyst onto a supplied mixing pad, mix them together for 20 to 30 seconds using a small spatula or tongue depressor, and coat the nasal surface of the pseudopalate. It is important to coat the pseudopalate with sufficient material to fill all voids between it and adjoining palatal and dental surfaces. The surfaces of the teeth that will be in contact with the material may be coated with hand cream or a petrolatum such as Vaseline to avoid having the material stick to them. Then simply place the pseudopalate in the subject's mouth, press it upward against the palate and teeth, and hold it in place until the material sets. The total working time after beginning to mix the material is only 2 minutes so the clinician must work rather quickly. After at least 5 minutes have elapsed from the beginning of the mix, the pseudopalate can be carefully pried loose, slipped down from the palate and teeth, and removed from the mouth. Excess material can them be trimmed with scissors or a sharp knife.

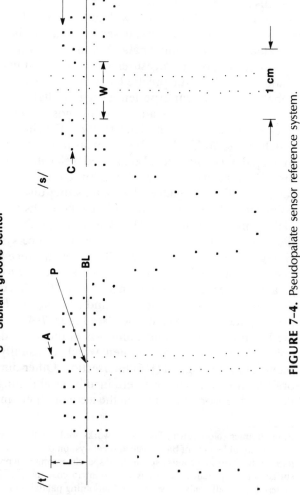

Legend:
• sensor location
■ contacted sensor
BL bicuspid line
A anterior contact
P posterior contact
L contact length
W Sibilant groove width
C Sibilant groove center

FIGURE 7–4. Pseudopalate sensor reference system.

alveolar border and rugae on the palate. Tongue contact height was established by measuring vertical distances between the origin electrode and landmarks such as the peak of the palatal vault or level of the occlusal plane of the maxillary teeth. The ability to define spatial relationships in precise quantitative terms enables the scientist and clinician to establish linguapalatal contact place, pattern, and area or extent meaningfully and use that information practically. These key capabilities set the palatometric system apart from "electropalatographic" devices.

As illustrated in the two pseudopalates of Figure 7–5, sensors may be located across a pseudopalate surface in different patterns. The

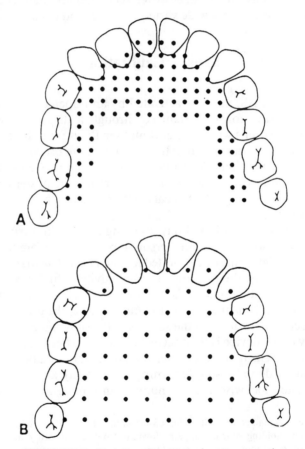

FIGURE 7–5. Variations in sensor locations on the pseudopalate. The sensor distribution on the left was designed to compare sibilant groove width during sibilant sound production. The one on the right provides opportunity to measure more global aspects of linguapalatal contact.

usual way is to place the sensors at equal intervals across the pseudo-palate in front-to-back columns and side-to-side rows. The sensors may, however, be concentrated within a particular region of the pseudopalate to increase measurement precision in that location or area of the articulatory surface.

The sensor distribution used with a particular talker depends on the type of information desired. Figure 7–5A illustrates a pattern in which the sensors are concentrated on the front third of the palate. This pattern is useful for assessing and modifying sibilant sound production and front consonant articulation. The "blanket pattern," shown in Figure 7–5B, is usually preferred, however. It enables articulatory comparisons to be made across a wide variety of vowel and consonant sounds.

Sensor Calibration

Palatometric measurement is activated by an imperceptible body signal (voltage wave form) introduced through a disposable electrode attached to the user's wrist. The current then flows from the wrist to the tongue where it is transferred to the sensors on the pseudopalate when the tongue touches them. This information is then relayed to the palatometric circuitry via fine wires that pass around the posterior borders of the gingavae, through the buccal cavities, and out the mouth at each corner of the lips.

The conductivity of the body, the tongue, and the surfaces of the mouth all vary somewhat from person to person; therefore the sensors on a pseudopalate must be calibrated for each user. The first step in this process is to adjust the palatometer's sensitivity to fit the conductivity present in the individual user's mouth. This is is done in two stages. First, the subject is instructed to raise the tongue to the pseudopalate so that it touches all or most of the sensors at the same time.[2] The general sensitivity of the device is then set as the tongue is held in this position. Normally the sensitivity level is set at a point that is at about 50% of its range. This is done by simply turning a sensitivity knob on the palatometer panel clockwise until the number on a numerical display and a

---

[2]Raising the tongue to contact all of the sensors at the same time can be explained to a young child by holding your hand, palm down, in front of you with your mouth open rather widely so the tongue can be seen to be well below the pseudopalate. The lower hand is then raised toward the pseudopalate at the same time as the lower hand is raised toward the upper one. The subject can then see that the lower hand touches all along the upper one as they come together. The tongue does the same against the pseudopalate. Repeat the action several times to be sure that the child mimicks the tongue raising and complete palate contact procedure. Demonstrate to the subject that the tongue is to be kept in touch with the pseudopalate until the palatometer sensitivity level is set.

line on a bar graph reaches "50."[3] If later usage indicates that some channels are activated without being touched, or if sensors that are touched do not show the contact in the pattern displayed, the general percentage threshold value can be raised to a higher or lower number by returning to the calibration procedure. Otherwise, the 50% default level set initially with the sensitivity knob may simply be accepted.

Individual sensor threshold levels must be set by using a routine that compares signal levels when the tongue is touching and not touching sensors (McCutcheon, Smith, Kimble, & Fletcher, 1983). Briefly, in this procedure the subject is asked to raise the tongue to the pseudopalate then move it around, striving to touch each of the sensors. The following instructions have been found to help:

> The instructions on the screen tell you to touch all of the sensors on the pseudopalate. To do this, raise the tip of your tongue and touch sensors all around the sides, down the middle, and way to the back of the pseudopalate. When you think you have touched all of them, swallow to clear the saliva from your pseudopalate then open your mouth widely and hold your tongue down so it is not touching the pseudopalate anywhere. *Check to be sure your tongue is not touching anywhere.*

Swallowing helps the subject bring the tongue into contact with sensors that may not have been touched as the tongue is moved around on the pseudopalate and clears the saliva from its surface. Holding the tongue down is essential to produce a clear field for registering no-contact voltage levels. The operator must be certain that the tongue is *not* touching any sensor at this time. To verify this the operator is queried about whether the number of sensors that fail to meet the sensitivity criterion is acceptable. If not, the data are discarded and the no-contact procedure is repeated. This procedure continues until four contact–no-contact data sets have been derived. Four sets of these data have been found to provide stable voltage reference levels.[4] Contact versus no-contact voltage differences are then calculated from the data and used to establish threshold levels for each of the pseudopalate sensors (usually 96).

The final step in the calibration routine is to certify the responsiveness of the individual sensors. This is done by having the subject hold the tongue so it is not touching any sensor on the pseudopalate then

---

[3]The threshold sensitivity of the system may be changed if needed to optimize the signal transfer conditions for a particular subject's mouth. This is typically done later in the calibration routine when the operator is given the option of entering any percentage threshold value between 0 and 100%.

[4]Computer software is used to maintain a record of the number of responses that have been accepted. It allows any new set of measurements to be discarded and the no-contact evaluation recycled until the operator indicates completion of the routine.

activating the palatometer to scan individual sensor responses as the tongue is moved systematically around on the pseudopalate touching all of the sensors again. This time, the count on the video screen drops as sensors are touched. The goal is to reduce the count to "0" or close to it. A "0" indicates that none of the sensors have failed to meet the contact–no-contact calibration criteria. When the count reaches "0," or stops decreasing despite the subject's continuing efforts to touch additional sensors on the pseudopalate, the action is stopped and the results evaluated. The program lists all sensors that fail to meet the calibration standards. The list of these sensors should be written in the user's log for future reference. The operator then determines whether the number and location of sensors that fail to meet the calibration standards are acceptable for monitoring the sounds to be assessed or taught. If not, possible problems such as procedural errors or electrode cleanliness may be checked and rectified and the calibration process repeated. If the calibration data are acceptable, the information can be stored on disk for later recall from memory. Disk storage of the calibration data allows a clinician or scientist to proceed rapidly into palatometric assessment and training sessions without recalibrating the system each time it is used with that individual. The system will then be ready to calibrate a second user's pseudopalate or begin evaluation and/or training routines.

Obtaining Parallel Acoustic and Physiologic Measures

The ability to manipulate articulatory actions through palatometric procedures adds a new dimension to the clinician's armamentarium. Specifically, it enables a deep pool of spatial information regarding imaging and other facets of motor skill learning that has been accumulating during the past decade to be tapped in speech training routines. Being able to manipulate spatial attributes of articulatory actions rather directly also provides an opportunity to use converging acoustic and physiologic principles that can shed new light on how speech skill is acquired and how it may be modified when it is deviant.

The ability to provide parallel acoustic and physiologic displays is a particularly important consideration in training. Acoustic information can provide a rather direct link between phonetic and physiological data as well as a time-line reference for interpreting dynamic phonetic events unfolding during speech production. Parallel physiologic data from measures such as speech articulation place, precision, and movement rates can then be used to isolate speech distortion sources and document deviations underlying abnormal phonetic patterns. Systematic developmental measures can be used to help differentiate changes from innate mechanisms that cause learners to be responsive to identifiable *sign stimuli,* which function as *releasers* to activate change through either clinician-initiated or self-regulated actions and to identify sensitive periods during which specific speech characteristics may have unusual potential for change.

Static Articulation Target (.TGT) Patterns

Talkers are presumed to manipulate, integrate, and smooth actions across standard postures that distinguish each sound from all others that are not members of the same phonetic class in a speaker's language. The goal of physiologic articulatory training is to link oral sensations of a talker who is speech impaired directly with spatial and temporal properties of normal speech. Speech is thus viewed as the actualization of temporally controlled sequences of targeted normal articulatory gestures. The orosensory goals selected to guide training should therefore be specifiable in terms of positions, configurations, and actions that underlie the production of normal sounds. For target patterns to contribute most in assessing and modifying articulation, a "relevant and optimum" (Peterson & Shoup, 1966) set of parameters must be used to capture important contrasts in articulatory features such as place, magnitude, movement patterns, and linguapalatal contact timing. The set of parameters needed to specify all critical dimensions of speech articulation is still evolving as deeper physiologic understanding develops. The reader is referred to articles such as those by Fletcher (1989a, 1990, and under review); Fletcher and Newman (1991); and Fletcher, Dagenais, and Critz-Crosby (1991b) for information and procedures that promise to be helpful.

Each articulation target must have a phonetic purpose. It is important to note, however, that in the current physiological framework, articulatory target patterns would not be expected to correspond one-to-one with phonemes and features derived from acoustic observations. For example, contact along the outer margins of the palate anchors or stabilizes the bulk of the tongue and enhances accurate, rapid execution of articulation sequences to distinguish sounds from each other. The normal palatometric model target for /t/, for instance, is thus drawn from the briefly sustained linguapalatal contact position just *before* production of the stop sound. At that time the tongue is in contact with the palate around the entire outer border of the alveolar ridge. Air pressure built up behind this linguapalatal obstruction is then abruptly released. The [−continuant], [+anterior], [+consonantal] features of the [t] thus represent a complex acoustic summation from all physical events along the vocal tract of the talker plus the auditory sensations and experiences of listeners. Humans appear to be congenitally designed to be responsive to specific auditory signals. Despite the complexities of the speech listening task, humans demonstrate a remarkable consistency in their auditory impressions of spoken sounds. Among other things these signals appear to function, at least in the young child, as phonetic sign stimuli or *releasers* which can activate articulatory change. If our earlier assumption is correct that visual stimuli serve a role that is similar to audition in early speech development, then visual exposure to normal articulatory actions could serve a similar role in phonetic learning.

With the palatometer calibrated, the speech clinician is ready to prepare target patterns for visual articulatory modeling and feedback routines designed to promote rapid, efficient acquisition of standard vowel and consonant postures. Two types of palatometric target patterns may be extracted automatically from talker's articulation gestures. One is a *static model* target pattern extracted in 10 msec slices from dynamic speech gestures. The other is a *dynamic model* target pattern extracted across an interval of speech.

The procedure used in the original palatometer developed by Fletcher and his associates will be used to illustrate how static and dynamic model target patterns may be derived automatically from normal talker utterances.[5] In each instance, the procedure begins with the talker being careful to lower the tongue so that it is not in contact with any sensor on the pseudopalate. The operator then activates data collection and the talker is notified to produce the chosen sound in the standard phonetic frame sentence, "Have a (bVb or C_1aC_2)," where V = the test vowel, C_1 = the test consonant, and C_2 a bilabial consonant. The sounds that frame the key element in this sentence were chosen so that when the sentence is spoken normally, the tongue will contact the palate only during the key vowel or consonant sound (between the [b] consonants in the "...bVb..." or "...a Ca..." nucleus word, as in "Have a beeb" for [i] or "have a top" for [t]). Locating the key sound in a stressed word, neutral phonetic environment reduces the probable influence from other articulatory gestures that might involve linguapalatal contact. After the sentence is spoken, the operator presses the E key on the keyboard to End data collection, and the program automatically detects and displays the linguapalatal contact pattern at its "maximum contact" moment (at the single 10 msec peak sample period during the response). It is important to note that only core articulation contacts are included in the static target patterns extracted automatically from a

---

[5]A similar set of routines has been implemented in the palatometer that is now commercially available through Kay Elemetrics Corporation, 12 Maple Avenue, P. O. Box 2025, Pine Brook, NJ 07058-2025.

talker's utterances. Dynamic gestural details regarding movements to and from the static target postures are not retained. Only the peak pattern is extracted and used to identify the static target pattern. If the operator feels that the pattern is not a good representation of the key sound, or would like to verify the adequacy of the pattern before beginning to save responses, provision has been made to discard the identified pattern and collect another one to replace it.

When a response is accepted, the program transfers the pattern to a special buffer where it can be used to produce an averaged pattern for the target sound. The provision for averaged measures across repeated productions of the same articulatory gesture is important. Even a carefully selected single response is unlikely to represent the way a person usually produces a particular sound. For this reason, provision was made in the palatometer software to continue collecting responses until a series of six to ten utterances are accumulated[6] on which to base the target pattern. The operator then enters a command to compute and display a final averaged contact pattern. This pattern is then stored as a "target" (.TGT) pattern with sensors identified for linguapalatal contact during training routines. A typical .TGT name would include the talker's initials, pseudopalate number, and phoneme represented by the contact pattern.

In standard palatometric displays sensors on the right side of the pseudopalate are mirrored on the right side of the video screen and sensors in the front of the mouth are at the top of the screen. These conventions help observers focus their attention on essential articulatory actions that tend to culminate in contrastive front and back linguapalatal contact patterns. Intraoral landmarks such as the teeth, borders of the alveolar ridge, and the major and minor rugae on the alveolar process are not portrayed. A border display can be used, to point out how the sensor locations are related to the teeth as clinicians acquaint their clients with the target patterns.

The second type of target pattern that could be built automatically is a *baseline articulation* pattern. This pattern is used to document current misarticulation, track spontaneous articulatory changes over time, and assess changes in response to articulation modeling and feedback intervention. The procedures outlined above for obtaining normal model patterns are also used to obtain samples of a talker's misarticulation. The clinician simply elicits vowel and/or consonant responses in the standard frame sentence then uses normative data to assess deviation from usual articulation patterns. If the person's language level is

---

[6]An even number is stipulated because when the accumulated patterns are processed, the sensors portrayed on the target must have been contacted at least half of the time to meet the 50% contact criterion for a representative response during the utterances. An even number permits selection of a real midpoint value.

inadequate for the sentence context, the sound can be sampled in isolation. A series of baseline tests may be elicited periodically during training to help document changes in the core articulatory postures across time. Differences between baseline misarticulation patterns elicited and normal model patterns may also be used to probe articulatory variability, isolate and describe error consistency, and evaluate influences from specific types of disability and/or intervention. Results from the baseline articulation tests may also be used to construct *Goal Articulation* target patterns manually to guide speech handicapped persons toward specific articulatory gestures. This option has the advantage of defining precisely how the action must specifically change to achieve a normal pattern.

Manual construction of a set of goal target patterns based on current patterns of misarticulation begins with identifying differences between the linguapalatal contact patterns of normal talkers, such as those shown for [i] in Figure 4–2 and [t] and [s] in Figure 4–7, and those of the talker who is speech impaired. These patterns must, of course, be adjusted to fit the palate configuration and sensor locations of the person who is speech impaired. It is done by using a computer mouse to highlight sensors identified as not contacted in the baseline articulation test that should be contacted to produce the sound correctly and unhighlight those that are currently contacted but should not be. This file is then used in early training to guide the subject toward the specific locations on the pseudopalate which must be contacted to produce the desired sound.[7]

Oftentimes the clinician will want to use stimulus words, phrases, or sentences to demonstrate articulation patterns dynamically without overlaid target patterns clouding the stimulus field. A "null target" may be prepared for this purpose. A null target is one which shows sensor locations but no specific sensors are highlighted in the display. This option has been found to be particularly helpful in live modeling situations after a client has learned to recognize and mimic tongue contact patterns and no longer needs a static reminder showing the goal pattern. The client simply discerns the critical articulatory parameters directly from live model displays. Practice can then focus on dynamic articulatory modeling and feedback routines designed to establish specific articulatory skills and produce accurate responses with smooth articulatory transitions in a variety of contrasting phonetic contexts.

---

[7]The CREFILE menu in the prototype device included options for creating files manually, assigning numbers to each pseudopalate sensor, and identifying their location on the pseudopalate. In the Kay Elemetrics palatometer, this information is now included on a diskette supplied by them with the pseudopalates. Similar diskettes are sent as other pseudopalates are supplied.

Creating Dynamic Target Files

Dynamic target files are created to demonstrate moving linguapalatal contact patterns and/or practice specific articulatory gestures in naturally contrasting phonetic environments. To do this using the prototype palatometer, the operator simply selected the appropriate option on the menu and stored response strings from single or repeated sounds, words, phrases, or sentences. For instance, a dynamic target string planned to contrast production of the /u/ vowel gesture with other point-vowel gestures might include a set of words such as "pool-peal, Luke-lock, who'd-had." For example, the file SF3OOc1 could be from a normal talker, Sharon Fowler, who used her pseudopalate #3 to demonstrate [oo] in a contrastive vowel stimulus set #1. Dynamic files thus provide opportunity for clients to practice stored stimulus patterns in independent drill sessions or for the clinician to expose a learner to the same words spoken by different talkers.

Files can also be created to relieve clinicians of routine housekeeping chores so their attention can be focused on using the instrumentation effectively and efficiently in diagnostic and training activities. These files contain such information as the locations of the pseudopalate sensors, users' names, .TGT patterns and files, and special stimulus materials for baseline testing and training use in articulatory modeling and shaping routines. This information, coded in a file name, can identify the users, the phonetic stimulus class (e.g., glide = C1, front stop = C2, back stop = C3, alveolar groove fricative = C4, postalveolar groove fricative = C5, laminar fricative = C6, affricate = C7, retroflex liquid = C8, lateral liquid = C9), the context in which the sounds will be presented (Wd = word, Ph = phrase, Sn = sentence), and the stimulus number[8] or the clinician may simply want to conduct articulation modeling and shaping routines "on the fly." In this instance, the articulation actions would presumably be modeled in live demonstrations by the clinician or via stored dynamic displays from other talkers. In the next chapter, we will discuss specifically how this might be done.

---

[8]Following this protocol, the name SF_JN24Sn3 would be assigned to Susan Fisher helping James Nelson develop front stop and alveolar sibilants using sentence set #3. Notations such as James Nelson. Consonant Training. 6/14/91. 7th training session may be included in the "comments" section.

CHAPTER 8

APPLYING ARTICULATION TRAINING PRINCIPLES

In previous chapters, emergence of motor skills was charted through the developmental years, and characteristics of the sensory and motor systems that support articulate speech development were examined. A central processing model was then presented to help conceptualize some of the basic principles that govern development of gestures, movements, and sensorimotor control. The premise of that review was that the structure and organization of speech articulatory tasks follow a route paralleling the development of the individual's other skilled motor responses. In other words, principles learned from studies of other motor activities may be expected to apply to those involved in speech developmental processes.

The aim of this chapter is to review previous approaches to speech articulation training and outline a treatment system that can be used to maximize speech articulation skill development and foster normal speech intelligibility. As the most demanding physiologic act performed by man, speech articulatory skill building may be expected to place unique demands on the motor system. An integrated approach to speech articulation training must therefore draw from information about general motor skill development and performance strategies. Special requirements apply uniquely to speech production skills.

As training procedures are outlined, care will be taken to point out the many ways in which practices that have long been part of speech training routines are now able to be subsumed and extended in the proposed motor skill approach to articulation assessment and treatment. New concepts will also be introduced. They will be based on firm experimental evidence that has demonstrated their utility in nonspeech as well as speech motor skill functions. The rationale for their inclusion in the speech training protocol will be presented along with examples of their possible utilization in training routines. The strategy outlined will thus be based firmly on systematically applied motor skill and learning theory concepts with underlying principles proposed to bring predictable and efficient change in speech performance.

The advantages and disadvantages of several general approaches are evaluated with the foregoing stipulations in mind. Based on the available information a general strategy will then be proposed to foster rapid, controlled development of new or modified speech articulatory skills within a physiological modeling and shaping framework.

ARTICULATION TRAINING APPROACHES

Two general approaches may be identified in past clinical speech training routines. The more traditional one has been based on building new or improved skills during production of single phonetic elements, such as /s/ and /r/. The sounds to be treated were identified through tests that classified articulation errors by the degree of deviation from normal sound development schedules. Training routines also followed a developmentally dictated progression. Sounds were selected and training sequences ordered according to their appearance in the developing sound repertoire of normal children. The sounds chosen for initial attention in a remediation regimen were therefore those normally acquired earliest in the developmental process. Treatment then focused on modification of single sounds determined to be sufficiently deviant from the normative standard that clinical intervention was deemed necessary. Each phonetic element was thus viewed as an isolated disturbance and training routines were based on the assumption that the talker was simply unable to perform the complex motor skills required for articulating the selected sound(s). Thus, the instructional routines focused on developing specific motor skills needed to produce specific sounds in isolation then in syllables, words, and phrases. During the training program, the context in which the sounds were presented was gradually expanded as the level of phonetic skill achieved progressed. The phonetic complexity of the stimuli was thus allowed to approximate the linguistic complexity of normal speech only after basic articulatory skills were firmly established in less demanding contexts.

More recently, a cognitive-linguistic approach has been adopted by many speech clinicians. This approach is based on the assumption that articulation errors are evidence of a phonological disorder. The individual has not learned how to use certain sound classes contrastively. This approach assumes that rules required for appropriate sound production and phonemic contrast have not been acquired. The instructional routines for this phonological approach thus differ sharply from those in the developmental phonetic approach. The phonological approach is designed to develop patterns that overcome an underlying phonemic deficiency signaled by individual articulation errors. This approach does not dismiss the physiologic demands that enable the phonological system to function. Rather, it emphasizes that disturbances are primarily reflections of phonological rule-based errors, not motor deficiencies.

The remediation procedures in the phonological approach treat misarticulated sounds as members of classes with common phonetic feature errors. The features are themselves based on rules derived from acoustic observations translated rather intuitively into articulatory functions. Many of the terms used are therefore difficult to understand from a strictly physical viewpoint. Typically, critical phonetic skills are taught through minimal word pairs selected to develop sound production through distinctive phonetic feature contrasts. The treatment routines are thus based on an assumption that when the phonetic feature is established in an appropriately selected exemplar, the articulation improvements attained will generalize to other sounds in the targeted phonetic feature class (McReynolds & Bennett, 1972). The general recommendation is that if the deficiency involves two or more feature differences, training should focus on segments with the least number of differences (McReynolds & Engmann, 1975). The ultimate goal of this approach is thus to improve speech intelligibility by mastery of feature contrasts, which are then transferred throughout the client's repertoire.

The *maximum contrast* procedure is a recently proposed extension of the phonological approach to speech remediation. This procedure is based on a top-down adaptation or extension of the phonological approach (Dinnsen & Elbert, 1984; Elbert, Dinnsen, & Powell, 1984; Gierut, 1985). The assumption is made that basic articulation skills are embedded within more complex articulatory gestures. From this it is reasoned that learning the more complex gestures which demand more intricate movements and motor control skills will automatically improve execution of other, less demanding gestures. For example, articulation of the more physically demanding sibilants and affricates should result in parallel improvements in stop sound production. This more global attack on articulatory disturbances thus presumes that new articulatory skills established in complex, physically demanding gestures will transfer automatically, or at least rapidly, to the basic maneuvers underlying the gestures taught. This approach thus predicts considerable savings in both time and effort as new, more broadly based motor skills, syllable shapes, and articulation patterns are introduced and established.

Gierut (1989a) demonstrated use of the maximum contrast phonological procedure with a child whose consonant phonetic inventory was initially limited to [m, b, w, j], primarily in postvocalic positions. The treatment program was initially directed toward establishing the sibilant [s] in contrast with [m, b, w]. Training was given in eight treatment sessions. Post-training tests indicated that the child had added [n, s, h] to his inventory. He was then taught the affricate [tʃ] in contrast with [m, b, s] during five sessions. These skills were reported to generalize to [t, d, z, ʃ, tʃ, dʒ, l], although these sounds were not always produced with 100% accuracy. Finally, the subject was taught [f] in contrast with [m, b, s, tʃ] during four sessions. One week later, a generalization probe showed consistent errors in conversational speech only on postvocalic [f, v], [l] clusters, and [r]. The [r] was the untreated control sound. Thus, this single child study supported the hypothesis that training focused on complex sound production can instigate broad generalization to less complex, untrained sounds without necessarily increasing treatment time.

The data from Gierut must be treated cautiously for a number of reasons. The most obvious reason is that the observations were from a single subject who may well have been exceptional. McReynolds (1989) has observed that children often begin to generalize after a new structure has been established in only a few exemplars. Others require many exemplars to be introduced before they initiate the generalization process. Unusual progress in therapy following relatively brief exposure to demanding phonetic contrasts can also result from many other factors, including newly awakened interest in spoken sounds which activates previously dormant but latent articulatory interests and skills.

In a rebuttal to a later critical review of her study (Fey, 1989), Gierut (1989b) provided some important details on the child's speech sound production that were not included in the initial article. Examination of those data showed that the child already had glide and stop gestures in his phonetic repertoire. The front grooved sibilant was also present in a number of words although it was not always used appropriately. The labiodental slit fricative [f] was also present as an [s] substitute — for example, [sit → fit]. On the other hand, [s] was used as an [f] substitute in the word "food," for example, [fu → su]. The errors thus showed that although the child had not achieved complete control of the groove versus slit gestural differentiations during intended frictional noise production, the underlying articulatory skills were present.

The [ʃ] sibilant, affricates, and linguadental slit fricatives were missing, however. From a physiological point of view, Gierut's selection of [s] as her starting point is thus seen to be well justified from a consonantal hierarchy viewpoint since that is the dividing point between the child's established and nonestablished articulatory gestures. After targeting the [s], the treatment regimen moved to developing the affricates and to the introduction of the slit fricative concept in [f] production during the final sessions. Thus, the success the child met in acquiring skills rapidly would be predicted from a physiologically based treatment order standpoint. The efficacy of the physiological approach is thus also supported by Gierut's results.

It should be noted that a central feature of the maximum contrast approach is use of variable practice. Our earlier review indicated that variable practice can lead to the discovery of explicit actions that consistently produce acceptable matches between targeted and actual motor skill patterns across a range of possible variations. At the same time, the variations across sounds could help localize sources of change, such as acoustic contrast arising from different movements within articulatory gestures. Variations within a set of articulatory responses may also permit the perceived acoustic consequences from articulatory trial responses to help isolate movements that are physiologically easiest to produce and also contribute most to the desired high phonetic contrast as the articulatory repertoire expands. This, in turn, could help weed out articulatory actions that are unsuccessful and stabilize those linked with successful performance in different phonetic contexts and speaking situations. From these observations, we can predict rather surely that future research with multiple subjects and comparisons across alternative procedures using individuals with different types of disorders would likely support the posited advantages of the maximum contrast approach if the choice were limited to it and the more traditional articulation training routines.

The ability to imitate unfamiliar sounds from the environment is an important consideration in evaluating the possible efficacy of using the maximum contrast approach with individual children. A review of findings from previous investigators by Kelly and Dale (1989) suggests that the ability to imitate unfamiliar sounds may not be fully established until about the time when children begin to use multi-word utterances. Skillful imitation also appears to be associated with emergence of the ability to engage in symbolic play activities. This would seem to mean that basic articulatory skills should be formed very early in the normal developmental process. Certain individuals such as those with severe language deficits from profound hearing losses or physical impairments that seriously limit their ability to execute the complex motor sequences demanded in basic articulatory gestures may be less likely to succeed in negotiating the multiple tasks and motor skills required in the maximum contrast approach. Such persons may need a more gradual introduction to the intricacies of natural speech articulatory gestures which normally provide opportunity to develop the basic motor skills involved in speech articulation rather directly.

A third approach to speech training has been proposed by Dinnsen, Chin, Elbert, and Powell (1990). This approach emphasizes the natural hierarchy of consonant sound production. These writers hypothesize that speech training may be most successful if it progresses systematically through the hierarchy of phonetic complexity shown in the left column of Table 4-2. The most limited inventory consisted of obstruent stop, nasal and glide consonants contrasted with syllabic glides. Initially only labial and alveolar obstruents were distinguished within this highly limited group of consonants. Obstruents were distinguished from nasal consonants by the [sonorant] feature. In other words, all of the early sonorants were nasals. The labial obstruents were distinguished from alveolars by the [coronal] feature and all obstruents were produced with an anterior contact point and without a voice distinction. The next contrasts developed were the [voice] and [anterior] features. The posterior obstruent thus entered at this level. The fricatives and/or affricates arrived next as the [continuant] and [delayed release] features were added. Both of these features were necessary to distinguish stops from affricates. Nasal versus liquid consonants were distinguished by the [nasal] feature. Finally the strident and nonstrident fricatives were distinguished by the feature [strident] and the lateral and retroflex consonants by the feature [lateral].

The goal of the developing child is to "fill out" the articulatory table for missing elements in the phonetic system. Specific rules are drawn from the hierarchical order. For example, fricative gestures may be more easily established after both the [consonantal] and [anterior] features paved the way for front and back stop gestures to be acquired. A later distinction, such as voicing, is predicted to be easier to establish if it is introduced in conjunction with phonetic features located higher than itself in the hierarchy. Voiced/voiceless distinctions would thus be likely to be learned more easily in a stop consonant than a fricative consonant environment. Data to test these assumptions clinically are still lacking.

It is convenient to dichotomize training into traditional phonetic motor skill versus cognitive-linguistic phonological approaches. At the clinical level it is often difficult or impossible, however, to determine whether particular articulation errors result from lack of articulatory motor skills, phonological knowledge, or deficiencies in both (Bernthal & Bankson, 1988). For this reason, instructional programs typically include procedures that could be derived from either orientation. Clinicians tend to be pragmatic. They use whatever techniques are proven to facilitate the development of desired articulation skills that are generalizable across a range of spoken messages.

The goal of the palatometric visual articulatory training approach is to link oral sensations directly with spatial and temporal properties of normal speech articulation. The aim is to help the individual first gain an accurate perception of articulatory postures and gestures that enable intelligible speech. From this information, the individual is guided toward understanding how specific gestures may be physically executed as the talker is taught strategies and actions that can lead to the required motor skills he or she will need to execute those actions spontaneously and naturally. In the process of instruction, the individual is helped to eradicate articulation errors systematically and integrate the essential gestures and movement patterns into new, skillfully executed articulatory sequences demanded in natural speech.

Our earlier review of maturational processes that influence development of vocal activities indicated that skilled movements extend from basic motor processes. The articulation skill level of a talker is thus evidenced by the degree of motor control attained, the validity and repeatability of articulatory gestures executed in a variety of phonetic contexts, and most importantly by the degree of speech intelligibility achieved through controlled and manipulated articulatory contrast within the gestures.

In palatometric training, articulatory information is extracted by mimicking visually displayed action models. Phonetic percepts and concepts are then extrapolated from this experience. The emerging articulatory gestures are accorded phonetic *salience* as they are executed in combinations that differentiate word meanings. The concepts that govern the development of new or improved articulatory skills through palatometric technology thus depend upon extensive and intensive use of clinician modeling and response shaping through joint clinician and subject feedback. An important assumption of the palatometric approach is that the clinician has normal speech. That fact needs to be verified in the process of preparing to use a palatometer clinically.

Up to this point, emphasis has been principally on assessment and development of new motor skills involved in speech production. Speech has been described as a *manifestation of language*, not just an arbitrary set of acoustic signals produced by the human vocal tract and perceptible to our auditory system (Halle & Stevens, 1979). The goal of speech treatment is to "abstract, describe, and classify as neatly as we can the recurrent sound units used to build up the spoken forms of a given language and to state the rules for their use" (Henderson, 1971, p. 36).

As we examine articulatory movements, we will seek to identify principles that govern actions that enable talkers to achieve particular target states (Halle & Stevens, 1979) or dynamic gestural goals (Bell-Berti & Harris, 1981). Movements toward a goal posture will thus be treated as an integral part of the gesture (see Figure 8–1). Speech production will then be viewed as the actualization of a temporally related sequence of targeted gestures or states of the articulatory structures (cf. Fletcher, 1989a). For a given articulator, the onset of the gesture will be treated as temporally independent of the preceding gesture if there is no articulatory conflict between them (Bell-Berti & Harris, 1981).

A fundamental characteristic of speech production is smoothly integrated, progressive actions, organized within response sets. The often-cited lip rounding gesture during an [u] vowel provides an appropriate example of the articulatory integration concept. In vowels, the gesture begins a constant time before the acoustic onset of the vowel, and vowel associated lip rounding occurs in conjunction with the tongue activity in labial consonants. Nonlabial consonants do not acquire the rounding feature.

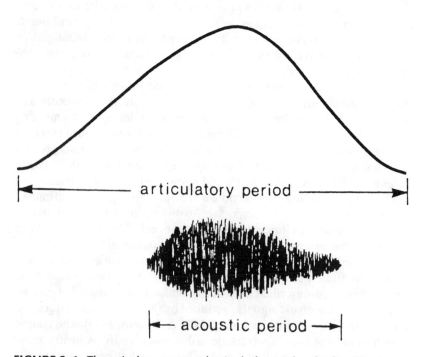

FIGURE 8–1. The articulatory gesture begins before and ends after the acoustic period. From Bell-Berti, F., & Harris, K. S. (1981). A temporal model of speech production. *Phonetica, 38,* 9–20. Reprinted by permission.

The orosensory goals of speech are logically specified in terms of positions, configurations, and contact surface relations between articulators (Perkell, 1979). During most of a connected speech utterance the articulators are moving between states, but not all of the structures involved in a given articulatory gesture arrive at the target configuration at the same moment. Different articulators move somewhat independently. This enables the movement to be adapted for phonetic content differences — such as conflicting gestures that involve the same articulator — while the elementary gesture of the syllable nucleus remains relatively invariant (Fugimura, 1986). Articulation actions are adapted to gain movement efficiency as the critical articulatory postures are executed within the allocated time span. These adjustments are largely accomplished by smoothing nontargeted parts of the actions. Articulatory "undershoot" in the nonessential phases of the gestures is thus a natural property of action integration. Timing of the gestures may likewise be treated as a basic parameter of the speech motor plan (Bell-Berti & Harris, 1981; Tuller & Kelso, 1984).

APPLYING MOTOR SKILL STRATEGIES

The ultimate goal of articulatory intervention is to change motor performance. The search for the keystones in this endeavor points to seven basic processes that underlie success in articulatory skill development: attention, focusing, imaging, goal setting, executing, feedback, and rehearsing. Each of these processes involves underlying principles, rules, and motor skill strategies that bear directly on the tasks and maneuvers involved. These functions will be discussed as variables that influence the development of specific motor skills. Specific procedures will also be outlined for their inclusion in the articulatory motor skill training program.

Goal Setting

Setting goals that motivate achievement is a central concern in the process of changing articulation motor behaviors. Care given to establishing hard, specific goals and performance standards and outlining the relevant tasks that lead to goal achievement has been shown to contribute directly to the success attained in gaining new motor response patterns and modifying old ones. The *objective* in speech articulatory training is normal speech achieved within a predictable time period. This objective is in keeping with the hypothesis that specific, difficult goals lead to higher levels of task performance than easy goals, no goals, or do-your-best goals. Individual tasks may, of course, be expected to vary with respect to the rapidity of achievement. Those articulatory gestures that require higher levels of skill and knowledge and are more physically demanding may be acquired more slowly and normal performance achieved with more difficulty than those which include less demanding articulatory sequences. Initial performance may thus be less successful on certain tasks or in certain phases of the training even if the subjects try hard. More complex tasks require time to develop strategies that lead to desired accomplishment.

It should be noted that the notion that failure will undermine motivation and performance has not been supported empirically in motor skill studies. Rather, the experiments cited earlier indicated that improved performance may be expected despite goals that may be beyond the participant's reach. Most individuals appear to experience repeated failure with no evidence of a decline in either motivation or performance. This finding has been replicated in a variety of studies. Participants do not necessarily cease to try hard nor drop in their performance despite repeated failure to reach assigned goals.

The most important explanation suggested to account for the apparent lack of performance decrement despite repeated failure to achieve targeted goal standards seems to be the individual's self-belief. Lofty goals appear to be motivating for most participants. They remain unshaken in their self-efficacy despite failure to achieve difficult goals. Others may become less sure of themselves when faced with failure, however, and still others seem to lose faith in their capabilities as an outgrowth of failure. Since the reaction to lofty, unattainable goals seems to be conditioned by the personality of the individual, this factor must be given careful consideration as articulation training routines are planned and as performance is monitored when the plan is implemented. The preparation of a specific, challenging goal should be treated as an extremely important factor in the training protocol. "Do your best" is no better than no goal at all. Individuals given specific, challenging goals may be expected to outperform those trying to do their best and surpass their own previous accomplishments in the process.

Modeling

The next step in the articulation motor skill training routine is using modeling and imaging strategies to organize and rehearse key properties, gestures, and intergesture movement patterns in goal-directed actions.

In speech training through palatometry, modeling is intentionally employed to elicit controlled imitation. The clinician uses speech production demonstrations as stimuli to induce images of desired articulatory actions, increase understanding of action sequences, and shape changes in the subject's articulation skills. Sequential modeling is introduced early in the training to build skills in functionally integrated speech production patterns. Success of the responses is then defined by the emergence of new articulation patterns that had no probability of occurrence prior to the training despite motivational inducements. Modeling is also used along with goal-directed social prompts to weaken inhibitions that subjects such as children who are deaf have developed in response to repeated failure in prior efforts to learn articulatory skills.

In the following paragraphs a set of theory-oriented demonstration, modeling, and shaping procedures will be outlined that, when applied systematically, will help foster efficient development of new or improved articulatory gestures and movement patterns. These patterns will then be used as the substrata to foster intelligible, socially acceptable speech.

The Clinician Model

A clinician's social attributes may be particularly influential in developing speech articulatory skills where individuals are commonly uncertain about their capabilities, lack task familiarity, or have self-doubts from difficulties in previous tasks they tried to perform well. Studies cited previously suggest that individuals who observe a skilled clinician model may be expected to outperform those who view either an unskilled teacher or skilled peer models. A series of studies have shown that model competence overrides any effect of model age. Nevertheless, it should be noted that failure on the part of a high status model, such as a clinician, may be expected to have a greater detrimental effect than failure on the part of a peer. Conversely, individuals are likely to be aided by performing modeled behavior they judge to be successful. Given equal competence, learners seem to pay closer attention to a higher status adult teacher model and gain more benefit from a skilled adult demonstration than anyone else. Peers may be helpful in improving feelings about self-efficacy, particularly among low-achieving children and others who are uncertain about their own capabilities or wonder whether they are capable of becoming as competent as the clinician. Because of this possibility, the clinician may wish to supplement instruction of low-achieving children with peer model demonstrations to enhance learning self-efficacy.

The timing when the clinician demonstrates an articulation task also influences the learning process. Seeing a task modeled before they began to learn it has been shown to help subjects "get the idea of the movement." But seeing the pattern modeled again after they have had an opportunity to practice is even more beneficial.

The age of the subject is an important consideration in the timing of modeling. Some evidence has been found that modeling halfway through a training program may lower performance of younger children (below 7-year-olds) but raise it for older ones. This difference has been interpreted as evidence that older subjects can adapt their motor response strategies to take advantage of opportunities to observe the modeled patterns at different times in the training program. Younger children may experience difficulty in changing their strategy once it has been set into play. It is also possible that younger children simply require additional time to deduce new possible strategies that can help them identify the critical aspects of modeled performances and translate that information into controlled responses. They may also be aware of differences that are noticeable but require a longer series of trials to discover how to implement them successfully. Patience and perseverance in providing additional trials over time would be expected to overcome these possible age-related limitations. Opportunity to observe a clinician is likely to help any child master new articulatory skills, but younger subjects may need more extended exposure than older ones to benefit fully from the same amount of experience.

Focusing

The process of establishing an environment that motivates change in articulatory skills and changing speech performance through palatometric training is centered on establishing attention via a dominantly vision-oriented speech perception plan. Visual articulatory displays are used to focus the learner's attention specifically on the physiological details of speech articulation. This information is then used to teach the individual how to arrive at specific postures within moving articulatory gestures. The subject is led to discover that when the gestures are perceived correctly and imitated accurately, desired speech outputs may be expected. The displays themselves are designed to activate formation of an oral spatial map that relates movements to articulator contact patterns which in turn can lead to intelligible speech. Attention is maintained by demonstrating speech production in sufficient detail that as the subject imitates the actions, the special properties of normal speech skills can emerge rather naturally. To make the greatest progress in this endeavor, the talker must realize that each step of the training program contributes to achieving the sought after normal communication skills.

Semantic meaning is essential in articulatory learning to integrate oral and visual sensations and phonetic percepts. In watching video display of an articulation pattern, the subject is guided to perceive, recognize, and extract properties that contribute meaning as the articulatory skills are modeled. This enables the actions to take on new salience as basic oral motor skill is demonstrated, mimicked, and eventually mastered. The ultimate goal of the modeling is to have articulatory perception become not merely the registration of objective linguapalatal contact form, but to have it "laced" with interpretation. What the subject "sees" must become the phonetic interpretations assigned to the palatometric displays. She or he should not only begin to see different things in the displays, but see things differently as phonetic patterns and word meanings emerge.

A fundamental requirement for skilled articulatory learning to take place is helping the subject focus on key actions. Focusing is specifically defined as presetting a subject's responses by spotlighting a relevant articulatory feature such as the location of the groove within a targeted sibilant production task explicitly. In general, studies have shown poor transfer from practice to performance when activity is not focused on a specific task. In other words, regardless of the comparative energy expended by the clinician and client and use of similar phonetic structures in different tasks, an essential criterion in training is that performers focus on the specific skill the exposure is designed to develop. In a speech articulation training routine this means that attention must be focused keenly on articulatory postures and gestures, usually embedded in actual sounds or words as an individual is being guided to produce the motor responses in a different way. In achieving this attentional focus, the subject must be taught to *attend selectively to activities taking place in one part of the action field and ignore, at least temporarily, other things that are taking place.* Both the locations and the operations performed at that location must be identified and used by the subject to establish controlled and coordinated actions. The aim of the attentional focus is to reduce the negative influence that competing events transpiring at the same time have on each other. The aim also includes eliciting the desired set of specific articulatory movements in the action sequences required to differentiate sounds from each other acoustically.

Attentional focus is achieved by priming the subject for the specific task through instructions that are designed to fit the individual's age and articulatory capabilities. Repetition and task simplification are especially important with younger children. Regardless of age, however, it is wise to keep explanations brief and explicit. Overexplaining can cause confusion. For example, simply point to the location where an important part of an essential movement will be taking place and say little more than "watch here." Then allow the subject to discover the most salient characteristics of the action. Such simplified guidance is likely to be more helpful in achieving a desired articulation pattern than providing a mass of verbal descriptions that may be confusing. The goal is to help the learner concentrate the gaze on visual field areas that contain the essential stimulus elements. As this information is absorbed, the scanning patterns can be expanded to encompass multiple action functions. The goal of the watchful effort is to prime the subject to perceive a particular target pattern or a sequential set of contrasting patterns.

Evidence was cited earlier that, in vision, inputs from the central foveal field of the eye are processed preferentially and detected more quickly than stimuli that are not in the direct field of attention. The subject's position with respect to the screen should therefore be carefully established. This dictates that the subject be seated in a position that enhances the ability to shift back and forth easily between the model and feedback portions of the video screen as attention is directed to sites of critical articulatory actions within the visual fields. As indicated by the visual sensory hierarchy, locations of actions within the stimulus field should be accorded preferential consideration in the initial modeling activities. Later, the attentional focus can be expanded to include features such as shape or area of linguapalatal contact at other locations. Attentional focus is thus applied to help the subject discern *core attributes* of the articulatory patterns as other attributes are rejected, ignored, or filtered out of perceptual awareness in the process of deriving a unified, meaningful percept of the actions and a *preparatory set* that can foster efficient, well modulated articulatory responses.

Imaging

One of the major goals of articulatory modeling is to develop a clear mental percept or *abstract visual image* that represents the core elements of the postures, gestures, and movement patterns to be performed. To accomplish this, three distinctive and sequential stages are thought to contribute. In the initial stage the learner is guided to scan the actual linguacontact pattern displayed and identify the focal sources of articulation change. In the second stage the person is encouraged to extract the parameters that appear to govern the changes observed and create an internalized spatial representation of the pattern perceived. In the final stage he or she is guided toward forming a general conceptualization of the core properties that are constant through a process of comparing what is seen with what is remembered from a series of similar and different utterances. The final stage thus includes a decision operation in which articulatory displays become categorized with respect to what is seen when a targeted sound is and is not present in a particular utterance.

Mental imagery is a natural outgrowth of watching with attentional focus. The facilitation of motor learning through mental imagery is based on the principle that abstract perception paves the way for correct production. Success in physical skill learning through feedback is a predicted outcome of careful mental imagery preparation. Toward this end, basic maneuvers should be modeled in palatometric displays that can be systematically repeated in dynamic, rapid, smoothly executed articulatory gestures. This experience can thus provide the varied opportunities needed to discern the underlying processes that govern perception of the modeled gestures and movement patterns.

The learning rate of beginners has been found to be particularly enhanced when they have been taught explicitly how to image patterns by a skilled model. When cognitive and motor components of a modeled task have been studied separately, the findings indicate that a major source of benefit is from the cognitive process rather than simply the motor skill learning. Paivio (1985) suggested that the principal beneficial effects of imagery arise from a combination of increased desire to achieve specific goals and cognitive insight gained through covert practice of imagined actions and strategies.

In the initial exposure to palatometric displays, the imaging may need to be focused on isolated submovements within specific articulatory gestures. Accurate representations may conceivably be developed more easily in a nonspeech, phonetically oriented context. But children have been shown to be more attentive to real speech patterns. Previously stored patterns from other talkers can be particularly helpful in developing a realistic image of sound-relevant articulatory contact patterns. In all imaging practice, the subject should be specifically instructed to form a picture in the mind of what the contact pattern looks like at the time when the key posture is portrayed on the video screen. The clinician can gain insight into the subject's internal processing and the actual representations stored in the subject's brain by having him or her describe or point to the key element or location of the critical change in the display as the sounds or words are spoken.

Finally, it is worth noting that it is not necessary to devote a large amount of time to any single mental imaging task. Three to 5 minutes spent in mental practice at one time may produce the best results.

Rehearsing

Rehearsal consists of a silent exercise or drill designed to establish a formal linkage between visual images and oral postural sensations through preliminary mental and motor practice. Rehearsal in the articulatory skill-training program emphasizes the need to isolate the specific tasks that training routines are intended to improve. Sage (1984) noted that mental practice seems to help correct execution errors, increase concentration, and develop improved motor strategies. The goal of motor rehearsing is to isolate and teach the sensations that may be expected when postures and movements produce desired linguapalatal contact patterns. In other words, the subject is guided to sense relationships between how certain articulatory acts are represented on the screen and felt in the mouth when the learner's own tongue is placed in desired locations within the oral cavity and moved to positions shown in the video display. Pattern generation can thus be used to verify image perception by giving the subject opportuntity to engage in trial practice as he or she strives to translate perceived images into preliminary articulatory postures.

A common tactic in speech training is to have a subject mentally review an erroneous response before trying it again. A critical component of this review is to determine whether the errors observed result primarily because the individual has not yet acquired an accurate image of the articulatory pattern, lacks essential physical skills needed to achieve targeted articulatory postures and movement patterns, or lacks skill in transferring articulatory gestures into highly constrained phonological contexts during speech production. The image deficit hypothesis would presume that the subject needs additional experience aimed at strengthening pattern recognition skills and establishing an accurate concept of the pattern to be expected when a particular sound is produced. The motor deficiency hypothesis would presume that rehearsal should concentrate on practicing how to picture and review the explicit spatial and temporal properties of a targeted sound. The speech context hypothesis would dictate that rehearsal should concentrate on conceptualizing the linkage found between sounds produced in the intricately connected sequences of spoken words. In this instance, attention should likely be directed toward imaging and rehearsing sound production in carefully constructed, contrasting word or sentence contexts. Additional research is needed to test all of the ramifications of these hypothesized processing stages encompassed in imaging and rehearsing strategies.

It should be remembered that the ability to imitate simple motor acts is inborn, but imitation skill increases with age. When working with subjects who are young or physically disabled, it may be necessary to model articulation postures and movements initially in very simplified action patterns that can be easily imaged and rehearsed. The actions can then be expanded to increase the complexity of rehearsal for motor skill development. Recall, however, that the best strategy even when motor responses appear to be deficient is likely to be to rehearse actions in varied and demanding contexts. This is consistent with the predictions from research on the use of hard goals and variable practice. To transfer motor skill learning to natural speech contexts, practice on isolated sound production to reduce possible conflicting motor activities and simplify the motor requirements of the task should therefore be strictly limited. Better long-term results may be attained through nonsense syllable and real-word rehearsal than in isolated sound production. The intent is to simulate a more natural speech context. The reader should be cautioned that although direct extensions of techniques derived from motor skill studies may appear to be very logical, their effectiveness in speech motor skill learning tasks should be scrutinized closely until their effectiveness has been directly documented in speech skill learning routines.

Opportunity to rehearse isolated parts of upcoming speech patterns are likely to be particularly helpful for younger children as they strive to focus their attention and efforts on specific aspects of the task at hand. Imaging and rehearsing would be expected to help them as well as more experienced learners sort through different aspects of complicated articulation routines and refine their response strategies.

Finally, it is worth noting that it is not necessary to devote a large amount of time to any single mental imaging and rehearsing task. Shick (1970) reported that 3 to 5 minutes spent in mental practice at one time seemed to produce the best results. It is likely that in most speech articulation applications even shorter periods of mental practice would contribute beneficial results.

Executing

One of the major benefits from mental and motor rehearsal may be that they prime the system for maximum proficiency in the speech motor execution activities that follow. The goal of the preliminary training is to enable the performer to block disrupting thoughts during execution of the patterns imaged and rehearsed. Once the articulatory task has been defined, imaged, and rehearsed, the sequences should be executed smoothly without conscious thought about articulatory motor details. The movement should thus be treated as a complete response that is a natural extension of the preparatory "set" as perceived patterns are translated into central commands and relayed to the motor system. The motor program may then be expected to organize and implement articulatory actions to achieve the specified phonetic goals without apparent oversight.

The rules that govern control of coincident motor actions and facilitate effective time sharing across the different articulators involved in a given utterance are thought to be applied at the physiological processing level. In initial training, potential movement conflicts during the active responses may still be circumvented by selecting articulatory tasks that have actions that are located far apart in oral space. Some uncertainty may still be expected, however, whenever motor tasks require unfamiliar actions to be directed toward unfamiliar targets or when novice speakers attempt nonhabitual postures and movement transitions "on the fly." These conflicts may be expected to continue until the articulation functions become more fully coordinated, integrated, and habituated in standard articulatory sequences.

The dominant symptom to be sought in developing articulatory skill is increasingly consistent, precise gestures with their elements tightly integrated into unified whole patterns. As a specific articulatory task is encountered repeatedly, routines may be expected to be developed that merge the actions together as a single response unit with the path of the movement less important than the goal that is achieved. The building of such units depends upon establishing a clear conceptual image of the outcome and practice until the individual movements and gestures are executed smoothly and accurately without interruptions to make physical corrections. The movement patterns are thus conceived as largely formulated internally on the basis of a backlog of experience with movements executed to achieve similar goals. Longer and more intricate programs may be expected to evolve as basic phonetic skills become automatic. Factors such as disturbances or distractions that tend to break up the routines and necessitate a return to dealing with smaller articulatory units should be avoided. This allows the movement execution to be paced largely by the subject rather than being driven by external forcing. Global rather than piecemeal processing should be emphasized. The goal of articulatory execution is to establish thoroughly practiced actions that become "automatic" in the sense that they are performed without conscious detailed monitoring or control.

Actions must be automatically programmed if performance is to keep in step with the person's rapidly developing vocabulary, expanding syntactic complexity, and desire to express increasingly intricate and complex thoughts. A characteristic of automatic actions is that performance becomes faster, smoother, and more accurate. In speaking, an additional evidence of desired automatic articulation accuracy and useful skill habituation is that the output remains fully intelligible as the individual becomes less aware of the physical actions transpiring.

Repetition is an important aspect of speech habituation. Pew (1974) notes that increased motor precision occurs with practice even without the sequence being consciously specified or coded. He described an experiment in which the subjects tracked an irregular course across several trials. Part of the course remained the same across trials while the rest varied. Accuracy increased for those parts that were repeated more than for the rest although the subjects were unaware, or imperfectly aware, that any portion of the track had recurred.

Automatic execution of motor action patterns permits talkers to maintain the meaning they are striving to convey in their attentional foreground during vocal communication. When difficulties arise in executing particularly difficult passages or talking under particularly difficult speaking conditions, the speaker may be expected to drop back temporarily to consciously monitoring the action pattern. This should be possible without necessarily invading the physical automaticity of the integrated movement patterns. This would be evidenced by an ability to shift from a foreground perception to a background motor frame of reference. In other words the characteristic qualities of accurately and efficiently executed motor response patterns and a sense that through automaticity each action can be initiated automatically without the need to observe outcomes of previous ones should be retained during such motor scanning periods. Such accurate, habitualized performance may be expected to engender a feeling of being unhurried since the entire foreground attention is essentially available for communicating and perceiving meaning. Only rarely would shifts to consciously monitoring articulation activities at the motor level then be necessary.

Verifying

One of the most salient predictions of training is that accurate feedback will increase interest in speech learning, enhance skill in achieving targeted behaviors, accelerate the rate of change in articulation patterns, and reduce both clinician and client fatigue during the learning process. The importance of feedback is undisputed. Studies of feedback have repeatedly shown little or no improvement without feedback, progressive improvement with it, and deterioration after its withdrawal.

In the current discussion, the term *feedback* refers to both internal and external sources of information that permit a subject to monitor, verify, and adjust his or her own articulatory postures and movements. Internal feedback is from *tactile* (touch) or *kinesthetic* (position and movement in space) receptors within the speech mechanism. For example, the position of the tongue within the oral cavity is sensed tactually during periods when it is in contact with other structures such as the palate and teeth and kinesthetically as it moves from one position to another in oral space. The output from these actions is sensed through auditory (hearing) and visual (sight) *teloreceptors. Self-reporting* of this information is relayed to the central nervous system where it is integrated with that from previous experiences stored in memory. Skill assessment is thus an outgrowth of current sensations and previous experiences. *Articulation success* is judged in terms of congruence between the speech patterns modeled as a standard, the talker's innate physical abilities and capacities in oral motor control tasks, and the level of emerging skill in using visual and auditory feedback to match what they see and hear as they strive to match the model. A crucial aspect of that success is thus how well they use the feedback in the speech learning process as they seek to develop the necessary articulation skills.

Two types of external, or *augmented*, feedback were described in Chapter 3. Feedback that provides a quantitative measure of the degree of success achieved in seeking the specifically targeted goal articulation postures is termed *knowledge of results* or, in abbreviated form, simply KR. KR may be from another person or an instrumental device such as the palatometer. Feedback that focuses on qualities of performance in the process of seeking to execute the stipulated articulatory movements or gestures is termed *knowledge of performance*, or simply KP. KP provides *kinematic* or touch- and movement-related evaluations to help the talker assess how well the articulatory actions involved in the response are performed. For example, the accuracy of producing a targeted stop articulation pattern would be indicated by the KR comment "Your score was 92" and a KP description "Your tongue was too far forward." KR would thus be used to provide an objective measure of articulation while KP describes the dynamics of the articulatory postures and gestures involved in the articulatory actions, generally with respect to the normal, standard pattern modeled. It may be evident that, except in the very earliest stages of articulatory training, the two sources of augmented feedback provide important foreground information for guiding articulatory change. The two types of augmented feedback clearly complement one another. For instance, KR provides a general measure of the response accuracy that could also be used by a speech clinician to measure and compare improvements from session to session or across a stipulated training period. KP provides a way to guide the articulatory actions toward explicitly defined goal positions and gestural patterns. Both KR and KP would thus supplement the information the speaker derives from internal tactile/kinesthetic feedback and self-evaluations.

On many occasions, speech is executed so rapidly and continuously that the information cannot be sensed, processed, and modified or scaled during ongoing activities. Fortunately, the key muscle contraction sequences and forces involved are monitored and controlled primarily at the *motor program* level via information stored in memory. KR and KP feedback information is fed into the system to instigate changes in the motor program and bring the response patterns into congruence with modeled goal patterns via visual articulatory modeling and shaping routines. Accurate internal and external feedback to guide and stabilize articulation patterns is a hallmark of the palatometric training approach.

Practicing

Principles of massed, spaced, and variable practice need to be applied systematically to maximize speech change, enhance training effectiveness, and foster articulation skill transfer into daily life activities. Our earlier review of motor skill learning indicated that goal motivated, performance directed practice is essential for acquiring and retaining complex motor skills. The question specifically raised at this point is what should be practiced to facilitate speech articulatory motor skill learning and retention?

Two opposing viewpoints are raised in answer to this question. The *specificity of learning principle* indicates that training should focus upon specific aspects of speech production to change articulation skills. A central assumption of that principle is that practice should focus on one and only one task. In its purest sense, this assumption would mean that changing a motor task even slightly would mean implementing a new motor program. This assumption seems to be most nearly applied in speech articulation training routines where clinician efforts are focused exclusively on a specifically missing or defective articulatory skill. It was observed earlier that this may be helpful with certain children who need highly structured, specifically targeted training routines, but probably not in most situations. If this type of speech articulation training were used, the procedure would consist of reinforcing responses in the presence of a specific stimulus until each response pattern is established and stabilized. Expansion of new skills through variable practice would thus be delayed until later training stages.

The variable practice hypothesis emphasizes the continuous use of contrastive sensory experiences in articulatory training. This would permit hypotheses to be formed, tested, and rejected as conditions are varied until action patterns are found that consistently produce acceptable responses across a range of possible actions. Variations around a central articulatory task would thus be used to form the basis of flexible speech skills within a broad scope of possible actions. This approach is well supported by motor skill studies. Such studies have consistently shown that the greater the variety of experiences in a motor act, the more flexible is the set of responses that develop.

Variety in speech articulation stimulus materials must also be sought to raise the likelihood that the articulatory training will result in skill transference to spontaneous speech conditions. Enhanced intelligibility in a variety of speaking contexts would be one of the predictable outcomes of a varied training program.

Errors also play an important role in variable practice theory. During the articulation concept development stage of speech development, learners appear to enter a search mode for a brief time after errors are made. At that time, the speaker is thought to be making decisions about which specific articulatory parameters should be varied to achieve the modeled normal speech pattern. As the talker strives to match the model pattern, he or she is presumed to set values on the dimensions of the parameters as they are identified and manipulated. Certain articulatory dimensions are assumed to be more noticeable (more *salient*) than others. These dimensions are likely to be tested first in the process of developing viable hypotheses and guiding action patterns. When a response is identified by either the subject or the clinician as correct (receives positive feedback during a trial), the hypothesis that dictated that response would be confirmed and the action retained. Through such hypothesis testing, the subject would be expected to narrow the articulatory possibilities and actions down until only correct maneuvers and response patterns remain. Those functions would then be stabilized and automatized.

It is important to note that no response in the emerging repertoire would be unchangeable. If on subsequent trials an articulation distortion or error is still manifest, the search mode could be reactivated and the testing operation re-entered to recheck and refine the action pattern. Speech articulatory skill is thus postulated to be directly related to the variations practiced as a subject works within a particular class of phonetic responses.

A number of motor skill studies have shown that variable practice during early learning activities enhances later transfer of learning to a novel task. Syllable content is one of the parameters that can be systematically varied to improve speech performance. Consonant and vowel alternation is a fundamental aspect of sound sequencing in speech. The consonant-vowel (CV) combination is the single most common syllable type across languages (Clements & Keyser, 1983), and a number of phonological observations point to CV and consonant-vowel-consonant (CVC) combinations as early preferred word shapes. Ingram (1978) concluded from a review of data across a series of single subject and small group studies that CV combinations dominate the use of monosyllables at the onset of spoken words. Wepman & Hass (1969) reported that about 40% of the 50 most common words spoken by 5- to 7-year-old children are CVC utterances, 20% are CV, 20% VC, and 10%

CVCV. The remaining 10% of the words identified in their study were a mixture of consonant and vowel combinations with CVCVC words rarely found (but see Ingram, 1978). Thus, all other things being equal, CV and CVC words appear to be among the most important phonetic units to include in initial speech training routines. Benefits from practice with verbal units that vary more widely in length and complexity are also possible but as yet less well explored.

The facility for sound acquisition also differs with the position of sounds in words. The articulatory hierarchy of sound acquisition described earlier postulates that stops should be learned most easily when they are in an initial position within a word. This is supported by Ingram's (1978) observation that stops tend to devoice in final position. Conversely, fricatives and affricates may be easier to learn in the final position within a word. The relative difficulty of initial fricative production is indicated by Ferguson and Farwell's observation (1975) that those in the initial position are more likely to be misarticulated by stop replacement than final ones. The phonetic context best suited for articulatory training may therefore need to be adapted to fit the sensitivities of targeted consonants within words to enhance success as attention is focused on production of particular sounds in a training sequence.

Establishing temporally significant contrasts within basic articulatory gestures is also essential for building accurate and flexible speech production concepts. Clinical evidence for this is found in the utility of maximally rather than minimally contrastive articulatory gestures (Gierut, 1989a). Maximally contrastive gestures differ along articulatory dimensions that generate phonetic outputs with multiple distinctive properties, as in teaching a voiced bilabial stop in contrast with a voiceless postalveolar fricative.

Finally, to achieve desired articulatory skills that contribute directly to word meanings, the child must be able to identify word boundaries in the speech stream in which they occur. This task is normally made easier in early speech learning by engaging in "naming games," an activity that all children seem to play with their parents or other caregivers (Brown, 1958). Ninio and Bruner (1978) observed that the repetitive and ritual character of word games makes relations between varied word and object meaning salient.

C H A P T E R   9

VISUAL
ARTICULATORY
MODELING AND SHAPING

In this chapter, we will move directly into speech assessment and training procedures. As pointed out by Wells (1947), the traditional assessment routines depend primarily on the human ear to discern normality and abnormality of spoken sounds:

> A purely phonemic transcription, by definition, records all and only the significant distinctions that can be heard. If two utterances or parts of utterances sound perfectly alike to native speakers of the language to which they belong, their phonemic transcription is identical . . . . Phonemics takes the point of view of the hearer. (pp. 270–271)

Because two phonetic elements sound alike, or have the same phonologic features, they are not necessarily produced alike. Talkers can produce perceptually equivalent vowels by manipulating articulatory parameters in different ways. Equivalent vowels can be generated either by manipulating the height of the tongue body (Gay, Lindblom, & Lubker, 1981) or the place and degree of linguapalatal contact along the lateral borders of the tongue (Fletcher, 1992). Normal sounding sibilants result from channeling the phonic stream through a narrow groove at the front (Christensen, Fletcher, Hasegawa, & Mc-

Cutcheon, in press; Fletcher, 1985) or farther back on the alveolar ridge (Fletcher, 1988; Fletcher & Newman, 1991). And the groove may be produced with the tip of the tongue behind the upper or lower incisors (Weinberg, 1968). Thus, although certain gestures and movements have rather direct and predictable acoustic properties, and most talkers produce sounds in roughly the same way, auditory sensations produce inferences, not facts, about articulatory patterns. From a speech production viewpoint, auditory impressions are far from infallible.

Straight (1980) observed that imitation consists of:

> .... the conversion of an auditory input form into an abstract representation that can serve as the basis for articulatory output processing .... [The relationships between auditory input and articulatory output features] .... may vary greatly in complexity and in specificity, but in no case will they be so simple and specific as to be univocal. (p. 65)

Since the human articulation system is fundamentally the same from one talker to another, it may be presumed that basic physical principles exist that help us achieve standard acoustic outputs easily and naturally. Although adaptations would be expected, based on specialized structure and function needs, the principles governing speech postures and movements may also be expected to be essentially the same as those that govern development of other motor skills.

The review of motor skill processes and maturation in Chapter 1 suggested that one of the basic principles in motor skill development is that nucleus postures and movements exist that provide stability and mobility for actions. That is, movements extend from, and revolve around, basic body postures. The postures serve, in part, to balance the forces of action and reaction in goal-directed movements. In articulate speech, special postures of the jaw and lateral margins of the tongue were found to stabilize the finely integrated, overlaid motions required to produce specific sounds. These actions were also observed to function within a motor control hierarchy. For example, the vowel system develops around lateral linguapalatal contact. The lateral contact is then used to stabilize front and back consonant gestures.

Basic physical capabilities that govern actions such as walking and talking are identifiable at birth. They are initially present in reflexively performed activities. Maturation brings refinement, not elimination, of these basic reflexes. As new skills emerge, different control modes are applied that span a continuum of movements within their functional hierarchies. And different functional demands cause shifts from one posture-movement synergy to another. In speech, actions of the slower moving jaw help position the tongue for nucleus vowel postures. Lateral linguapalatal contact is then manipulated precisely to help differentiate the different vowels. The talker then learns to locate the tongue in positions that can foster rapid, precise consonant articulatory actions at the front and back margins of the palate. The basic vowel posture thus fuses the syllable movement together and helps free the anterior and posterior extremities of the tongue for the discriminant movements of the consonants. Consonants are thus seen to be anterior and posterior refinements of basic vowel postures. Stetson (1951) called attention to an important distinction between the consonant-vowel (CV) combination which opens a (CVC) syllable and the vowel-consonant (VC) which closes it. He noticed that the actions consist "primarily of taking-positions and holding-positions" (p. 45). Translated into more current physiologic phonetic terms, the tongue is conceived as being anchored in postures that enhance stability of the preceding consonant, foster balanced articulation of the vowel, then steady execution of the final consonant.

Conflicting stabilization and articulation postures across sounds require reductions in the movement rate. This relationship is illustrated by Stetson's observation that the maximum rate of CV syllable repetition drops from 8 to 12 syllables per sec for "ta, ta . . . ta" to about 5 syllables per sec for repetitions of "ti-tu-te."

The articulatory system usually compensates for increased speech rate demands by reducing movements of certain articulators. Gross jaw and tongue movements are suppressed as speech rate and/or articulation precision increases. This jaw and tongue motion limitation is used to free actions of the tongue extremities as rapidity and precision demands of higher speech rates are met. Motor disabilities require a slower speech production rate. New skill learning is also enhanced by adopting a slower articulation rate. Movement rate is thus sacrificed for intelligibility, which is the pre-eminent goal of speech production.

Automaticity in a motor event allows actions to be triggered without explicit attention being devoted to the motor processes. In speech and other repetitive activities, rhythmical automatization fosters smooth transitions between adjacent elements and expands the range of skilled, executable maneuvers that can be carried out in tandem. An automatic act is also typically performed unconsciously. This prevents the actions from interfering with attended activities and with other automatic functions (Shiffrin & Grantham, 1974). One of the prices paid for this loss of oversight control is that once started, automatic actions usually cannot be stopped intentionally. In speech, automatization frees the talker's attention from the physical actions of articulation so it can be directed toward producing and listening to spoken messages. Automatization thus allows the major focus of speech to be on communicating meaning through the words uttered.

Of direct clinical significance are three levels of motor skill automaticity distinguished by Kahneman and Treisman (1984). They suggested that an act should be classified as *strongly* automatic only if it is neither facilitated by focusing attention on it or impaired by diverting attention from it. The act would be classified as *partially* automatic if it is normally completed even when attention is diverted from it but can be speeded or facilitated by attention. It is *marginally* automatic if it generally requires attention but can sometimes be completed without it. Strong automaticity of articulation action patterns that result in intelligible speech output is the ultimate goal of speech modification and training.

VOWEL MISARTICULATION

The vowel has long been recognized as the core of the syllable nucleus. The term consonant (con = with, sonant = vowel) reflects the important role vowel postures play in consonant production. In the past, vowel production skills have been thought to be rarely disturbed. This is a misconception. Vowel misarticulation disorders are often simply overshadowed by associated consonant disturbances. Renfrew (1966) called attention to a group of individuals that did not respond to conventional, consonant-oriented articulation therapy. She noted that the speech of these individuals, and a similar group described earlier by Morley (1957), revealed systematically deviant vowels *and* consonants. The vowels tended to be distorted and the consonants reduced in number. This joint disability limited the articulation base to only 6 to 10 consonants. The consonants that were present were typically correctly articulated only in the initial position within words. The vowel effect was highlighted by the observation that many medial and virtually all final consonants were omitted. Although most children start out with the limited CV syllable construction, in less than 3 years they normally add the final consonant. Based on her clinical observations, Renfrew outlined a series of 10 maturation stages that such children seemed to pass through on their road to normal speech. These stages are listed in Table 9-1. It may be seen that as final consonant production skills develop, they follow a systematic progression from omitted consonant, to mastery of nasals, then stops, and finally fricatives. She observed that the "open syllable" group seemed unable to "make the transition from vowels to consonants within the same syllable" (p. 372). They apparently had not learned to use the tongue for the joint stabilization and articulation functions that normally accompany maturation of vowel production skills.

    In 1974, Panagos described a group of 10 children with "largely unintelligible speech" that showed speech patterns similar to those identified by Renfrew. As summarized in Table 9-2, these children had

TABLE 9-1. Stages of articulation development by individuals with persistent open syllables. From C. A. Renfrew (1966). Persistence of the open syllable in defective articulation. *Journal of Speech and Hearing Disorders, 31,* 370–373. Reprinted by permission.

Stage 1. When the child is seen initially at about 4 or 5 years old, there is a reduced base of consonant articulation with perhaps only six to ten consonants being used. Medials are used only when duplicating the initial consonant in familiar words, e.g., "mummy," "baby." No blends or final consonants are used. *Vowels are frequently distorted* [italics added].

Stage 2. All consonants except /θ/ and /r/ are used consistently in the initial position, and occasionally in the medial position. (Stage 2 may not be reached until after Stage 4 if no speech therapy is given.)

Stage 3. Two-syllable words are correctly articulated if neither blends nor finals are required, e.g., "coffee" will be correctly articulated, but bækə will be said for "blanket." When attempting to imitate a word with a final consonant, two syllables are produced, e.g., dɔ-gə for "dog" and bʌ-s for "bus."

Stage 4. Nasal consonants only are used at the ends of words where appropriate; /m/ is used correctly as a final but /n/ and /ŋ/ vary.

Stage 5. Nasal finals are all used consistently and appropriately; /l/ finals and blends are used and attempts are made at /r/ blends.

Stage 6. Glottal stops are used for all final plosives; /r/ and /θ/ are correctly articulated initially and medially.

Stage 7. In the final position /p/, /b/, and /d/ are used consistently and appropriately; glottal stops are still used for /k/, /g/, and /t/, but the *length of the vowel preceding the stop indicates which of the three plosives was intended* [italics added].

Stage 8. Final /t/ is used consistently and appropriately; sometimes several attempts are made at fricative finals before the correct one is selected.

Stage 9. All final consonants, including fricatives, are used consistently and appropriately except /k/ and /g/.

Stage 10. Articulation normal.

---

no errors during production of isolated vowels nor of consonants in elementary CV syllables. Errors began to appear in VC syllables (14%). The errors involved 23% of the consonants in CVC syllables and 100% of them in the physically more complex VCC, CCV, and CCCVC syllables. These observations indicate that as the phonetic complexity of the sounds uttered expanded to multiple consonants balanced by a single vowel, the system broke down. In most instances, the subjects simply reduced the phonetic complexity of the words to the CV syllable structure they could handle. Panagos cited similar data in single subject studies reported earlier by Van Riper and Smith (1954), Simms (1963), and Haas (1963).

TABLE 9-2. Frequencies of intelligible syllables produced spontaneously by 10 children with largely unintelligible speech. Based on J. M. Panagos (1974).

Syllable Shape	Example	Number in Sample	Percent Correct	Percent Reduced
V	a	4	100	0
CV	to	11	100	0
VC	all	7	71	14
CVC	car	21	76	23
VCC	and	6	0	100
CCV	try	1	0	100
CCVC	stop	4	50	50
CVCC	doors	4	50	50
CCCVC	street	1	0	100

Speech articulation disabilities occur when physical or mental conditions exist which prevent persons from expanding, refining, and automatizing the processes, gestures, and movements that govern articulation action patterns. Misarticulation can thus be traced to factors, such as auditory deficits, that cause a talker to be unable to sense or control the basic physical elements in speech. Talkers normally learn to raise the jaw and bulk of the tongue to bring their tongue into contact with the outer borders of the palate, block the air stream for air pressure buildup within the oral cavity, and produce sounds at preferred sites within the oral cavity by listening to and mimicking speech of other talkers. Speech impairments result when talkers are unable to sense accurately what is happening when other talkers speak or what is happening in their own mouths when they attempt to duplicate patterns heard and seen. Impairments are also associated with deficits in central representations of the postures and movements required for articulation; difficulties in translating central representations into appropriate motor commands that govern the use of postures and movements; and disturbances in integrating actions into automatic, dynamic articulatory maneuvers that produce perceptually distinct utterances.

Automaticity is a major goal in speech motor skill development. One of the barriers on the road to development of normal, automatic speech skills is that it is difficult to maintain voluntary attention until skills are mastered. To help lessen that problem and achieve automaticity systematically, a six-step training routine is proposed. The routine includes focused attention, pattern recognition, mental imaging, response rehearsal, and systematic practice as precursors to automatic execution. Verification and evaluation procedures are applied to maintain progress and help prevent slips and lapses in motor skill development. The sequence of steps outlined for motor skill training are appealing because they acknowledge the most salient features of habitual actions. Speech performance becomes an outgrowth of highly practiced, routinized activities.

Erroneous actions usually take the form of automatized behavior that is unsuited for the prevailing intention. In the training routines, repeated performance of specifically modeled, normal motor patterns are used to promote errorless sound production under control of the central motor system. As largely automatic subroutines are developed, they foster actions that are sequenced and timed by the emerging executive programs.

The penalty one pays for attentional deficits is that intended actions may be diverted to errant pathways and produce erroneous responses (Reason, 1984). The resulting errors may be mild, as in slips of the tongue in normal everyday living, or debilitating, as in unintelligible speech resulting from multiple misarticulations. To a large extent, the integrity of a talker's output is a function of the switching system that seeks to regulate the different facets of present, past, and future articulatory events. Errors are therefore identified with specific failures. For example, input failures are traceable to dysfunctions such as misdiscrimination of modeled patterns. Misperceived articulatory features counter movements required to produce intended patterns. In applying the motor skill training routines, attention failures may thus be traced to learners not using imaging and rehearsing activities effectively, or exiting from them prematurely. Execution failures could indicate diversion by learners as they attempt to "spot check" actions in the middle of marginally automatized sequences. Central mode failures might be identified with unintended actions triggered or pre-empted by more familiar, earlier-established routines. It may be evident that such possibilities stem from hypotheses that now seem most probable. Further study is likely to reveal additional hypotheses or rejection of those presented. The key point is that specific classes of errors should be identified with specific hypotheses about causes. Failure to progress should be just as predictable as success.

A number of tests have been devised to identify phonetic processing dysfunctions and disabilities through auditory analyses of spoken words (Goldman & Fristoe, 1969; Kahn & Lewis, 1986; Secord, 1981; Shriberg & Kwiatkowski, 1980). Efforts to develop procedures that can yield parallel data about sensory-motor functions and disabilities are now increasing. Together, such information can potentially provide powerful insight into speech perception, central processing functions and phonological knowledge, and motor skill levels. All three sets of information are essential for accurate diagnosis of articulation disorders and effective treatment planning. Gierut, Elbert, and Dinnsen (1987) and Tyler, Edwards, and Saxman (1990) have provided evidence that articulation knowledge predicts progress in articulation skill development.

The first step in establishing a client's current speech production skill as a function of phonological knowledge is to develop an accurate description of a talker's actual articulation patterns. This requires assessment of vowel and consonant production in a phonetic environment that can be controlled and systematically manipulated. We have found palatometric tests with key sounds repeatedly produced in a carrier sentence to be useful for this purpose. Production of speech in a controlled phonetic environment is required to define central tendencies and variabilities that bear directly on articulation proficiency and disorders. Procedures involved in such testing will now be described in some detail to provide practical examples of how palatometric assessment procedures may be used for diagnosis and treatment planning.

In palatometric tests, a pseudopalate is placed in the client's mouth, and he or she is given at least 20 minutes to adapt to it. During this time the client can be introduced to the procedures involved in the test and instructed concerning the production of key sounds in a standard frame-sentence. A typical vowel testing routine may include repetitions of /i, ɪ, ɛ, æ, ʌ, ɑ, o, ʊ, u, ʒ, eɪ, aɪ, ɔɪ, aʊ/ with each vowel embedded in the frame-sentence "Have a bVb away" (e.g., "Have a beeb away" where V is the /i/vowel). Placing the nuclear vowel between bilabial consonants and schwa vowels effectively isolates it from competing linguapalatal manipulations in the frame-sentence environment. This circumvents the limitations of citation form testing and adds the power of the contextual, connected speech environment to the evaluation of the utterances. Speech pathologists have long realized that interactions occur between connected speech phones that are not found in isolated sound production (Faircloth & Faircloth, 1970).

The use of a standard frame-sentence in speech testing enables precise descriptions to be made about articulation repeatability and variability in sound production and explicit comparisons across sounds. The effects of special coarticulatory demands can also be assessed within a standard frame-sentence environment. The frame-sentence testing procedures are not limited to single sound sampling. For instance, the influence of overlapping and conflicting movements on articulation can be assessed by embedding more than one sound, syllable, or word in a carefully constructed sentence, then examining the differences between the phones in competing versus noncompeting settings. To be specific, the influence of voiceless, front-back and stop-sibilant consonants on [i] sound production could be assessed by embedding the [i] in words such as "pea-peep," "peace-seep," "peak-seep," "keep-peak," and "cease-keek."[1] These articulatory data, along

---

[1]"Keek" is a non-real-word exception. Such words can be used occasionally to illustrate phonetic rules being taught.

with those from nonconflicting phonetic environment tests and listener perceptual scores, could then be used to assess the client's degree of skill in manipulating specific physical parameters to produce phonetic contrast. Such information can help the clinician determine the extent to which each phonetic parameter is incorporated into the client's current phonetic system. Attention can then be directed to isolating specific types and patterns of misarticulation and devising modeling and shaping strategies and routines to overcome those limitations. The aim of the training routines can thus be directed pointedly toward establishing easily and naturally executed articulatory gestures and movements in finely coordinated, rhythmical sequences.

To prepare a client for palatometric data collection, he or she is given a short practice session to familiarize him or her with each sound as it will appear in the spoken sentence. Responses are then evoked at approximately 2.5 sec intervals. The practice should be continued until the client's response timing and articulation patterns are stable. The sentences are then usually elicited in randomized 10-utterance response sets. If the client becomes confused or shifts to a different sound during a set, the responses should be terminated. The subject can then be reinstructed, and the data on that vowel or consonant re-collected. As the responses are elicited, they may be audiotaped as well as palatometrically recorded. The audiotape recording can then be used later to verify clinician phonetic transcriptions and to generate grouped-listener perceptual ratings. For example, sounds identified may be summed across listeners and entered as percentage scores in a confusion matrix from which percentage error patterns and vowel intelligibility ratings may be derived (see Fletcher, 1983, 1990). The audiorecordings are also needed for acoustic analyses which can help document significant but possibly nonperceptible phonetic characteristics that can influence treatment planning and success achieved.[2]

Palatometric data analysis routines have been described by Fletcher (e.g., 1985, 1989a). Briefly, these procedures make use of parallel acoustic intensity, acoustic frequency, and linguapalatal contact displays to identify utterance boundaries and segment the key word from its carrier phrase. The nucleus phonetic element, in this instance the vowel, is then segmented from the word, for example, "beeb." Measures of the minimum, maximum, and mean number of sensors contacted and X-Y plots of the contact patterns may then be extracted from the data using available computer software.

---

[2] For example, Tyler, Edwards, and Saxman (1990) found that a subject with perceptually identical stop consonants but significantly different voice-onset-time (VOT) values progressed significantly more rapidly in developing voice/voiceless contrasts in speech production than two subjects with no VOT pretreatment differences.

The following parameters, illustrated in Figure 7–4, have been found to provide meaningful numerical descriptions of vowel articulation patterns:

1. *Anterior point (AP) of linguapalatal contact.* AP is the most forward sensor contacted at least 50% of the time during each vowel in the 10-utterance sets.
2. *Median row of sensors contacted (MdP).* The MdP identifies the row of sensors within which the linguapalatal contact midpoint occurs across the 10 utterances of each vowel.
3. *Mean contact magnitude (MM).* MM is the average number of sensors contacted. It is calculated from the interval between the vowel acoustic onset and offset, then averaged across the 10 responses for each vowel.
4. *Maximum (MX) and minimum (MN) contact magnitude.* The MX and MN scores represent a pooled average of the frames in which the contact reaches its high (MX) and low (MN) points across each vowel.
5. *Contact movement (Mvmt).* Mvmt is defined as the difference between the maximum and minimum (MX–MN) number of sensors contacted as the vowel is repeated.

As described in Chapter 4, a similar set of data analysis procedures may be used to define consonant production patterns. The ultimate goal is, of course, to use the assessment information to help learners acquire articulation skills. Accurate information can be used to develop new ways to signal differences in verbal meaning and enable the talker to communicate comfortably through intelligible, spontaneous, normal speech. The rest of this chapter will be devoted to detailing how that might be accomplished.

ESTABLISHING BASIC ARTICULATORY GESTURES

Recall that in Chapter 2, six basic properties that contribute toward development of a motor schema were identified. It is rule based, practice motivated, experience expanded, information ordered, reality stored, and temporally differentiated. The first property suggests that a learner will distill rules from perceptual experiences and success in achieving response goals. The use of rules reduces the number of details that must be accessed when a response is activated. The practice-motivation property indicates that progress in motor skill based training may be accelerated by repetitive, carefully constructed routines from which rules may be extracted. The extraction of meaningful information may also be enhanced in training by using mental imagery and rehearsal to create a clear percept of postures and movements needed to differentiate a particular sound from all others. This is done by using demonstrations that illustrate and develop subphonetic articulatory gestures and movement patterns. These patterns can then be transferred later to natural, connected speech contexts. The ultimate goal of articulatory training is to establish articulatory gestures and movements that are executed easily and accurately by the talker in finely coordinated, rhythmical, connected speech patterns.

As indicated in earlier chapters, many of the competencies that underlie the processes of speech articulation development are inborn. Skills normally develop which use these innate competencies in complex articulatory combinations. Normal talkers provide a natural model to activate and stimulate natural speech patterns. New technologies such as palatometry may be used to provide special opportunities to help talkers who are speech impaired become familiar with skills that may not otherwise be easily perceived and mimicked.

The first step in the presently proposed physiological approach to speech remediation is to introduce the client to how the palatometer translates linguapalatal contact information into spatial images. Visual articulatory modeling and mimicry can then be applied to help the learner build a visual/oral spatial map of tongue positions within the oral cavity.

Palatometry uses dynamic pictorial displays combined with clinician and subject evaluations to channel actions toward model-defined articulatory goal postures and movement patterns. This information is supplemented by clinician and client observations, ratings, and evaluations. Success in the speech learning task is judged by accuracy and consistency in mimicking the modeled patterns and by the degree to which the skills gained are transferred to social speaking conditions both inside and outside the clinic.

Two cautionary matters must be considered in the process of using palatometry as a training tool. First, the clinician must be thoroughly familiar with the physiological indices of normal speech production. Feedback is in vain if it is insufficient or, worse, erroneous. Failure consumes resources, including time, and risks negative results. On the other hand, accurately perceived errors can provide one source of change in motivation. Appropriate feedback enhances motivation to overcome misarticulation problems. It also enables variations around a central task to be used meaningfully to test and refine emerging motor control rules. Flexible skills with a broad scope of possible actions develop as rules are verified, applied, and extended, and errors are eliminated. Care in establishing the proper training conditions, in applying motor-skill learning principles, and assessing sources of errors is essential to prevent errors and assure systematic progress in speech articulation skill development.

The second precaution deals with attaining *automatic* speech articulation patterns. When the training has reached the connected speech level of performance, too much conscious monitoring is likely to be detrimental. The learner must use internal feedback to achieve rapid, accurate, and smoothly integrated movements. The motor program must be free to coordinate the key muscle contraction sequences and to balance and time the motor forces involved in the speaking process without being encumbered by the necessity of reporting during the stream of ongoing articulation activities. This is why emphasis is given in the training protocol to delaying analysis and verification of responses until after actions are completed.

The first step in introducing palatometry to a user is to point out that each sensor on the pseudopalate is represented by a small dot on the palatometric video display. The dots are located on the screen in a pattern that mirrors the sensor locations on the person's pseudopalate. The left side of the pseudopalate is represented by dots on the left side of the video screen. When the tongue touches sensors on the pseudopalate, the associated dots on the video screen are expanded or "brightened." The subject's goal is to use the information provided by linguapalatal contact patterns from a normal clinician talker to learn to touch the roof of the mouth with his or her tongue in ways that emulate the normal patterns demonstrated.

TEACHING ORAL MIMICRY
IN SUBPHONETIC GESTURES

Basic articulation skills are established initially in subphonetic tongue postures, gestures, and actions. As these skills are taught in early training sessions, phonetically dictated vowel and consonant postures and movements are defined and developed. This paves the way to establishing desired articulatory competencies in dynamic speech contexts.

The use of subphonetic oral gestures is based on the principle of component learning (see Parker & Fleishman, 1961). The routines introduce the subject to basic linguapalatal contact patterns that reflect tongue height, front-back, and medio-lateral gestural components. This information is used later to develop specific vowel and consonant production skills in speech contexts. Initially the gestures are modeled and mimicked at a slow, methodical movement rate. Later they are accelerated to approximate movements found in normal speech. Extensive and intensive clinician modeling and response shaping are used to build specific speech skills throughout the palatometric routines.

Developing Vowel Production Skills

Vowel production training starts with subphonetic gestures for the [i, æ, u, ɑ] point vowels. These vowels define the extreme vertical and horizontal positions of the tongue within oral space. High-low, front-back, and medio-lateral linguapalatal contact parameters are then added to refine the positional contrasts within oral space. An articulatory feature representation of the nondiphthong American English vowel positions is shown in Table 9–3.

From a linguapalatal contact standpoint, the most basic subphonetic gesture is that of the /i/ vowel. The high-front-tense position required for [i], or [i]-like vowels, is used physiologically as a common referent for all of the other intraoral articulation patterns. It is initially developed in contrast with a low-back-relaxed [ɑ]-like subphonetic gesture. The concept of tongue forwardness and backwardness in [i]-like and [u]-like postures ± lip rounding is then introduced and skill in contrasting production of these postures is established. Control of tongue height is introduced next. This ability is fostered through developing contrasts between [i]−, [ɛ]−, and [æ]-like postures. Control of tongue height leads to control of medio-lateral contact magnitude needed to differentiate the tense/lax [i−ɪ] and [u−ʊ] vowels. Finally, diphthongs, such as [eɪ−aɪ], are taught. These near-neighbor and far-neighbor dipthongs are used to solidify the significant concept of dynamic movement across time in vowel production.

If the client already produces /i/ contrastively with other vowels and a normal linguapalatal contact pattern is evident during its production, palatometrically guided modification of its articulatory pattern would not be necessary. Conversely, if the /i/ is not in the client's repertoire, the initial training goal should be directed toward establishing a subphonetic posture that can yield accurate, consistent, well-timed [i]-like gestures.

TABLE 9–3. Vowel contrasts by tongue contact height (vertical axis), placement (horizontal axis), and medio-lateral magnitude (** = strong, * = medium, no asterisk = no contact). Spread vs. rounded lips and rhotic tongue movements are indicated parenthetically.

| Tongue | Tongue Placement | | |
Height	Front	Mid	Back
High	i** (spread)	ɝ** (rhotic)	u** (round)
	ɪ*	ɚ* (rhotic)	ʊ* (round)
Intermediate	ɛ*	ð	o (round)
Low	æ	ʌ	ɑ

The subphonetic posture for the [i] vowel is introduced by having the client hold the teeth a few millimeters apart, spread the lips widely, then bring the tongue into extensive contact with the lateral and mediolateral surfaces of the pseudopalate. The movement into an [i]-like posture may be demonstrated by having the clinician open his or her mouth widely so the client can see the tongue with its outer edges curled upward in the "spoon-shaped" configuration (described in Chapter 1). The jaw and tongue are then raised to bring the outer borders of the tongue into contact with the pseudopalate. As this is done, the linguapalatal contact will cause dots along the outer edges of the video display to "light up." That is, the dots representing sensors along the outer borders of the pseudopalate are expanded and brightened when the sensors they represent are contacted. In the tongue raising maneuver described, a central channel forms and narrows as the tongue continues to move upward and inward across the palate. The upward movement is continued until a long, rather narrow channel is evident along the central part of the palate. This channel characterizes the [i].[3] The jaw and tongue may then be lowered to demonstrate that as the tongue drops away from the palate, the central channel expands and finally disappears. The action required to bring the tongue into extensive contact with both lateral alveolar shelves of the palate should be repeated several times. As this is done, it should also be pointed out that as the tongue is raised, the contact is first established against the back, outer borders of the palate. It then moves forward and inward from there. The progressive rear-to-front and lateral-to-medial movements help provide support for the tongue as it progresses toward its high, forward, [i]-like vowel posture. This contact support and shaping principle is identified repeatedly in both vowel and consonant phonetic functions during sound production. The clinician should urge the client to watch the display intently as the actions are repeated to gain an accurate impression of just what the movements and ultimate tongue posture should look like when the targeted sound is produced correctly. The clinician should then switch the display to the client's side of the video screen to teach him or her how to mimic the jaw and tongue raising and lowering actions demonstrated. The initial goals in this task are to connect the display with the client's own oral movements and sensations, and, at the same time, develop skill in controlling tongue postures by mimicking specific patterns modeled. Accuracy in mimicking the clinician model patterns should be stressed as the display is switched back and forth between the clinician and the client.

The client's attention should also be directed toward oral sensations that accompany the intentionally contrasted high-front-tense

---

[3]To achieve this pattern, the tongue also must curl a bit more as it is raised upward within the palatal vault.

and low-back-relaxed [i]- and [ɑ]-like tongue postures invoked as the tongue raising and lowering actions are alternated. Formulation of accurate articulatory percepts begins during this period.

As the client mimics the tongue raising and lowering action, the clinician should introduce the concepts of focal attention, mental imagery, and subvocal rehearsal. In introductory comments, the clinician should stress the importance of learning to visualize mentally *exactly* how the normal pattern *looks* on the video screen and how it *feels* inside the mouth when it is mimicked correctly. Practice should then be given in watching, imaging, and rehearsing the oral sensations before any sound is overtly vocalized. Emphasis can then be directed toward executing the response without conscious oversight. This will thus begin the process of developing automatic control of the basic posture and movement patterns in contrasting vowel-like actions.

With the tongue in the high-front-tense position, simply turning on the voice should generate an [i]-like vowel output. Vocalizing with the tongue in the low-back-relaxed non-contact posture should produce a contrasting [ɑ]-like vowel.

As soon as the client has given evidence that he or she is able to mimic high-front-tense [i]-like versus low-back-relaxed [ɑ]-like vowel contrasts, a KR scoring procedure can be introduced. This is done by notifying the learner that one of the major goals in palatometric training is to help him or her learn to mimic tongue postures and actions *exactly*. With older children the scoring may include assigning numerical scores to the client's responses. A 10-point scale is suggested.[4] A score of "10" in this scale would mean that the client has matched the model linguapalatal contact pattern perfectly. A score of "0" would mean that the two patterns have no resemblance, and a "5" would indicate that about half of the contacts in the client's display are the same as those in the clinician's model pattern. The goal is to have all of the responses receive ratings of "9" (very similar to the clinician's model) or "10" (exactly matches the model). After the preliminary explanation of the scoring or rating procedures are given, follow the instructions outlined earlier to produce a set of scored responses.

The second vowel quality to be established stems from learning to position the tongue in a front-to-back continuum along the lateral alveolar shelves on each side of the palate. This quality is demonstrated by starting with the already established high-front-tense tongue posture then sliding the tongue backward along the outer margins of the pseu-

---

[4]Children less than 5 to 6 years old are unlikely to be able to make use of the 10-point performance scaling procedure now described. For them, simple descriptive labels of "OK," "good," or "real good" may be sufficient to set high performance standards and be less confusing to the younger child.

dopalate. As this is done, the lips should be rounded.[5] The tongue movement causes the number of contacted sensors in the palatometric video display to drop systematically. Alternating forward and backward actions can then be modeled, mimicked, and scored. The movements are introduced first with the actions in slow motion. The rate can then be increased to that found in normal speech. Finally, the actions can be demonstrated and practiced at contrasting slow, medium, and fast movement rates.

The tongue-height vowel quality can be uniquely demonstrated through modeling tongue positions for the front vowels [i, ɪ, ɛ, æ]. These vowels form a series with progressively lower jaw positions and less linguapalatal contact.[6] On the display, the contact is seen to drop medio-laterally first, then front-to-back as the subphonetic postures for these vowels are demonstrated and mimicked.

The American English vowel gestures can also be divided into groups by medio-lateral contact magnitude. The magnitude of the contact is closely associated with lingual muscle tenseness and midline tongue height which differentiate the [i-ɪ], [eɪ-ɛ], and [u-ʊ] vowel pairs.[7] Only the higher-contact member of these pairs can occur in stressed, open syllable English words, such as "he," "hay," and "who." The less intensive member must be followed by a syllable-closing consonant, as in "hid," "head," and "hood." Perhaps because of the effort required to produce the more extensive medio-lateral linguapalatal contact, the [i] and [u] vowels have longer durations than their more relaxed counterparts.

Medio-lateral contact magnitude contrasts may be demonstrated in subphonetic gestures by producing a sustained [i]-like pattern then consciously relaxing the tongue to produce an [ɪ]. Similarly, the tense [u] may be produced by moving the tongue into a strongly velarized posture toward the back of the palate and rounding the lips. Con-

---

[5]In the English language all high back vowels are produced with lip rounding. Wolfe and Blocker (1990) described overgeneralization of this principle by certain individuals who had impaired speech. For example, with few exceptions the person they studied produced labial consonants with back vowels and alveolar consonants before front vowels. Similar findings were reported by Grunwell (1981) and Stoel-Gammon (1983).

[6]The acoustic frequency of the first formant (F1) is raised as the space above the tongue and between the teeth is systematically increased across these sounds. The distance between the tongue root and the posterior pharyngeal wall decreases as the tongue is lowered within the oral cavity. This also tends to raise the F1 resonant frequency. On the other hand, pharyngeal constriction increases as the tongue is moved lower within the oral cavity. This increased constriction lowers the F2 frequency. Conversely, the F2 frequency is raised by increasing the front tongue constriction. The F2 frequency is lowered when the constriction is moved back within the oral cavity, as in production of the /u/ vowel.

[7]These three vowel pairs are also distinguished by the tense-lax phonetic feature.

sciously relaxing the lips and tongue results in production of a lax [ʊ]-like vowel. Similar reduction in muscle tension thus allows the tongue to drop and the linguapalatal contact to recede in the second member of the [i-ɪ] and [eɪ-ɛ] vowel pairs.

Tongue actions for the rhotic vowels are similar to those for the rhotic consonants; therefore they will not be discussed at this time. As indicated in the Table 9–3 summary of vowel articulatory features, the other vowels are not differentiated by linguapalatal contact. The [o] is produced with rounded lips, a rather low, back tongue posture, and no linguapalatal contact. The low central [ʌ] is produced by simply relaxing all of the articulators, opening the mouth, and generating the vowel with the tongue in a low, central position within the oral cavity. The jaw opening is about half that of the low front [æ] and low back [ɑ] vowels.

Developing Diphthong Production Skills

Diphthongs are characterized by movement from one vowel-like posture toward another as illustrated in Figure 9–1. For example, in the near-vowel diphthong [eɪ], the action starts from a tongue position near [ɛ] and moves toward one near, but not quite to the [i]. During production of the far-vowel diphthong, [aɪ], the movement starts from a position near the low, back [ɑ] and progresses up and forward to a position near the [i]. Since the terminal position for both of these diphthongs is beyond that of [ɪ], the [i] vowel posture is used as a reference to guide their production. The precise position of the tongue at the termination of the diphthong may be left somewhat fuzzy. This permits attention to be concentrated on the progressive movement, which is the key characteristic of the diphthongal vowels. The starting position for the [ɔɪ] diphthong is that of the [o]. In this instance, the movement modeled also includes a change from rounded- to spread-lip postures. The two remaining American English diphthongs, /aʊ/ and /oʊ/, are produced by movements from low-front and mid-to-low back tongue positions to a posture near but not quite to the /u/. The diphthongs tend to consume about 350 ms during their production; therefore, the movement is more rapid in those diphthongs that have greater distances for the tongue to travel. In connected speech, the movement is less than in isolated sound production, but the characteristic of moving from little or no contact to positions with medium to strong contact is retained.

In the subphonetic modeling and shaping routines, the difference in contact magnitude, or muscle tenseness, is also used to help develop the movement distance and rate concepts. The motor skill modeling, imaging, rehearsing, executing, evaluating, and practicing routines should continue until the client's responses are consistently close to the clinician's.

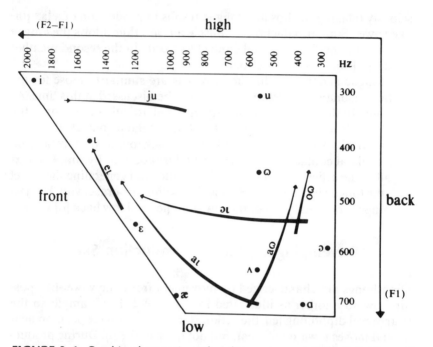

FIGURE 9–1. Combined acoustic and auditory representation of diphthongal movement in some of the American English vowels. (From Ladefoged, P., 1975. *A course in phonetics* [p. 194]. New York: Harcourt Brace Jovanovich. Reprinted with permission.)

Developing Consonant Production Skills

Consonants are differentiated from vowels by where and how the vocal tract is constricted, by frictional noise generated through narrowed passageways, and by the use of voiced versus unvoiced sounds. All vowels are voiced. The glides /w, j, h/ are produced like vowel diphthongs but with more rapid movements. Glides are normally juxtaposed next to the vowels in syllables and words (Clements & Keyser, 1983). This facilitates movement contrast as the actions progress to the more open vowel gestures. The glides are the only consonants that require that they be followed by a vowel. The [j] starts from an [i]-like contact position. The [w] originates from an [u]-like linguapalatal contact position. The [h] has no preparatory posture.

The anterior stop and sibilant articulatory gestures serve as common referents for all of the other intraoral consonant articulation patterns. During production of the intraoral stop consonants /t/ and /k/ and their voiced cognates /d/ and /g/, the air stream is completely blocked by the tongue then abruptly released to produce an explosive noise. The "groove" fricatives /s/ and /ʃ/ are produced by forcing air through a narrow channel formed between the blade of the tongue and the alveolar ridge at its front and rear margins. The turbulent noise from the groove is then amplified in a resonant cavity formed between the tongue and the teeth. This produces a noise with a frequency emphasis above 3500 Hz for /s/ and above 2500 Hz for /ʃ/.

The "slit" fricatives, [θ] (as in "thin") and its voiced cognate [ð] (as in "then"), are produced by channeling a continuous flow of air through a channel formed between the blade of the tongue and the front teeth. The laminar air flow from this slit produces a broad band frictional noise.

The affricates, [tʃ] (as in "chaw") and its voiced cognate [dʒ] (as in "jaw"), are produced by moving the tongue quickly from stop to groove fricative postures. Finally, the sonorants [w, r, l] are produced by routing voiced sound through vowel-like, moving constrictions. All of the consonants except the sonorants have voiced and voiceless cognates.

Contrastive complete versus partial linguapalatal contact around the outer borders of the palate serves as the common referent for stop and sibilant sound production. The *front stop gesture* is demonstrated by placing the upper and lower teeth about 3 mm apart and bringing the tongue into contact with the pseudopalate around its entire outer margins. As the front stop posture is achieved, the display will show brightened points around the entire outer margin of the alveolar ridge. The front stop *movement* is then demonstrated by lowering and raising the tip and blade of the tongue to and from the alveolar ridge at the front of the mouth. This action is facilitated by maintaining lingua-alatal contact along the lateral margins of the pseudopalate. This posture stabilizes the bulk of the tongue and frees movements along its anterior and posterior margins. In other words, the lateral alveolar process and molar teeth are used to anchor the sides of the tongue and free the tip and blade for the precisely articulated movements that follow. After these actions are demonstrated several times, switch to the client's side of the screen to practice the front stop gesture and movement pattern. The role that complete contact around the palatal periphery plays in stop sound production can be illustrated by having the subject feel the burst of air as the blockage is suddenly released to generate the [t] sound.

The *back stop* subphonetic gesture is similar to the front stop except the back of the tongue is raised and lowered to and from the velum and back margin of the palate. The lateral contact also moves back somewhat to stabilize the tongue posture in the back-contact position. To demonstrate this gesture initially, the clinician may wish to open his or her mouth widely with the tongue tip held down so the client can see the back of the tongue. The back of the tongue is then raised slowly to the back of the palate as the action is demonstrated. As this is done, the location and pattern of posterior linguapalatal contact shown in the palatometric display may be pointed out.

The next step in subphonetic training is to introduce the concept that lingual gestures may be facilitated by jaw position, but tongue actions are not totally dependent on jaw support. To do this, the clinician may place an 8- to 10-mm bite-block between the molar teeth then produce front and back linguapalatal stop gestures. As the client mimics this action, he or she learns that both front and back linguapalatal contact can be achieved and released easily at different response rates without changing the jaw position. Note again that as these actions are practiced in alternating movements, the lateral edges of the tongue stay in contact with the sides of the psuedopalate. The scores assigned should rise quickly as these actions are imaged, rehearsed, executed, scored (KR), evaluated (KP), practiced, and stabilized.

The fricatives /s, z, ʃ, ʒ/ and afficates /tʃ, dʒ/ are grouped together as "sibilant" sounds. Sibilants are among the most commonly misarticulated sounds. They are not normally mastered until the elementary school years although children as young as two or three years old may produce them. Sibilants are characterized physiologically by air pressure buildup behind a groove formed between the tongue and the alveolar process. Acceleration of the air particle movement occurs as the phonic stream is forced through the groove. The particle acceleration generates a turbulent air flow which becomes a hissing noise when the air stream strikes the teeth or the major rugae on the back of the alveolar ridge. The hissing noise is then amplified in a small resonance chamber between the tongue and the teeth. During [ʃ] the chamber is usually expanded by lip protrusion. Pressure behind the groove, the cross sectional area of the groove, and the length of the resonant cavity are all used to differentiate the sibilants from other sounds (Fant, 1960; Fletcher & Newman, 1991; Hixon, Minifie, & Tait, 1967; Meyer-Epplar, 1953; Rubin, House, & Stevens, 1955; Shadle, 1985; Stevens, 1971).

The *front groove* subphonetic sibilant-like gesture is taught next. To do this, the clinician should start with the tongue in the front-stop position. The tip of the tongue should then be lowered to produce a 5- to 10-mm groove just behind the upper central incisor teeth. This action is enhanced by maintaining the linguapalatal contact along the outer borders of the pseudopalate except where the groove is formed. The importance of contacting the palate all around its outer border except for the groove can be demonstrated by having the client feel the fine stream of air on the back of his or her hand as it flows through the groove and passes between the teeth and lips. The gesture may then be taught by switching back and forth between the clinician's model and the client's as this basic presibilant subphonetic gesture is watched, imaged, felt, executed, scored (KR), evaluated (KP), practiced, and stabilized. The *back sibilant* gesture can then be introduced.

The back sibilant gesture is taught by reestablishing the front groove posture then drawing the tongue backward until the groove is shifted to the rear margin of the alveolar ridge. When this is done as lateral lingua-palatal contact is maintained, the groove naturally widens to 10- to 15-mm. As the tongue is pulled back, the clinician should also round his or her lips to lengthen the resonant cavity anterior to the groove. Air channeled through this groove will then produce an [ʃ]-like sound for the client to mimic. Alternating the front and back subphonetic groove gestures may be added later to contrast [s]- and [ʃ]-like noise production. Note that as these noises are alternately produced, only the contact along the alveolar ridge changes. The contact along the lateral margins of the palate which stabilizes the tongue action is held essentially constant. By now, the display can usually be switched back and forth between the clinician and the client rather quickly as the subphonetic front and back groove gestures and movements are watched, imaged, felt, executed, scored (KR), evaluated (KP), practiced, and stabilized.

Subphonetic gestures for the remaining consonants are taught as variants of the stop and groove gestures. The preaffricate gesture is, for example, taught by blocking and opening the flow of air through the back alveolar groove. This is done by generating a prolonged [ʃ]-like sound through the groove formed at the rear margin of the alveolar process. The tip of the tongue is then raised to and from the back edge of the alveolar ridge to stop then release air flow through the groove. As this alternating movement becomes more rapid, [tʃ]-like sounds are heard. The action may then be switched back and forth between the clinician and client as repetitive, then isolated [tʃ]-like actions are observed, imaged, rehearsed subvocally, executed without conscious control, scored, evaluated, and practiced. The practice should continue until the [ʃ]-like and [tʃ]-like contrasting sound production patterns are at least partially habituated.

The /r/ sound is produced with a moving tongue action. Its pre-movement posture is established by bringing the tongue into a lateral linguapalatal contact position near that of the [ɛ] vowel. The movement which generates its rhotic sound quality may then be done in two ways. Some speakers curl the tongue tip upward and somewhat backward in a retroflex movement as they produce the sound. This upward, backward flexing tongue movement will actually produce an [r] from any vowel. Other talkers drop the tip down and bunch the tongue as they move the tongue rearward in the mouth to produce the rhotic sound. The special rhotic acoustic effect is the result of active expansion of the resonant cavity formed between the blade and undersurface of the tongue as the tongue is elevated or depressed and slid a bit rearward along the lateral palatal shelves. The amount of backward curl or *retroflexing* varies across speakers and phonetic contexts. The use of the rhotic rather than retroflex label de-emphasizes the notion that the posterior sliding movement must have a strong backward tongue tip curling component.

In an early phase of normal articulation development, children often substitute lip rounding for front tongue actions as the tongue moves backward in attempting rhotic sound production. This results in an [ɛɔ]-like [r]. This possible difficulty may be circumvented in palatometric training by emphasizing the unrounded lip posture as the forepart of the tongue is elevated or depressed during its rearward move.

The sonorant, [l], is also characterized by a moving articulatory action. In this instance the action starts from a preparatory posture with linguapalatal contact all around the periphery of the palate except for a gap along one or both front corners of the alveolar ridge.

The slit fricatives consist of sounds produced when air is channeled through a broad, narrow space between two articulators. The voiceless [f] and voiced [v] labiodental fricatives are visually observable slit fricatives produced by air passing between the lower lip and upper incisor teeth. Their intraoral, linguadental counterparts are the voiceless [θ] and voiced [ð] sounds. They are taught by first placing the tongue in the front stop posture with contact completely around the outer borders of the palate. The tongue is then slid forward until it touches *lightly* against the inner surfaces of the upper incisor teeth. Since sensors are not usually located near the occlusal surfaces of the incisors, the palatometric display may reveal only the contact along the lateral borders of the pseudopalate when the tongue is in this posture. As a flow of air is generated with the tongue in this position, it pushes past the tongue blade and exits through a narrow slit between the tongue and the incisor teeth. The laminar air flow that results can be detected by placing the back of the subject's hand just in front of the lips and feeling the wide, rather delicate flow of air passing through the slit between the tongue and teeth. This air flow produces a broadband frictional noise, which has the least acoustic intensity of all sounds in the English language (Fletcher, 1953). In ordinary speech, the [θ] is barely audible to a normal listener 10 feet away.

Movement Constraints

Languages such as English that allow multiple consonants before or after the vowel in a syllable tend to impose movement constraints to and from the vowel. For example, movements toward the vowel often progress from stop consonants through semi-vowels or liquids before reaching the vowel posture. Movements away from the vowel progress in the reversed order (Clements & Keyser, 1983). When an /r/, or where permissible /l/, is used before a vowel in a consonant cluster, it must be preceded by a stop consonant (as in "price," "tree," "clod"). After the vowel, the order reverses (as in "burp," "hurt," "milk"). This fosters a monotonic movement during both actions opening into the vowel and those closing it into syllable-final consonants (Keating, 1983).

The Utility of Subphonetic Gesture Reviews

A brief subphonetic review period may be used fruitfully at the beginning of each treatment session to reorient the subject to linguapalatal contact positions and movements and refresh familiarity with the palatometric displays. This activity can also be used by the clinician to assess the degree to which fundamental skills are moving toward automatic control. For this last purpose the basic gestures should be presented in a randomized order and the actions judged on a 10-point, closeness-of-fit scale. These scores can then be entered into the clinical log book to maintain a running record of articulatory skill development and response habituation. Modeling should not be used during collection of these data since it would negate their usefulness as a measure of motor skill learning. The session-to-session trend measures may also be used to reveal possible systematic change toward a consistently close fit between modeled and mimicked basic articulatory gestures.

APPLYING ARTICULATORY
SKILL-BUILDING STRATEGIES

You will now be led through a preliminary set of procedures that illustrate how to establish specific articulatory patterns in speech contexts using motor skill building, theory-based palatometric modeling and shaping routines. The training will begin with VC versus CVC maximally contrasting words then progress to other phonetic units. To accentuate contrastive comparisons across sound sequences, the linguapalatal contact patterns are demonstrated without specifically targeted sensor patterns.

The training will start with the two contrasting CVC and VC stimulus words, "beet" and "ahs," produced three times each (e.g., beet ... ahs, beet ... ahs, beet ... ahs). Note that the more physically demanding sibilant gesture is presented in a nonsense word context. In this example, the sibilant gesture is introduced with [ɑ] so it will contrast maximally with linguapalatal contact in "beet." The use of the nonsense word context will allow the learner to extract the targeted sibilant sound perceptually and begin to form rules unhampered by meaning and by previously established speech production habit patterns.[8] Finally, the [s] is set in a word-ending position. This follows the "natural constraint" hierarchy rule that predicts that fricates will be developed most readily in postvocalic positions within syllables. Practice in developing the [s] will be illustrated by following the series of steps outlined in Chapter 6 and described above to provide a general framework for motor skill training.

The first step in the motor-skill development training program is to arouse the learner's attention, identify a focal action location within the planned set of words, and prime the subject for a particular type of response. In the "beet...ahs" example, the initial training goal is to have the subject identify the sibilant groove in contrast with the front stop gesture. In other words, focal attention is directed toward detecting the difference between complete contact around the outer borders of the palate and the groove formed just behind the incisor teeth.

It was pointed out earlier that skill in searching for informational cues is age-related. The defining characteristic of the [s] is a 6- to 8-mm groove formed on the central, front surface of the alveolar ridge. Having the client fix the gaze on this precise location for the [s] in "ahs" will help him or her ignore other movements within the articulatory field. The following monologue, which may be adapted for individual learner and training situations, illustrates instructions that might be used for this purpose:

Focusing

Watch the screen closely (point to upper, central location on the screen where the [s] groove will appear when you say "ahs"). I'm going to show you how the [s] is made in the word "ahs." You will see that it is different from the [t] in "beet." I'll say "beet" first then "ahs" three times. Notice exactly how the points on the screen light up when my tongue touches the palate to make each word.

The clinician should pause briefly between each word in the "beet ...ahs" pairs and a bit longer between each of the pairs in the set. The clinician can also enhance the palatometric contrast by lowering the tongue to remove all linguapalatal contact between the words.

Interspersed modeling and responding should be used to overcome inhibitory reactions in information storage and retrieval during the learning process. Provision for spaced learning in preliminary

---

[8]See Johnson, Goldberg, and Mathers (1984) for a discussion of the merits of possible extended training with nonsense syllables as stimuli.

mental imaging may be built into the routine by using a random-order-ed stimulus word presentation, as in "beet-ahs, ahs-beet, ahs-beet, beet-ahs, ahs-beet, ahs-beet, beet-ahs, beet-ahs, ahs-beet." To solidify the developing articulatory percepts, the subject can be instructed to point to the screen each time the [s] or the [t] sound is produced by the clinician.

Imaging

In mental imagery, the subject is specifically taught to imagine what the tongue must do to capture articulatory contact differences between sounds as actions move into and out of modeled and mimicked iso-lated gestures. The specific goal of mental imagery is a cognitive link-age between imagined and actual actions. This produces increased awareness on the part of the subject of precisely what he or she is to do to achieve stipulated articulatory goals.

Mental imagery in articulatory modeling is based on the principle that all things are created twice, first mentally then physically. A key factor in speech motor imaging is that learners be familiar with the specific motor pattern they intend to replicate. In speech articulatory training, this points to the need to isolate the targeted articulatory ges-ture from other movements.

Imaging instructions are planned to develop an accurate cognitive image of the critical articulatory parameters the subject will be expect-ed to control. For example, the sibilant groove in [s] and the stop posi-tion for [t] are distinguished by a complete versus partial constriction formed around the outer borders of the palate. The unique parameter is presence or absence of a groove in the contact shown just behind the incisors.

In the imaging process, the [s] in "ahs" is tied to the earlier intro-duced subphonetic lingual grooving gesture as its functional role in speech sound production is taught. Instructions for this purpose are il-lustrated in the following monologue:

Now I'm going to say the words "ahs" and "beet" again. During "ahs" you will be able to see how the [s] looks because the tongue doesn't touch the palate during "ah." Notice the groove right here (point to the top, central part of the screen) for the air to pass through for the [s]. During the [t] in "beet," the tongue touches all around the edges of the palate (touch around the outer margins of the sensor display on the video screen). No groove is formed and air can't pass through. Try to form a picture in your mind of exactly what the pattern should look like on the screen for the [s] and for the [t] sounds. Then try to imagine air flowing through the groove for the [s].

Rehearsing

After a mental image of an action is established, touch sensations are coupled with it. The subject is taught to imagine how the sounds should feel inside the mouth as they are formed. In other words, the subject's attention is focused acutely on oral sensations anticipated as the sounds are articulated within a real word. Rehearsal has been shown to become an increasingly effective tool in motor-skill learning as experience in using it accumulates. Movements observed and practiced mentally have been consistently shown to enhance motor performance. The benefits appear to come from insight gained through strategies that arise during the observation and covert practice of the intended action and from an increased desire to achieve specific performance levels that this rehearsal engenders as the anticipated actions are modeled and rehearsed.

Mental rehearsal again emphasizes the need to isolate the specific gestures and movements that must be established in the training. The rehearsal helps the subject translate imagined movements into oral sensations. With more mature subjects these sensations may be formed in connected speech contrasts. Younger subjects may need experience in imaging and rehearsing single-word utterances before they are able to hold more than one pattern in memory long enough for multiple-word comparisons.

A "trial-by-number" system may be used to bind the perceptual and motor facets of sound production together in motor-skill learning. In this procedure a specific number is assigned to subcomponents of the skill-mastery process. The numbers are then used to trigger perceptual and motor functions as the motor-skill subcomponents are systematically presented. The following instructions illustrate the use of focusing, imaging, and rehearsing using numbers to prime the system for maximum performance:

> Now I'll say the number *"1"* then the words "beet" then "ahs" three times each. The number *"1"* will alert you to notice *exactly* how the points on the screen light up when my tongue touches the palate to make each word. Then I'll say the number *"2."* When I do that, close your eyes and try to see an image in your mind of just what the screen should look like in "beet" and in "ahs." When I say *"3"* think about how it should *feel* in your mouth when you actually say "beet" and "ahs," but don't say anything yet. Just concentrate on what the sounds should feel like inside your mouth when you make them correctly.

The time devoted to specific instances of imaging and rehearsing should be kept relatively brief so that the client's attention can be steadily channeled toward the speech production task they are preparing to perform. For most benefit, careful attention needs to be devoted to creating and sustaining clear images and sensations of the anticipated actions.

Executing

Execution refers to the translation of articulation images and movements rehearsed into spatiotemporally coordinated actions driven by the respiratory system. The spoken word is thus treated as a lawful consequence of an integrated series of imaged and rehearsed articulatory gestures and movements that are used to achieve specific phonetic goals. Rules that govern these actions are presumed to be dictated and integrated at the central processing level. The intent is to have the actions become automatic in the sense that they are performed without conscious control.

In our earlier discussion, examples were cited of multitask activities, such as simultaneous talking and knitting, that may be executed in tandem with no evidence of cross interference. These observations suggest that both the preparatory and current facets of a motor response are normally programmed and carried out out at a subconscious, physiological level. In the training, an attempt is therefore made to bypass conscious monitoring as a planned movement is executed. This should allow the motor control program to devote full energy to generating concurrent, intricately interwoven action sequences. The freedom from reporting is instituted to foster a dependable set of automatic articulatory actions. In conversations, this also permits the speaker to focus his or her attention on communicating ideas rather than on the mechanics of respiration, phonation, articulation, and speech timing. The general trends of spoken sequences to become longer with age of the talker and for speech quality to deteriorate with fatigue point to the complex nature of the motor integration task.

Despite the advantages of motor automaticity, the imposition of brief, periodic sensory monitoring seems to be retained throughout life. The discomfort typically felt by talkers following dental anesthetization attests to ongoing use of at least some physiological monitoring during speech. Conversely, the *usual* automatic nature of on-line monitoring is suggested by the difficulty that even trained phoneticians have in localizing sources of disruption when speech errors are made. Undetected slips of the tongue and the comment "I didn't say that" highlight the automatic nature of motor control in natural talking situations. In articulation training, the achievement of automatic speech execution is sought through instructions such as the following:

Now we are going to add another new task. At the count of *"1"* watch closely what happens when I say "beet" then "ahs" three times each. At the count of *"2,"* close your eyes and picture in your mind exactly what appears on the screen as each word is spoken. Focus particularly on the patterns for the [t] and the [s] sounds. At the count of *"3"* rehearse in your mind how it should *feel* in your mouth when you say each word, but don't say anything yet. Rehearse especially the differences in how the [t] and [s] should feel when they are spoken correctly. At the count of *"4"* say "beet" then "ahs" three times each. Don't think about what is happening inside your mouth this time. Just watch the patterns on the screen and notice how close they are to the patterns when I say them.

Verifying

Verifying focuses on evaluating changes in targeted articulation patterns and judging progress toward preset goals and standards of performance. In the process of try-assess-revise-try again, verification plays a central role in maintaining progress and assessing the extent to which training objectives are being met. Learners distribute their efforts in proportion to the rewards offered through successful achievement. In a real sense, appropriate and accurate modeling, valid mimickry, authentic rehearsal, and effective reinforcement of successful responses are all verified by the output accuracy. Successful actions are likely to be repeated.

Feedback is used to inform the subject of the response accuracy. It includes both personal, internalized spatial and tactile-kinesthetic biofeedback and clinician- and instrument-provided augmental feedback. Augmental feedback must be linked closely with response contingent consequences used to enhance performance. Experimental studies have repeatedly shown that the more accurate and meaningful the feedback and reinforcement of positive change, the more rapid and predictable is the progress toward goal driven behaviors. Feedback and response contingent reinforcement are thus natural extensions of verification. "Success" is largely dictated by the combined quality of the biofeedback and augmented feedback available to the learner. For maximum progress, feedback must be connected with hard, specific goals.

In motor-skill training, feedback is particularly helpful in monitoring and evaluating performance attributes that a person is normally unable to sense accurately. Much of this inability may be an outgrowth of inexperience in sensing particular properties of his or her responses. One of the most important aspects of speech articulation training is thus bringing information such as the place and patterns of linguapalatal contact into a learner's sensory field. This is done by providing accurate, timely instrumental displays and clinician originated quantitative knowledge of results (KR) and qualitative knowledge of performance (KP) assessments to augment the person's own biofeedback evaluations. The following instructions provide an example of how this might be done.

Now I'm going to teach you how to judge your success in learning how to say words correctly. At the count of *"1"* watch exactly what happens when I say "beet" then "ahs" three times each. At the count of *"2,"* close your eyes and picture in your mind what you saw on the video screen. At the count of *"3"* rehearse in your mind how it should *feel* in your mouth when you actually say the words, but don't say anything out loud. Just rehearse what it should feel like as you say each word. At the count of *"4"* say the words three times each. Don't think about what is happening inside your mouth as you say them though. Just watch the pattern on the screen and try to make the words so they are closer to my model each time you say them. At the count of *"5,"* we will judge how well you did in matching my model. If the patterns are *exactly* like mine, we will give you a "10." If they look almost like mine, we will give you an "8" or a "9." If one word is right on target but the other word isn't, the score will be about "5." If neither word is close, the score should be "2" or "3." After we have assigned scores, I'll replay both patterns so we see just how close my pattern and yours match. We will also decide what needs to be changed to improve. The goal is to have all "10"s. You should try for a "10" every time you imitate what I say.

After the subject has followed the motor skill training protocol and received the KR feedback information, review the dynamic articulation patterns in slow motion and stop frame displays to provide knowledge of performance (KP) information. After this preliminary review, return to the normal display mode and repeat the same procedures as you rotate back and forth between your modeled and his or her mimicked productions of the words. Continue doing this until the subject produces at least three response sets (18 consecutive words) with each utterance having an 8 or higher rating and performance that is very similar to the modeled pattern. As soon as that level of competency is achieved, the words should be elicited in short phrase contexts to encourage their generalization to natural speech.

After the targeted groove fricative versus labial stop gestures are consistently produced correctly in the VC and CVC syllables, you can introduce a new set of stimulus words. For example, paired CV and CVC words such as "moose ... bee, seem ... bub, boss ... moo, Sue ... Bob" could be used. In this set the targeted [s] consonant is in maximally contrastive point vowel and voiced labial stop phonetic environments. The stimuli need not always be single contrastive words. A set of words in a phrase like "I ... buy ... my ... pie" could be used to develop a diphthong-like [aɪ] in a connected speech context.

It is important that as each set of new words is introduced, a record be made of the client's pretreatment production patterns. After that has been done and the data stored as baseline patterns, the words should then be modeled in real time and a set of similar responses elicited from the subject with a brief pause between each word. These data should be stored as a record of the client's pretraining mimicry skills. These responses can then be reviewed with the subject in slow motion and stop frame displays to ascertain the status of critical articulatory properties such as contact sequences, positions, and linguapalatal contact shapes as the articulatory actions move into and out of the modeled target consonant postures. Then return to the normal display mode and again rotate back and forth between your modeled and the subject mimicked productions of the new stimuli, again following the motor skill modeling and shaping procedures. Practice should continue until both the clinician and the client assign ratings of 8 or higher to the responses and the KP evaluations indicate that both the contact patterns and timing are "very close" to the pattern modeled for all consonants and vowels across the response sets (16 consecutive words in the exemplary set of CV and CVC words listed).

The training could then move to another set of CV and/or CVC words or move to a new set of paired word combinations with CVCV maximal consonant and high-low vowel contrasts (e.g., peace-so ... so-bee, bossy ... see-boss, bass-sue ... sue-bass). The general speech training goal is phonetic mastery. Phonetic mastery means that the information is accessed rapidly and efficiently in speech contexts whether or not the articulation patterns have been established class by class. The importance of speed and accuracy in achieving targeted phonetic postures becomes increasingly evident as talkers progress from isolated sounds to words in connected speech contexts where actions "downstream" are anticipated and articulatory adjustments built into the speech production system. In this process, articulatory boundaries and end point postures become blurred, and extreme postures within the vocal tract are smoothed as combined, rapidly moving gestures are partially overlapped during their execution.

As mastery of articulation patterns in isolated words is evidenced, the skills should be transferred to short phrases that contrast the articulatory patterns and clarify sound-to-sound movements. It should be emphasized that the particular sounds and sound sequences in the training routines described are to be considered only illustrative. Actual choices concerning sounds to be treated and treatment scheduling must be made on the basis of individual articulation skills and proficiencies. The ultimate goal is intelligible, connected speech performance. This goal may not be fully realizable for particular speech impaired individuals.

Words or word-like syllables should be used in all palatometric training beyond the subphonetic articulatory gestural level. A beginning phonetic repertoire can be built by contrasting the subphonetic gestures in random ordered responses during articulatory drill. The articulatory percepts and skills can then be systematically introduced into words which contain sounds in contrastive phonetic contexts then generalized in phrase and natural speech contexts. Varied practice and phonetic content must be emphasized throughout the training routines. As palatometric procedures are used to accomplish each of the goals outlined, finer and finer lingual motor control should likewise be expected.

In Chapter 3 it was observed that massed practice techniques may yield superior results in isolated articulatory skill training designed to establish a particular gesture. Conversely, if a series of gestures are planned in naturally repeating articulatory movements during connected speech, then spaced practice will likely yield better and longer lasting results than massed practice.

Rest periods between trials are also important in motor-skill training. These periods do not require total inactivity, however. Rather, a rest interval can be provided simply by switching activities. For instance, in an articulation training task, the procedures could switch back and forth from connected speech to isolated sound drill as production of a particular articulatory gesture is established, refined and habitualized. In this example, "rest" simply means "diversion," and diversion may be achieved by introducing a different, nonconflicting articulatory task.

Another question is whether to practice an articulatory skill broken down into its component parts or to practice it in its entirety. The answer to this question depends on the nature of the task. In practicing isolated sounds where the gestures include different, critically related, highly integrated movements the *whole model* will likely be the better choice.

REFERENCES

Abd-El-Malek, S. (1939). Observations of the morphology of the human tongue. *Journal of Anatomy, 73,* 201–310.

Adams, J. A. (1971). A closed-loop theory of motor learning. *Journal of Motor Behavior, 3,* 111–150.

Adams, J. A. (1987). Historical review and appraisal of research on the learning, retention, and transfer of human motor skills. *Psychological Bulletin, 101,* 41–74.

Allen, G. L. (1972). The location of rhythmic stress beats in English: An experimental study I. *Language & Speech, 15,* 72–100.

Allen, G. L. (1985). Strengthening weak links in the study of the development of macrospatial cognition. In R. Cohen (Ed.), *The development of spatial cognition* (pp. 301–321). Hillsdale, NJ: Lawrence Erlbaum.

Andersen, R. A., Essick, G. K., & Siegel, R. M. (1985). Encoding of spatial location by posterior parietal neurons. *Science, 230,* 456–458.

Anderson, S. R. (1974). *The organization of phonology.* San Diego, CA: Academic Press.

Art, J., & Fettiplace, R. (1984). Efferent desensitization of auditory nerve fibre responses in the cochlea of the turtle *Pseudemys Scripta Elegans. Journal of Physiology, 356,* 507–523.

Atkinson, J. W. (1977). Motivation for achievement. In T. Blass (Ed.), *Personality variables in social behavior* (pp. 25–108). Hillsdale, NJ: Lawrence Erlbaum.

Baer, D. M. (1981). *How to plan for generalization.* Austin, TX: Pro-Ed.

Baer, T., Gore, J. C., Boyce, S., & Nye, P. W. (1987). Application of MRI to the analysis of speech production. *Magnetic Resonance Imaging, 5,* 1–7.

Bandura, A. (1969). *Principles of behavior modification.* New York: Holt, Rinehart & Winston.

Bandura, A. (1971). Vicarious- and self-reinforcement processes. In R. Glaser (Ed.), *The nature of reinforcement* (pp. 228–278). New York: Academic Press.

Bandura, A. (1986). *Social foundations of thought and action: A social cognitive theory.* Englewood Cliffs, NJ: Prentice-Hall.

Bandura, A., & Cervone, D. (1986). Differential engagement of self-reactive influences in cognitive motivation. *Organizational Behavior and Human Decision Processes, 38,* 92–113.

Baptista, L. F. (1975). Song dialects and demes in sedentary populations of the white-crowned sparrow (*Zonotrichia leucophryx nuttalli*). *University of California Publications in Zoology, 105*, 1–52.

Baptista, L. F., & Petrinovich, L. (1984). Social interaction, sensitive phases and the song template hypothesis in the white-crowned sparrow. *Animal Behaviour, 32*, 172–181.

Bartlett, F. C. (1932). *Remembering*. Cambridge, England: Cambridge University Press.

Bartlett, F. C. (1947). The measurement of human skill. *British Medical Journal, 1*, 835–838, 877–880. Reprinted in *Occupational Psychology*, (1948) *22*, 31–38, 83–91.

Bartley, S. H., & Chute, E. (1947). *Fatigue and impairment in man*. New York: McGraw-Hill.

Basmajian, J. V. (Ed.). (1979). *Biofeedback: Principles and practice for clinicians*. Baltimore, MD: Williams & Wilkins.

Beaubaton, D., & Hay, L. (1986). Contribution of visual information to feedforward and feedback processes in rapid pointing movements. *Human Movement Science, 5*, 19–34.

Bell-Berti, F., & Harris, K. S. (1981). A temporal model of speech production. *Phonetica, 38*, 9–20.

Bellezza, F. S. (1982). *Improve your memory skills*. Englewood Cliffs, NJ: Prentice-Hall.

Bellezza, F. S. (1983). Recalling script-based text: The role of selective processing and schematic cues. *Bulletin of the Psychonomic Society, 21*, 267–270.

Bellezza, F. S. (1987). Mnemonic devices and memory schemas. In M. A. McDaniel & M. Pressley (Eds.), *Imagery and related mnemonic processes* (pp. 34–55). New York: Springer-Verlag.

Berger, S. M. (1977). Social comparison, modeling, and perseverance. In J. M. Suls & R. L. Miller (Eds.), *Social comparison processes: Theoretical and empirical perspectives* (pp. 209–234). Washington, DC: Hemisphere.

Bernstein, N. (1967). *The coordination and regulation of movements*. New York: Pergamon Press.

Bernthal, J. E., & Bankson, N. W. (1988). *Articulation and phonological disorders*. Englewood Cliffs, NJ: Prentice-Hall.

Berry, J. K. (1971). *A study of lingual-palatal contacts during the production of selected consonant sounds*. Unpublished master's thesis, University of New Mexico, Albuquerque.

Berthoz, A., & Pozzo, T. (1988). Intermittent head stabilization during postural and locomotory tasks in humans. In B. Amblard, A. Berthoz, & F. Clarac (Eds.), *Posture and gait: Development, adaptation, and modulation* (pp. 189–206). Amsterdam, The Netherlands: Elsevier.

Bickley, C. (1984). Acoustic evidence for phonological development of vowels in young children. *MIT RLE Speech Group Working Papers, 4*, 111–124.

Bickley, C. (1986). Comment on C. A. Ferguson's paper on discovering sound units. In J. S. Perkell & D. H. Klatt (Eds.), *Invariance and variability in speech processes* (pp. 54–57). Hillsdale, NJ: Lawrence Erlbaum.

Biederman, I. (1986). Recognition by components: A theory of visual pattern recognition. *The Psychology of Learning and Motivation, 20*, 1–54.

Bilodeau, E. A., & Bilodeau, I. McD. (1961). Motor skills learning. In P. Farnsworth (Ed.), *Annual Review of Psychology,* 243–280, Palo Alto, CA: Annual Reviews.

Bindra, D. (1968). Neuropsychological interpretation of the effects of drive and incentive-motivation on general activity and instrumental behavior. *Psychological Review, 75,* 1–22.

Binford, T. (1971). *Visual perception by computer.* Paper presented at IEEE Conference on Systems and Control, Miami, FL.

Binford, T. (1981). Inferring surfaces from images. *Artificial Intelligence, 17,* 205–244.

Bjerner, B. (1949). Alpha depression and lowered pulse rate during delayed actions in a serial reaction test. *Acta Physiologica Scandinavica, 19* (Suppl. 65).

Blesser, B. A. (1969). *Perception of spectrally rotated speech.* Doctoral dissertation, Massachusetts Institute of Technology, Cambridge.

Bloomer, H. H. (1943). A palatopograph for contour mapping of the palate. *Journal of the American Dental Association, 30,* 1053–1057.

Boden, M. A. (1990). *The creative mind. Myths and mechanisms.* London: George Weidenfeld and Nicolson Ltd.

Bolinger, D. (1958). A theory of pitch accent in English. *Word, 14,* 104–149.

Bolles, R. C. (1970). Species-specific defense reactions and avoidance learning. *Psychological Review, 77,* 32–48.

Borden, G. J., & Harris, K. S. (1984). *Speech science primer. Physiology, acoustics, and perception of speech.* Baltimore, MD: Williams & Wilkins.

Bosma, J. F., Truby, H. M., & Lind, J. (1965). Cry motions of the newborn infant. *Acta Paediatrica Scandinavica,* (Suppl. 163), 61–92.

Bowman, J. P. (1968). Muscle spindles in the intrinsic and extrinsic muscles of the rhesus monkey's *(macaca mulatta)* tongue. *Anatomical Record, 161,* 483–487.

Bowman, J. P. (1971). *The muscle spindle and neural control of the tongue. Implications for speech.* Springfield, IL: Charles C. Thomas.

Bowman, J. P., & Combs, C. M. (1969). The cerebrocortical projection of hypoglossal afferents. *Experimental Neurology, 23,* 291–301.

Brodie, A. G. (1941). On the growth pattern of the human head from the third month to the eighth year of life. *American Journal of Anatomy, 68,* 209–262.

Brooks, V. (1983). Motor control: How posture and movements are governed. *Physical Therapy, 63,* 664–673.

Browman, C. P., & Goldstein, L. (1987). Tiers in articulatory phonology, with some implications for casual speech. In *Status report on speech research, SR-92* (pp. 1–30). New Haven, CT: Haskins Laboratory.

Browman, C. P., & Goldstein, L. (1989). Gestural structures and phonological patterns. In *Status report on speech research, SR-97/98* (pp. 1–23). New Haven, CT: Haskins Laboratory.

Brown, R. (1958). *Words and things.* Glencoe, IL: Free Press.

Bruner, J. (1964). The course of cognitive growth. *American Psychologist, 19,* 1–15.

Bruner, J. M. R. (1967). Hazards of electrical apparatus. *Anesthesiology, 28,* 396–425.

Burton, R. (1985). *Bird behavior.* New York: Alfred A. Knopf.

Butcher, A., & Weiher, E. (1976). An electropalatographic investigation of coarticulation in VCV sequences. *Journal of Phonetics, 4,* 59–74.

Campbell, T. F., & Keegan, J. F. (1987). A primary-secondary task paradigm for estimating processing capacity during speech production: Some preliminary data. *Psychological Reports, 60,* 1279-1286.

Carlson, B. M. (1988). *Patten's foundation of embryology* (5th ed.). New York: McGraw-Hill.

Carlson, R., Erikson, Y., Granstrom, B., Lindblom, B., & Rapp, K. (1975). Neutral and emphatic stress patterns in Swedish. In G. Fant (Ed.), *Proceedings of the Speech Communication Seminar, 2,* (pp. 209-218). Stockholm: Almqvist & Wiksell.

Carnahan, H., & Lee, T. D. (1989). Training for transfer of a movement timing skill. *Journal of Motor Behavior, 21,* 48-59.

Carron, A. V. (1969). Performance and learning in a discrete motor task under massed vs. distributed practice. *Research Quarterly, 40,* 481-489.

Carron, A. V. (1980). *Social psychology of sport.* Ithaca, NY: Mouvement Publications.

Chafe, W. (1968). *English questions.* PEGS Paper No. 26. Washington, DC: Center for Applied Linguistics.

Chase, W., & Ericsson, K. (1982). Skill and working memory. In G. Bower (Ed.), *The psychology of learning and motivation, Vol. 116* (pp. 1-58). New York: Academic Press.

Chi, M. T. H., & Glaser, R. (1980). The measurement of expertise: Analysis of the development of knowledge and skill as a basis for assessing achievement. In E. L. Baker & E. S. Quellmely (Eds.), *Educational testing and evaluation* (pp. 37-47). Beverly Hills, CA: Sage.

Christensen, J. M., Fletcher, S. G., Hasegawa, A., & McCutcheon, M. J. (in press). Esophageal speaker articulation of /s,z/: A dynamic palatometric assessment. *Journal of Communication Disorders.*

Chuang, C. K., & Wang, W. S. (1978). Use of optical distance sensing to track tongue motion. *Journal of Speech and Hearing Research, 21,* 482-496.

Clark, J. E. (1982). The role of response mechanisms in motor skill development. In J. A. S. Kelso & J. E. Clark (Eds.), *The development of movement control and co-ordination* (pp. 151-173). New York: John Wiley.

Clark, J. M., & Paivio, A. (1987). A dual coding perspective on encoding processes. In M. A. McDaniel & M. Pressley (Eds.), *Imagery and related mnemonic processes* (pp. 5-33). New York: Springer-Verlag.

Clements, G. N., & Keyser, S. J. (1983). *CV phonology: A generative theory of the syllable.* Cambridge, MA: MIT Press.

Cochran, R. (1977). *The acquisition of /r/ and /l/ by Japanese children and adults learning English as a second language.* Unpublished doctoral dissertation, University of Connecticut, Storrs.

Coleman, C. (1974). *A study of acoustical and perceptual attributes of isochrony in spoken English.* Doctoral dissertation, University of Washington, Seattle.

Coles, J. O. (1872a). A plan for ascertaining more accurately the physiology of speech. *Transactions of the Odontological Society of Great Britain, 4,* 189-217.

Coles, J. O. (1872b). On the production of articulate sound (speech). *Transactions of the Odontological Society of Great Britain, 4,* 110-124.

Colgan, P. (1989). *Animal motivation.* London: Chapman and Hall.

Condon, W. S., & Sander, L. W. (1974). Synchrony demonstrated between movement of the neonate and adult speech. *Child Development, 45,* 456-462.

Cooper, S. (1953). Muscle spindles in the intrinsic muscles of the human tongue. *Journal of Physiology, 122,* 193–202.

Costello, J. (1983). Generalization across settings: Language intervention with children. In J. Miller, D. Yoder, & R. Schiefelbusch (Eds.), *Contemporary issues in language intervention, ASHA Reports 12* (pp. 275–297). Rockville, MD: American Speech-Language-Hearing Association.

Crawford, A. (1961). Fatigue and driving. *Ergonomics, 4,* 143–154.

Crystal, D. (1973). Intonation and linguistic theory. In K.-H. Dahlstedt (Ed.), *The Nordic languages and modern linguistics* (pp. 267–303). Stockholm: Almqvist & Wiksell.

Crystal, D. (1980). The analysis of nuclear tones. In L. R. Waugh & C. H. van Schooneveld (Eds.), *The melody of language. Intonation and prosody* (pp. 55–70). Baltimore, MD: University Park Press.

Crystal, T. H., & House, A. S. (1988). The duration of American-English vowels: An overview. *Journal of Phonetics, 16,* 263–284.

Cutler, A. (1987). Speaking for listening. In A. Allport, D. MacKay, W. Prinz, & E. Scheerer (Eds.), *Language perception and production. Relationships between listening, speaking, reading, and writing* (pp. 23–40). London: Academic Press.

Cutler, A., & Isard, S. D. (1980). The production of prosody. In B. Butterworth (Ed.), *Language production* (pp. 245–269). London: Academic Press.

Dam, H. J. W. (1896). The new marvel in photography. *McClure's Magazine, 6,* 402–413.

Daniloff, R. G., & Hammarberg, R. E. (1973). On defining coarticulation. *Journal of Phonetics, 1,* 239–248.

Darwin, C. J. (1975). On the dynamic use of prosody in speech perception. In *Status report on speech research, SR-42/43* (pp. 103–115). New Haven, CT: Haskins Laboratory.

Davis, P. J., & Nail, B. S. (1988). The sensitivity of laryngeal epithelial receptors to static and dynamic forms of mechanical stimulation. In O. Fujimura (Ed.), *Vocal physiology: Voice production. Mechanisms and functions* (pp. 1–18). New York: Raven.

Denny-Brown, D. (1960). The general principles of motor integration. In H. W. Magoun (Ed.), *Handbook of physiology. Volume 2. Section I: Neurophysiology* (p. 393). Baltimore, MD: Williams & Wilkins.

Dickinson, J. (1978). Retention of intentional and incidental motor learning. *Research Quarterly. 49,* 437–441.

Dinnsen, D. A., Chin, S. B., Elbert, M., & Powell, T. W. (1990). Some constraints on functionally disordered phonologies: Phonetic inventories and phonotactics. *Journal of Speech and Hearing Research, 33,* 28–37.

Dinnsen, D. A., & Elbert, M. (1984). On the relationship between phonology and learning. In M. Elbert, D. Dinnsen, & G. Weismer (Eds.), *Phonological theory and the misarticulating child, ASHA Monographs, 22,* 59–68.

Disner, S. F. (1984). Insights on vowel spacing. In I. Maddieson (Ed.), *Patterns of sounds* (pp. 136–155). Cambridge, England: Cambridge University Press.

Dooling, R. J. (1989). Perception of complex, species-specific vocalizations by birds and humans. In R. J. Dooling & S. Hulse (Eds.), *The comparative psychology of audition* (pp. 423–444). Hillsdale, NJ: Lawrence Erlbaum.

Duncan, J. (1985). Visual search and visual attention. In M. I. Posner & O. S. M. Marin (Eds.), *Attention and performance XI* (pp. 85–105). Hillsdale, NJ: Lawrence Erlbaum.

Dyson, A. T. (1988). Phonetic inventories of 2- and 3-year old children. *Journal of Speech and Hearing Disorders, 53,* 89–93.

Earley, P. C., & Lituchy, T. R. (1991). Delineating goal and efficacy effects: A test of three models. *Journal of Applied Psychology, 76,* 81–98.

Easton, E. J., & Powers, J. A. (1986). *Musculoskeletal magnetic resonance imaging.* Thorofare, NJ: Slack.

Easton, T. A. (1972). On the normal use of reflexes. *American Scientist, 60,* 591–599.

Elbers, L. (1982). Operating principles in repetitive babbling: A cognitive continuity approach. *Cognition, 12,* 45–63.

Elbert, M., Dinnsen, D. A., & Powell, T. W. (1984). On the prediction of phonologic generalization learning patterns. *Journal of Speech and Hearing Disorders. 49,* 309–317.

Elkind, D., Koegler, R., & Go, E. (1964). Studies in perceptual development. Volume II. Part-whole perception. *Child Development, 35,* 81–90.

Ericsson, K. A., & Simon, H. A. (1984). *Verbal protocol analysis.* Cambridge, MA: MIT Press.

Estes, W. K. (1971). Reward in human learning: Theoretical issues and strategic choice points. In R. Glaser (Ed.), *The nature of reinforcement* (pp. 16–44). New York: Academic Press.

Fairbanks, G. (1960). *Voice and articulation drillbook* (2nd ed.). New York: Harper & Row.

Faircloth, M. A., & Faircloth, S. R. (1970). An analysis of the articulatory behavior of a speech defective child in connected speech and in isolated-word responses. *Journal of Speech and Hearing Disorders, 35,* 51–61.

Fant, G. (1960). *Acoustic theory of speech production.* The Hague, The Netherlands: Mouton.

Fantz, R. L. (1965). Visual perception from birth as shown by pattern selectivity. *Annals of the New York Academy of Science, 118,* 793–814.

Farnetani, E., & Kori, S. (1986). Effects of syllable and word structure on segmental duration in spoken Italian. *Speech Communication, 5,* 17–34.

Farnetani, E., Vagges, K., & Magno-Caldognetto, E. (1985). Coarticulation in Italian /VtV/ sequences: A palatographic study. *Phonetica, 42,* 78–99.

Faure, G., Hirst, D. J., & Chafcouloff, M. (1980). Rhythm in English: Isochronism, pitch, and perceived stress. In L. R. Waugh & C. H. van Schooneveld (Eds.), *The melody of language* (pp. 71–79). Baltimore, MD: University Park Press.

Feltz, D. L. & Landers, D. M. (1983). The effects of mental practice on motor skill learning and performance: A meta-analysis. *Journal of Sport Psychology, 5,* 25–57.

Ferguson, C. A. (1963). Assumptions about nasals: A sample study in phonological universals. In J. H. Greenberg (Ed.), *Universals of language* (pp. 53–60). Cambridge, MA: M.I.T. Press.

Ferguson, C. A. (1978). Phonological processes. In J. H. Greenberg (Ed.), *Universals of human language, Volume 2. Phonology* (pp. 403–442). Stanford, CA: Stanford University Press.

Ferguson, C. A. (1986). Discovering sound units and constructing sound systems: It's child play. In J. S. Perkell & D. H. Klatt (Eds.), *Invariance and variability in speech processes* (pp. 36–53). Hillsdale, NJ: Lawrence Erlbaum.

Ferguson, C. A., & Farwell, C. (1975). Words and sounds in early language acquisition. *Language, 51,* 418–439.

Fey, M. E. (1989). Describing developing phonological systems: A response to Gierut. *Applied Psycholinguistics, 10,* 455–467.

Field, T. M., Woodson, R., Greenberg, R., & Cohen, D. (1982). Discrimination and imitation of facial expressions by neonates. *Science, 218,* 179–181.

Findlay, A. (1965). *A hundred years of chemistry.* London: Duckworth.

Fischer, K. W., & Hogan, A. (1989). The big picture for infant development: Levels and sources of variation. In J. Lockman & N. Hazen (Eds.), *Action in social context: Perspectives on early development* (pp. 275–305). New York: Plenum.

Fitts, P. M. (1964). Perceptual-motor skill learning. In A. W. Melton (Ed.), *Categories of human learning* (pp. 243–285). New York: Academic Press.

Fitzgerald, M. J. T., & Alexander, R. W. (1969). The intramuscular ganglia of the tongue. *Journal of Anatomy, 104,* 587.

Flege, J. E. (1976). Plasticity in adult and child speech production. *Journal of the Acoustical Society of America, 79,* S54.

Flege, J. E. (1987). A critical period for learning to pronounce foreign languages? *Applied Linguistics, 8,* 162–177.

Flege, J. E., Fletcher, S. G., & Homiedan, A., (1987). Compensating for a bite block in /s/ and /t/ production: Palatographic, acoustic, and perceptual data. *Journal of the Acoustical Society of America, 83,* 212–228.

Fletcher, H. (1953). *Speech and hearing in communication.* Princeton, NJ: Van Nostrand.

Fletcher, S. G. (1962). Speech as an element in organization of a motor response. *Journal of Speech and Hearing Research, 5,* 292–300.

Fletcher, S. G. (1966). Cleft palate: A broader view. *Journal of Speech and Hearing Disorders, 31,* 1–13.

Fletcher, S. G. (1970). Processes and maturation of mastication and deglutition. *ASHA Report No. 5* (pp. 92–105). Rockville, MD: American Speech and Hearing Association.

Fletcher, S. G. (1973). Maturation of the speech mechanism. *Folia Phoniatrica, 25,* 161–172.

Fletcher, S. G. (1974). *Tongue thrust in swallowing and speaking.* Austin, TX: Learning Concepts.

Fletcher, S. G. (1982). Seeing speech in real time. *IEEE spectrum, 19,* 42–45.

Fletcher, S. G. (1983a). Dynamic orometrics: A computer-based means of learning about and developing speech by deaf children. *American Annals of the Deaf, 128,* 525–534.

Fletcher, S. G. (1983b). New prospects for speech by the hearing impaired. In N. J. Lass (Ed.). *Speech and language: Advances in basic research and practice, Volume 9* (pp. 1–41). New York: Academic Press.

Fletcher, S. G. (1985). Speech production and oral motor skill in an adult with an unrepaired palatal cleft. *Journal of Speech and Hearing Disorders, 50,* 254–261.

Fletcher, S. G. (1988). Speech production following partial glossectomy. *Journal of Speech and Hearing Disorders, 53,* 232–238.

Fletcher, S. G. (1989a). Palatometric specification of stop, affricate, and sibilant sounds. *Journal of Speech and Hearing Research, 32,* 736–748.

Fletcher, S. G. (1989b). Glossometric measurement in vowel production and modification. *Clinical Linguistics & Phonetics, 3,* 359–375.

Fletcher, S. G. (1989c). Visual articulatory training through dynamic orometry. *The Volta Review, 91,* 47–64.

Fletcher, S. G. (1990). Recognition of words from palatometric displays. *Clinical Linguistics & Phonetics, 4,* 9–24.

Fletcher, S. G. (under review, a). *Linguapalatal contact in vowels.*

Fletcher, S. G. (under review, b). *Speech adaptation and compensation in oncology.*

Fletcher, S. G. (under review, c). *Tongue and jaw position in vowel production and perception.*

Fletcher, S. G., Dagenais, P. A., & Critz-Crosby, P. C. (1991a). Teaching vowels to profoundly hearing-impaired speakers using glossometry. *Journal of Speech and Hearing Research, 34,* 943–956.

Fletcher, S. G., Dagenais, P. A., & Critz-Crosby, P. C. (1991b). Teaching consonants to profoundly hearing-impaired speakers using palatometry. *Journal of Speech and Hearing Research, 34,* 929–942.

Fletcher, S. G., & Hasegawa, A. (1983). Speech modification by a deaf child through dynamic orometric modeling and feedback. *Journal of Speech and Hearing Disorders, 48,* 178–185.

Fletcher, S. G., Hasegawa, A., McCutcheon, M. J., & Gilliom, J. D. (1980). Use of lingual contact patterns to modify articulation in a deaf adult. In D. L. McPherson & M. Schwab (Eds.), *Advances in prosthetic devices for the deaf: A technical workshop* (pp. 127–133). Rochester, NY: National Technical Institute for the Deaf.

Fletcher, S. G., McCutcheon, M. J., Smith, S. C., & Smith, W. H. (1989). Glossometric measurements in vowel production and modification. *Clinical Linguistics & Phonetics, 3,* 359–375.

Fletcher, S. G., McCutcheon, M. J., & Wolf, M. B. (1975). Dynamic palatometry. *Journal of Speech and Hearing Research, 18,* 812–819.

Fletcher, S. G., McCutcheon, M. J., Wolf, M. B., Sooudi, I., & Smith, T. L. (1975). Palatometric-gnathometric study of speech articulation. Final Report. (NIH Grant No. NS10540).

Fletcher, S. G., & Newman, D. G. (1991). /s/ and /ʃ/ as a function of linguapalatal contact place and sibilant groove width. *Journal of the Acoustical Society of America, 89,* 850–858.

Fletcher, S. G., Shelton, R. L., Jr., Smith, C. C., & Bosma, J. F. (1960). Radiography in speech pathology. *Journal of Speech and Hearing Disorders, 25,* 135–144.

Fletcher, S. G., Smith, S. C., & Hasegawa, A. (1985). Vocal/verbal response times of normal-hearing and hearing-impaired children. *Journal of Speech and Hearing Research, 28,* 548–555.

Folkins, J., & Abbs, J. H. (1975). Lip and jaw motor control during speech: Response to resistive loading of the jaw. *Journal of Speech and Hearing Disorders, 18,* 207–220.

Folkins, J. W., & Bleile, K. M. (1990). Taxonomies in biology, phonetics, phonology, and speech motor control. *Journal of Speech and Hearing Disorders, 55,* 596–611.

Folkins, J. W., Miller, C. J., & Minifie, F. D. (1975). Rhythm and syllable timing in phrase level stress patterning. *Journal of Speech and Hearing Research, 18,* 739–753.

Forssberg, H. S., Grillner, S., & Rossignol, S. (1975). Phase dependent reflex reversal during walking in chronic spinal cats. *Brain Research, 85,* 103–107.

Fourcin, A. J. (1981). Laryngographic assessment of phonatory function. In C. L. Ludlow & M. O. Hart (Eds.), *Proceedings of the conference on the assessment of vocal pathology, ASHA Reports 11* (pp. 116–127). Rockville, MD: American Speech-Language-Hearing Association.

Fowler, C. A. (1980). Coarticulation and theories of extrinsic timing. *Journal of Phonetics, 8,* 113–133.

Freedle, R., & Lewis, M. (1977). Prelinguistic conversations. In M. Lewis & L. A. Rosenblum (Eds.), *Interaction, conversation, and the development of language* (pp. 157–185). New York: John Wiley.

Frese, M., & Sabini, J. (1985). Action theory: An introduction. In M. Frese & J. Sabini (Eds.), *Goal directed behavior: The concept of action in psychology* (pp. xvii–xxv). Hillsdale, NJ: Lawrence Erlbaum.

Fugii, I. (1970). Phoneme identification with dynamic palatography. *Annual Bulletin* (Research Institute of Logopedics and Phoniatrics, University of Tokyo), *4,* 67–73.

Fugimura, O. (1981). Temporal organization of articulatory movements as a multidimensional phrasal structure. *Phonetica, 38,* 66–83.

Fugimura, O. (1986). Relative invariance of articulatory movements: An iceberg model. In J. S. Perkell & D. H. Klatt (Eds.), *Invariance and variability in speech processes* (pp. 226–234). Hillsdale, NJ: Lawrence Erlbaum.

Fugimura, O., & Kakita, Y. (1979). Remarks on quantitative description of the lingual articulation. In B. Lindblom & S. Ohman (Eds.), *Frontiers of speech communication research* (pp. 17–24). London: Academic Press.

Fujimura, O., Kiritani, S., & Ishida, H. (1969). Digitally controlled dynamic radiography. *Annual Bulletin* (Research Institute of Logopedics and Phoniatrics, University of Tokyo), *3,* 1–34.

Galef, B. G., McQuoid, L. M., & Whiskin, E. E. (1990). Further evidence that Norway rats do not socially transmit learned aversions to toxic baits. *Animal Learning and Behavior, 15,* 327–332.

Gallistel, C. R. (1985). Motivation, intention, and emotion: Goal directed behavior from a cognitive-neuroethological perspective. In M. Frese & J. Sabini (Eds.), *Goal directed behavior: The concept of action in psychology* (pp. 48–65). Hillsdale, NJ: Lawrence Erlbaum.

Gallistel, C. R., Brown, A. L., Carey, S., Gelman, R., & Keil, F. C. (1991). Lessons from animal learning for the study of cognitive development. In S. Carey & R. Gelman (Eds.), *The epigenesis of mind: Essays on biology and cognition* (pp. 336). Hillsdale, NJ: Lawrence Erlbaum.

Garland, H. (1983). The influence of ability, assigned goals, and normative information on personal goals and performance: A challenge to the goal attainability assumption. *Journal of Applied Psychology, 68,* 20–30.

Garland, H. (1985). A cognitive mediation theory of task goals and human performance. *Motivation and Emotion, 9,* 345–367.

Gay, T., Lindblom, B., & Lubker, J. (1981). Production of bite-block vowels: Acoustic equivalence by selective compensation. *Journal of the Acoustical Society of America, 69,* 802–810.

Gentile, A. M. (1972). A working model of skill acquisition with application to teaching. *Quest,* Monograph 17, 3–23.

Gibb, N. (1985). *An experimental investigation of novel bilingual vocabulary acquisition by four minority-language pre-school children.* Unpublished master's thesis, University of Arizona, Tucson.

Gierut, J. A. (1985). *On the relationship between phonological knowledge and generalization learning in misarticulating children.* Doctoral dissertation, Indiana University, Bloomington. (Distributed by the Indiana University Linguistics Club, 1986.)

Gierut, J. A. (1989a). Maximal opposition approach to phonological treatment. *Journal of Speech and Hearing Disorders, 54,* 9–19.

Gierut, J. A. (1989b). Describing developing phonological systems: A surrebuttal. *Applied Psycholinguistics, 10,* 469–473.

Gierut, J. A., Elbert, M., & Dinnsen, D. A. (1987). A functional analysis of phonological knowledge and generalization learning in misarticulating children. *Journal of Speech and Hearing Research, 30,* 462–479.

Gilfoyle, E. M., Grady, A. P., & Moore, J. C. (1990). *Children adapt* (2nd ed.). Thorofare, NJ: Slack

Gimson, A. C. (1972). *An introduction to the pronunciation of English* (2nd ed.). London: Edward Arnold.

Goldhor, R. S. (1985). *Representation of consonants in the peripheral auditory system: A modeling study of the correspondence between response properties and phonetic features* (Tech. Rep. No. 505). Cambridge, MA: MIT Press.

Goldman, A. (1986). *Cognition and epistemology.* Cambridge, MA: MIT Press.

Goldman, R., & Fristoe, M. (1969). *Goldman-Fristoe Test of Articulation.* Circle Pines, MN: American Guidance Service.

Gordon, T. G. (1987). Communication skills of mainstreamed hearing-impaired children. In H. Levitt, N. S. McGarr, & D. Geffner (Eds.), *Development of language and communication skills in hearing impaired children. ASHA Monograph No. 26* (pp. 108–122). Rockville, MD: American Speech-Language-Hearing Association.

Goss, C. M. (1954). *Anatomy of the human body by Henry Gray.* Philadelphia: Lea & Febiger.

Goss, S. A., Johnston, R. L., & Dunn, F. (1978). Comprehensive compilation of empirical ultrasonic properties of mammalian tissues. *Journal of the Acoustical Society of America, 64,* 423–457.

Greene, P. H. (1972). Problems of organization of motor systems. In R. Rosen & F. Snell (Eds.), *Progress in theoretical biology* (Vol. 2, pp. 303–338). New York: Academic Press.

Greer, W. H. (1970). *Development and fabrication of a linguapalatometer.* Unpublished master's thesis, University of New Mexico, Albuquerque.

Groll, E. (1966). Zentralnervöse und periphere Aktivierungsvariable bei Vigilanzleistungen. *Zeitschrift für experimentisch und angewandte Psychologie, 13,* 248–264.

Grossman, R. C., & Hattis, B. F. (1967). Oral mucosal sensory innervation and sensory experience: A review. In J. F. Bosma (Ed.), *Symposium on oral sensation and perception* (pp. 5–63). Springfield, IL: Charles C. Thomas.

Grunwell, P. (1981). *The nature of phonological processes.* London: Academic Press.

Grützner, P. (1879). Physiologie der Stimme und Sprache. In L. Herman (Ed.), *Handbuch der physiologie* (pp. 204–207, 219–221). Leipzig: Vogel.

Haas, W. (1963). Phonological analysis of a case of dyslalia. *Journal of Speech and Hearing Disorders, 28,* 239–246.

Halle, M., & Stevens, K. N. (1979). Some reflections on the theoretical bases of phonetics. In B. Lindblom & S. Öhman (Eds.), *Frontiers of speech communication research* (pp. 335–349). London: Academic Press.

Hamlet, S. L., & Stone, M. (1978). Compensatory alveolar consonant production induced by wearing a dental prosthesis. *Journal of Phonetics, 6,* 227–248.

Hammarberg, R. (1976). The metaphysics of coarticulation. *Journal of Phonetics, 4,* 353–363.

Hardcastle, W. J. (1970). The role of tactile and proprioceptive feedback in speech production. *Work in Progress, 4,* 100–112.

Hardcastle, W. J. (1972). The use of electropalatography in phonetic research. *Phonetica, 25,* 197–215.

Hardcastle, W. J. (1976). *Physiology of speech production. An introduction for speech scientists.* London: Academic Press.

Harley, W. T. (1972). Dynamic palatography — a study of linguopalatal contacts during the production of selected consonant sounds. *Journal of Prosthetic Dentistry, 27,* 364–376.

Harris, K. S. (1974). *Mechanisms of duration change.* Paper presented at Eighth International Congress on Acoustics, London, England.

Harshman, R., Ladefoged, P., & Goldstein, L. (1977). Factor analysis of tongue shapes. *Journal of the Acoustical Society of America, 62,* 693–707.

Hasegawa, A., Christensen, J. M., Fletcher, & McCutcheon, M. J. (1977). Articulatory characteristics of fluent esophageal speakers for selected English consonants. *Journal of the Acoustical Society of America, 62,* S5.

Hawkins, D. (1977). Probability, information, and inference. In A. Aykac & C. Brumat (Eds.), *New developments in the application of Bayesian methods* (pp. 11–37). New York: North Holland.

Head, H. (1920). *Studies in neurology. Vol. 2.* London: Hodder and Stoughton.

Heckhausen, H., & Kuhl, J. (1985). From wishes to action: The dead ends and short cuts on the long way to action. In M. Frese & J. Sabini (Eds.), *Goal directed behavior: The concept of action in psychology* (pp. 134–159). Hillsdale, NJ: Lawrence Erlbaum.

Hellebrandt, F. A., Schade, M., & Carns, M. L. (1962). Methods of evoking the tonic neck reflexes in normal human subjects. *American Journal of Physical Medicine, 41,* 89–139.

Helms, C. A., Richardson, M. L., Moon, K. L., & Ware, W. H. (1984). Nuclear magnetic resonance imaging of the temporomandibular joint: Preliminary observations. *Journal of Craniomandibular Practice, 2,* 220–224.

Henderson, E. J. A. (1971). Structural organization of language: Phonology. In N. Minnis (Ed.), *Linguistics at large* (pp. 35–53). London: Paladin.

Henneman, E. (1990). Comments on the logical basis of muscle control. In M. D. Binder & L. M. Mendell (Eds.), *The segmental motor system* (pp. vii–x). New York: Oxford University Press.

Henneman, E., & Mendell, L. M. (1981). Functional organization of the motoneuron pool and its inputs. In V. B. Brooks (Ed.), *Handbook of physiology. Section 1: The nervous system* (Vol. 1, Part 1, pp. 423–507). Bethesda, MD: American Physiological Society.

Herrnstein, R. J. (1970). On the law of effect. *Journal of the Experimental Analysis of Behavior, 13,* 243–266.

Hess, W. R. (1943). Das Zwischenhirn als Koordinations organ. *Helvetica Physiologica Pharmacologica Acta, 1,* 549–565.

Hillyard, S. A., Munte, T. F., & Neville, H. J. (1985). Visual-spatial attention, orienting, and brain physiology. In M. I. Posner & S. M. Marin (Eds.), *Attention and performance XI* (pp. 63–84). Hillsdale, NJ: Lawrence Erlbaum.

Hirano, M. (1975). Phonosurgery: Basic and clinical investigations. *Otologia Fukuoka, 21*(Suppl. 1) (Japanese).

Hirano, M. (1981). Structure of the vocal fold in normal and disease states. Anatomical and physical studies. In C. L. Ludlow & M. O. Hart (Eds.), *Proceedings of the Conference on the Assessment of Vocal Pathology, ASHA Reports 11* (pp. 11–30). Rockville, MD: The American Speech-Language-Hearing Association.

Hixon, T. J. (1966). Turbulent noise sources for speech. *Folia Phoniatrica, 18,* 168–182.

Hixon, T., Minifie, F. D., & Tait, C. A. (1967). Correlates of turbulent noise production for speech. *Journal of Speech and Hearing Research, 10,* 133–140.

Hockett, C. (1960). The origin of speech. *Scientific American, 203,* 89–96.

Hoffman, D. D., & Richards, W. (1974). Parts of recognition. *Cognition, 18,* 65–96.

Hollien, H., & Schoenhard, C. (1983). The riddle of the "middle" register. In I. R. Titze & R. C. Scherer (Eds.), *Vocal fold physiology: Biomechanics, acoustics and phonatory control* (pp. 256–269). Denver, CO: The Denver Center for the Performing Arts.

Holtzer, H. Sasse, J., Horwitz, A., Antin, P., & Pacifici, M. (1986). Myogenic lineages and myofibrillogenesis. In B. Christ & R. Cihák (Eds.), *Development and regeneration of skeletal muscles* (pp. 1–23). Basel, Switzerland: S. Karger.

Hudspeth, A. J. (1985). The cellular basis of hearing: The biophysics of hair cells. *Science, 230,* 745–752.

Huggins, A. W. F. (1978). Speech timing and intelligibility. In J. Requin (Ed.), *Attention and performance. VII* (pp. 279–297). Hillsdale, NJ: Lawrence Erlbaum.

Hughes, G. W., & Halle, M. (1956). Spectral properties of fricative consonants. *Journal of the Acoustical Society of America, 28,* 303–310.

Hull, C. L. (1943). *Principles of behavior.* New York: Appleton-Century.

Ingram, D. (1974). Phonological rules in young children. *Journal of Child Language, 1,* 49–64.

Ingram, D. (1978). The role of the syllable in phonological development. In A. Bell & J. B. Hooper (Eds.) *Syllables and segments* (pp. 143–155). Amsterdam, The Netherlands: North-Holland.

Ingram, D. (1985). On children's homonyms. *Journal of Child Language, 12,* 671–680.

Ingram, D., Christensen, L., Veach, S., & Webster, B. (1980). The acquisition of word-initial fricatives and affricates in English by children between 2 and 6 years. In G. H. Yeni-Komshian, J. F. Kavanagh, & C. A. Ferguson (Eds.), *Child phonology. Volume 1. Production* (pp. 169–192). New York: Academic Press.

Jackson, M. T. T. (1988). Phonetic theory and cross-linguistic variation in vowel articulation. *UCLA Working Papers in Phonetics, 71.*

Jakobson, R. (1938). Observations sur le classement phonologique des consonnes. *Proceedings of the 3rd International Congress on Phonetic Science, Ghent* (pp. 34–41).

Jakobson, R. (1968). *Child language, aphasia, and phonological universals.* The Hague, The Netherlands: Mouton.

Jakobson, R., & Halle, M. (1956). *Fundamentals of language.* The Hague, The Netherlands: Mouton.

Johnson, K. (1969). Mapping the movements of the human tongue. *The Atom, 6,* 12–16.

Johnson, P. (1982). The functional equivalence of imagery and movement. *Quarterly Journal of Experimental Psychology, 38A,* 349–365.

Johnson, R. G., Goldberg, L. R., & Mathers, P. L. (1984). Coarticulation: Theory to therapy. In R. G. Daniloff (Ed.), *Articulation assessment and treatment issues* (pp. 31–49). San Diego, CA: College-Hill Press.

Johnson, T. D. (1988). Developmental explanation and the ontogeny of birdsong: Nature/nurture redux. *Behavioral and Brain Sciences, 11,* 631–675.

Johnston, J. C., & Hale, B. L. (1984). The influence of prior context on word identification: Bias and sensitivity effects. In H. Bouma & D. G. Bouwhis (Eds.), *Attention and performance X. Control of language processes* (pp. 243–255). London: Lawrence Erlbaum.

Jones, D. (1972). *An outline of English phonetics.* Cambridge, England: Cambridge University Press.

Jürgens, U., & Ploog, D. (1988). On the motor coordination of monkey calls. In J. D. Newman (Ed.), *The physiological control of mammalian vocalization* (pp. 7–19). New York: Plenum.

Kahn, L., & Lewis, N. (1986). *Kahn-Lewis Phonological Analysis.* Circle Pines, MN: American Guidance Service.

Kahneman, D. (1973). *Attention and effort.* Englewood Cliffs, NJ: Prentice-Hall.

Kahneman, D., & Treisman, A. (1984). Changing views of attention and automanticity. In R. Parasuraman & D. R. Daview (Eds.), *Varieties of attention* (pp. 29–61). Orlando, FL: Academic Press.

Kahneman, D., Triesman, A., & Burkell, J. (1983). The cost of visual filtering.

Journal of Experimental Psychology: Human Perception and Performance, 9, 510–522.

Kanfer, F. H. (1965). Vicarious human reinforcement: A glimpse into the black box. In L. Krasner & L. P. Ullman (Eds.), *Research in behavioral modification* (pp. 244–267). New York: Holt.

Keating, P. (1983). Comments on the jaw and syllable structures. *Journal of Phonetics, 11*, 401–406.

Keller, E. (1989). Predictors of subsyllabic durations in speech motor control. *Journal of the Acoustical Society of America, 85*, 322–326.

Keller, E., & Ostry, D. (1983). Computerized measurement of tongue dorsum movement with pulsed echo ultrasound. *Journal of the Acoustical Society of America, 73*, 1309–1315.

Kelly, C. A., & Dale, P. S. (1989). Cognitive skills associated with the onset of multiword utterances. *Journal of Speech and Hearing Research, 32*, 645–656.

Kelsey, C. A., Minifie, F. D., & Hixon, T. J. (1969). Applications of ultrasound in speech research. *Journal of Speech and Hearing Research, 12*, 546–575.

Kelso, J. A. S. (1982). *Human motor behavior: An introduction.* Hillsdale, NJ: Lawrence Erlbaum.

Kelso, J. A. S., Saltzman, E. L., & Tuller, B. (1986). Dynamical perspectives on speech production: Data and theory. *Journal of Phonetics, 14*, 29–59.

Kelso, J. A. S., & Tuller, B. (1984). Converging evidence in support of common dynamical principles for speech and movement coordination. *American Journal of Physiology, 246*, R928–935.

Kelso, J. A. S., Vatikiotis-Bateson, E., Saltzman, E. L., & Kay, B. (1985). A qualitative dynamic analysis of reiterant speech production: Phase portraits, kinematics, and dynamic modeling. *Journal of the Acoustical Society of America, 77*, 266–281.

Kent, R. D. (1985). Developing and disordered speech: Strategies for organization. In J. L. Lauter (Ed.), *Proceedings of the conference on the planning and production of speech in normal and hearing-impaired individuals: A seminar in honor of S. Richard Silverman* (pp. 29–37). Rockville, MD: American Speech-Language-Hearing Association.

Kent, R. D., & Moll, K. L. (1972). Articulatory timing in selected consonant sequences. *Brain and Language, 2*, 304–323.

Kety, S. S. (1970). The biogenic amines in the central nervous system: Their possible roles in arousal, emotion, and learning. In F. O. Schmitt (Ed.), *The neurosciences: Second study program* (pp. 324–336). New York: Rockefeller University Press.

Kiernan, B., & Swisher, L. (1990). The initial learning of novel English words: Two single-subject experiments with minority-language children. *Journal of Speech and Hearing Research, 33*, 707–716.

King, M., Meyer, G. E., Tangney, J., & Biederman, I. (1976). Shape constancy and a perceptual bias toward symmetry. *Perception and Psychophysics, 19*, 129–136.

Kiritani, S., Itoh, K., Imagawa, H., Fujisaki, H., & Sawashima, M. (1975). Tongue pellet tracking and other radiographic observations by a computer controlled x-ray microbeam system. *Annual Bulletin* (Research Institute of Logopedics and Phoniatrics, University of Tokyo), *9*, 1–14.

Klatt, D. (1982). Speech processing strategies based on auditory models. In R. Carlson & H. Granstrom (Eds.), *The representation of speech in the peripheral auditory system* (pp. 181–196). New York: Elsevier Biomedical Press.

Klein, H. B., Lederer, S. H., & Cortese, E. E. (1991). Children's knowledge of auditory/articulatory correspondences: Phonologic and metaphonologic. *Journal of Speech and Hearing Research, 34,* 559–564.

Klein, R. M., & Posner, M. I. (1974). Attention to visual and kinesthetic components of skills. *Brain Research, 71,* 401–411.

Konishi, M. (1965). The role of auditory feedback in the control of vocalization in the white-crowned sparrow. *Zeitschrift für Tierpsychologie, 22,* 770–783.

Kuczynski, L., Zahn-Waxler, C., & Radke-Yarrow, M. (1987). Development and content of imitation in the second and third years of life: A socialization perspective. *Developmental Psychology, 23,* 276–282.

Kuzmin, Y. I. (1962). Mobile palatography as a tool for acoustic study of speech sounds. *Proceedings of the Fourth International Congress on Acoustics, Copenhagen, G35,* 1–3.

Kydd, W. L., & Belt, D. A. (1964). Continuous palatography. *Journal of Speech and Hearing Disorders, 29,* 489–492.

Kymissis, E., & Poulson, C. L. (1990). The history of imitation in learning theory: The language acquisition process. *Journal of the Experimental Analysis of Behavior, 54,* 113–127.

Ladd, D. R., Silverman, K. E. A., Tolkmitt, F., Bergmann, G., & Sherer, K. R. (1985). Evidence for the independent function of intonation contour type, voice quality, and F_0 range in signaling speaker effect. *Journal of the Acoustical Society of America, 78,* 435–444.

Ladefoged, P. (1957). Use of palatography. *Journal of Speech and Hearing Disorders, 22,* 764–774.

Ladefoged, P. (1975). *A course in phonetics.* New York: Harcourt Brace Jovanovich.

Lakshminarayanan, A. V., Lee, S., & McCutcheon, M. J. (1991). MR imaging of the vocal tract during vowel production. *Journal of Magnetic Resonance Imaging, 1,* 71–76.

Landers, D. M. (1975). Observational learning of a motor skill: Temporal spacing of demonstrations and audience presence. *Journal of Motor Behavior, 7,* 281–287.

Landers, D. M. (1980). The arousal-performance relationship revisited. *Research Quarterly for Exercise and Sport, 51,* 77–90.

Landers, D. M., & Landers, D. M. (1973). Teacher versus peer models: Effects of model's presence and performance level on motor behavior. *Journal of Motor Behavior, 5,* 129–139.

Larson, C. R., & Kistler, M. K. (1986). The relationship of periaqueductal grey neuronal activity associated with laryngeal EMG in the behaving monkey. *Experimental Brain Research, 63,* 596–606.

Larson, C. R., DeRosier, E., & West, R. (1991). Physiological analysis of the involvement of brainstem neurons in vocal mechanisms in monkeys. In J. Gauffin & B. Hammarberg (Eds.), *Vocal fold physiology: Acoustic, perceptual, and physiological aspects of voice mechanisms.* San Diego, CA: Singular Publishing.

Lashley, K. S. (1951). The problem of serial order in behavior. In L. A. Jeffress

(Ed.), *Cerebral mechanisms in behavior* (The Hixon Symposium) (pp. 112–136). New York: John Wiley.

Lauttamus, T. (1984). *Distinctive features and English consonants.* Joensuu, Finland: University of Joensuu.

Lavery, J. J. (1962). Retention of simple motor skills as a function of type of knowledge of results. *Canadian Journal of Psychology, 16,* 300–311.

Lavery, J. J. (1964). The effect of one-trial delay in knowledge of results on the acquisition and retention of a tossing skill. *American Journal of Psychology, 77,* 437–443.

Lee, T. D., & Genovese, E. E. (1988). Distribution of practice in motor skill acquisition: Learning and performance effects reconsidered. *Research Quarterly for Exercise and Sport, 59,* 277–287.

Lee, T. D., Magill, R. A., & Weeks, D. J. (1985). Influence of practice schedule on testing schema theory prediction in adults. *Journal of Motor Behavior, 17,* 283–299.

Lehiste, I. (1970). *Suprasegmentals.* Cambridge, MA: MIT Press.

Lehiste, I., & Peterson, G. E. (1959). Vowel amplitude and phonemic stress in American English. *Journal of the Acoustical Society of America, 31,* 428–435.

Leonard, E. L. (1990). Early motor development and control: Foundations for independent walking. In G. L. Smidt (Ed.), *Gait in rehabilitation* (pp. 121–140). New York: Churchill Livingston.

Leonard, J. A. (1953). Advance information in sensorimotor skills. *Quarterly Journal of Experimental Psychology, 5,* 141–149.

Leonard, L. B. (1981). Facilitating linguistic skills in children with specific language impairment. *Applied Psycholinguistics, 2,* 89–118.

Leopold, W. F. (1939). *Speech development of a bilingual child, Volume I.* Evanston, IL: Northwestern University Press.

Levelt, W. J. M. (1989). *Speaking. From intention to articulation.* Cambridge, MA: The MIT Press.

Lewin, K. (1935). *A dynamic theory of personality.* New York: McGraw-Hill.

Liberman, M., & Streeter, L. A. (1978). Use of nonsense-syllable mimicry in the study of prosodic phenomena. *Journal of the Acoustical Society of America, 63,* 231–233.

Lieberman, P. (1960). Some acoustic correlates of word stress in American English. *Journal of the Acoustical Society of America, 32,* 451–454.

Lieberman, P. (1967). *Intonation, perception, and language.* Research Monograph No. 38. Cambridge, MA: MIT Press.

Lieberman, P. (1975). *On the origins of language: An introduction to the evolution of human speech.* New York: Macmillan.

Lieberman, P. (1980). On the development of vowel production in young children. In G. H. Yeni-Komshian, J. F. Kavanagh, & C. A. Ferguson (Eds.), *Child phonology. Volume 1. Production* (pp. 113–142). New York: Academic Press.

Lieberman, P., Katz, W., Jongman, A., Zimmerman, R., & Miller, M. (1985). Measures of the sentence intonation of read and spontaneous speech in American English. *Journal of the Acoustical Society of America, 77,* 649–657.

Lindblom, B. (1983). Economy of speech gestures. In P. F. MacNeilage (Ed.), *The production of speech* (pp. 217–245). New York: Springer-Verlag.

Lindblom, B., & Lubker, J. (1985). The speech homunculus and a problem of phonetic linguistics. In V. A. Fromkin (Ed.), *Phonetic linguistics. Essays in honor of Peter Ladefoged* (pp. 169–192). Orlando, FL: Academic Press.

Lindblom, B., & Sundberg, J. (1971). Acoustical consequences of lip, tongue, jaw, and larynx movement. *Journal of the Acoustical Society of America, 50,* 1166–1179.

Little, W. S., & McCullagh, P. (1989). Motivation orientation and modeled instruction strategies: The effects on form and accuracy. *Journal of Sport & Exercise Psychology, 11,* 41–53.

Locke, E. A. (1968). Toward a theory of task motivation and incentives. *Organizational Behavior and Human Performance, 3,* 157–189.

Locke, E. A. (1982). Relation of goal level to performance with a short work period and multiple goal levels. *Journal of Applied Psychology, 67,* 512–514.

Locke, E. A., & Latham, G. P. (1985). The application of goal setting to sports. *Journal of Sport Psychology, 7,* 205–222.

Locke, E. A., Shaw, K. N., Saari, L. M., & Latham, G. P. (1981). Goal setting and task performance: 1969–1980. *Psychological Bulletin, 90,* 125–152.

Locke, J. L. (1983). *Phonological acquisition and change.* New York: Academic Press.

Löfqvist, A., & Yoshioka, H. (1981). Interarticulator programming in obstruent production. *Phonetica, 38,* 21–34.

Lorenz, K. Z. (1935). Der Kumpan in der Unwelt des Vogel. In K. Lorenz (Ed.), *Studies in human and animal behaviour,* 2 vols. (R. Martin, Trans., 1970). Cambridge, MA: Harvard University Press.

Luria, A. R. (1961). *The role of speech in the regulation of normal and abnormal behavior* (J. Tizard, Trans.). New York: Pergamon Press.

Maassen, B. (1986). Marking word boundaries to improve the intelligibility of the speech of the deaf. *Journal of Speech and Hearing Research, 29,* 227–230.

Maassen, B., & Povel, D-J. (1985). The effect of segmental and suprasegmental corrections on the intelligibility of deaf speech. *Journal of the Acoustical Society of America, 78,* 877–886.

MacDonald, J., & McGurk, H. (1978). Visual influences on speech perception processes. *Perception and Psychophysics, 24,* 253–257.

Mackay, D. G., & Bowman, R. W. (1969). On producing the meaning in sentences. *American Journal of Psychology, 82,* 23–39.

Macken, M. A. (1979). Developmental reorganization of phonology: A hierarchy of basic units of acquisition. *Lingua, 49,* 11–49.

Macken, M. A. (1980). Aspects of the acquisition of stop systems: A cross-linguistic perspective. In G. H. Yeni-Komshian, J. F. Kavanagh, & C. A. Ferguson (Eds.), *Child phonology. Volume 1. Production* (pp. 143–168). New York: Academic Press.

Macnamara, J. (1972). The cognitive basis of language learning in infants. *Psychological Review, 79,* 1–13.

Maddieson, I. (1984). *Patterns of sounds.* Cambridge, England: Cambridge University Press.

Magill, R. A. (1989). *Motor learning. Concepts and applications* (3rd ed.). Dubuque, IA: William C. Brown.

Mandler, J. M. (1979). Categorical and schematic organization in memory. In

C. R. Puff (Ed.), *Memory organization and structure* (pp. 259-299). New York: Academic Press.

Marchall, A. (1988). *La palatographie*. Paris: Centre national de la recherche scientifique.

Marlatt, G. A. (1968). *Vicarious and direct reinforcement control of verbal behavior in an interview setting*. Unpublished doctoral dissertation, Indiana University, Bloomington.

Marler, P. (1970). A comparative approach to vocal learning: Song development in white-crowned sparrows. *Journal of Comparative and Physiological Psychology, 71,* 1-25.

Marler, P. (1984). Song learning: Innate species differences in the learning process. In P. Marler & H. S. Terrace (Eds.), *The biology of learning* (pp. 289-309). Berlin: Springer-Verlag.

Marler, P. (1991). The instinct to learn. In S. Carey & R. Gelman (Eds.), *The epigenesis of mind: Essays on biology and cognition* (pp. 37-66). Hillsdale, NJ: Lawrence Erlbaum.

Marler, P., & Peters, S. (1988). Sensitive periods for song acquisition from tape recordings and live tutors in the swamp sparrow, *Melospiza georgiana. Ethology, 76,* 89-100.

Marler, P., & Sherman, V. (1985). Innate differences in singing behaviour of sparrows reared in isolation from adult conspecific song. *Animal Behaviour, 33,* 57-71.

Marr, D., & Nishihara, H. K. (1978). Representation and recognition of the spatial organization of three-dimensional shapes. *Proceedings of the Royal Society, London,* B200, 269-294.

Marshall, J. C., Morton, J., Bever, T. G., Brown, J. W., Estes, W. K., Grossman, K. E., Huber, M. G. H., Petersen, W. R., Squire, L. R., & Weinstein, S. (1984). Biology of learning in humans. Group report. In P. Marler & H. S. Terrace (Eds.), *The biology of learning* (pp. 687-795). Berlin: Springer-Verlag.

Marteniuk, R. G., & MacKenzie, C. L. (1980). Information processing in movement organization and execution. In R. S. Nickerson (Ed.), *Attention and performance VIII* (pp. 29-57). New York: Academic Press.

Martin, J. G. (1970). Rhythm-induced judgments of word stress in sentences. *Journal of Verbal Learning and Verbal Behavior, 9,* 627-633.

Martin, J. G. (1972). Rhythmic (hierarchical) versus serial structure in speech and other behavior. *Psychological Review, 79,* 487-509.

Massion, J. (1984). Postural changes accompanying voluntary movements. Normal and pathological aspects. *Human Neurobiology, 2,* 261-267.

Mavilya, M. P. (1969). Spontaneous vocalization and babbling in hearing impaired infants. Doctoral dissertation, Columbia University, New York City. (University microfilm No. 70-12879.)

McCarty, T. A., & Hamlet, S. L. (1977). Comparison of phonetic judgments and electropalatographic measurements of articulatory place of production. *Perceptual and Motor Skills, 44,* 115-118.

McClelland, D. C. (1965). Toward a theory of motive acquisition. *American Psychologist, 20,* 321-333.

McCracken, H. D., & Stelmach, G. E. (1977). A test of the schema theory of discrete motor learning. *Journal of Motor Behavior, 9,* 193-201.

McCutcheon, M. J., Hasegawa, A., Smith, S. C., & Fletcher, S. G. (1981). A sys tem for measurement and display of the hard palate and maxillary teeth. *Proceedings of the 14th International Conference on System Sciences, Honolulu, Volume II, Section I* (pp. 446–456). North Hollywood, CA: Western Periodicals.

McCutcheon, M. J., Lee, S., Lakshminarayanan, A. V., & Fletcher, S. G. (1990). A comparison of glossometric measurements of tongue position with mag netic resonance images of the vocal tract. *Journal of the Acoustical Society of America, 87,* S122.

McCutcheon, M. J., Smith, D. G., Kimble, S. O., & Fletcher, S. G. (1983). Micro processsor controlled instrument for tongue-palate contact measurement during speech. *Proceedings of the 2nd Southern Biomedical Engineering Con ference* (pp. 263–266). San Antonio, TX: Pergamon.

McCutcheon, M. J., Smith, S. C., Stilwell, D. J., & Fletcher, S. G. (1982, April). Development of instrumentation for tongue-palate·distance measurement during speech. *Proceedings of the Institute of Electrical and Electronic Engineers* (pp 571–572). New York: IEEE.

McGarr, N. S. (1987). Communication skills of hearing-impaired children in schools for the deaf. In H. Levitt, N. S. McGarr, & D. Geffner (Eds.), *Develop ment of language and communication skills in hearing impaired children* (pp. 91–107). ASHA Monograph No. 26. Rockville, MD: American Speech-Language-Hearing Association.

McGarr, N. S., & Lofquist, A. (1982). Obstruent production by hearing-impaired speakers: Interarticulator timing and acoustics. *Journal of the Acoustical Society of America, 72,* 34–42.

McGurk, H., & MacDonald, J. (1976). Hearing lips and seeing voices. *Nature, 264* (Suppl. 1), 746–748.

McNeill, D. (1987). *Psycholinguistics: A new approach.* Cambridge, MA: Harper and Row.

McReynolds, L. V. (1989). Generalization issues in the treatment of communi cation disorders. In L. V. McReynolds & J. E. Spradlin (Eds.), *Generalization strategies in the treatment of communication disorders* (pp. 1–12). Toronto, Canada: Decker.

McReynolds, L. V., & Bennett, S. (1972). Distinctive feature generalization in articulation training. *Journal of Speech and Hearing Disorders, 37,* 462–470.

McReynolds, L. V., & Engmann, D. (1975). *Distinctive feature analysis of misar ticulations.* Baltimore, MD: University Park Press.

Medress, M., Skinner, T. E., & Anderson, N. E. (1971). Acoustic correlates of word stress. *Journal of the Acoustical Society of America, 51,* 101.

Melzoff, A. N., & Moore, M. K. (1977). Imitation of facial and manual gestures by human neonates. *Science, 198,* 75–78.

Menn, L. (1978). *Pattern, control, and contrast in beginning speech.* Bloomington, IN: Indiana University Linguistics Club.

Menn, L. (1982). Development of articulatory, phonetic, and phonological capabilities. In B. Butterworth (Ed.), *Language production. Volume 2* (pp. 3–50). London: Academic Press.

Mento, A. J., Steel, R. P., & Karren, R. J. (1987). A meta-analytic study of the effects of goal setting on task performance: 1966–1984. *Organizational Behav-*

ior and Human Decision Processes, 39, 52–83.

Menzel, E. W., & Halperin, S. (1975). Purposive behavior as a basis for objective communication between chimpanzees. *Science, 189,* 652–654.

Metz, D. E. (1980). Morphological boundaries and the timing of stressed vowels by profoundly hearing impaired adults. *Journal of Phonetics, 8,* 63–68.

Metz, D. E., Schiavetti, N., Samar, V. J., & Sitler, R. W. (1990). Acoustic dimensions of hearing-impaired speakers' intelligibility: Segmental and suprasegmental characteristics. *Journal of Speech and Hearing Research, 33,* 476–487.

Meyer-Epplar, W. (1953). Zum Erzeugungsmechanismus der Gerauschlaute. *Zeitszhrift für Phonetik, 7,* 196–212.

Miller, G. A. (1956). The magical number seven, plus or minus two: Some limits on our capacity for processing information. *Psychological Review, 63,* 81–97.

Minas, S. C. (1978). Mental practice of a complex perceptual motor skill. *Journal of Human Movement Studies, 4,* 102–107.

Miner, J. B. (1984). The validity and usefulness of theories in an emerging organizational science. *Academy of Management Review, 9,* 296–306.

Moll, K. L. (1960). Cinefluorographic techniques in speech research. *Journal of Speech and Hearing Research, 3,* 227–241.

Moore, S. P. (1984). Systematic removal of visual feedback. *Journal of Human Movement Studies, 10,* 165–173.

Moray, N., & Fitter, M. (1973). A theory and the measurement of attention. In S. Kornblum (Ed.), *Attention and performance IV* (pp. 3–19). New York: Academic Press.

Morley, M. E. (1957). *The development and disorders of speech in childhood.* Edinburgh, Scotland: Livingston.

Morris, H. (1942). *Morris: Human anatomy* (10th ed.). Philadelphia, PA: Blakiston.

Morton, J. (1979). Facilitation in word recognition: Experiments causing change in the logogen model. In P. A. Kolers, M. Wrolstead, & H. Bouma (Eds.), *Processing of visible language* (pp. 259–268). New York: Plenum.

Moses, E. R. (1940). *Interpretations of a new method in palatography.* Ann Arbor, MI: Edwards Brothers.

Nadler, R., & Abbs, J. (1988). Use of the x-ray microbeam system for the study of articulatory dynamics. *Journal of the Acoustical Society of America, 84,* S124.

Navon, D. (1985). Attention division or attention sharing. In M. I. Posner & O. S. M. Marin (Eds.), *Attention and performance XI* (pp. 133–146). Hillsdale, NJ: Lawrence Erlbaum.

Nearey, T. (1978). *Phonetic features for vowels.* Bloomington, IN: Indiana University Linguistics Club.

Neisser, U. (1963). Decision time without reaction time: Experiments in visual scanning. *American Journal of Psychology, 17,* 376–385.

New, P. J. F., Rosen, B. R., Brady, T. J., Buononno, F. S., Kistler, J. P., Burt, C. T., Hinshaw, W. S., Newhouse, J. H., Pohost, G. M., & Taveras, J. M. (1983). Potential hazards and artifacts of ferromagnetic surgical and dental materials and device in nuclear magnetic resonance imaging. *Radiology, 147,* 139–148.

Newell, K. M., & Shapiro, D. C. (1976). Variability of practice and transfer of training: Some evidence toward a schema view of motor learning. *Journal of Motor Behavior, 8,* 233–243.

Newell, K. M., & Walter, C. B. (1981). Kinematic and kinetic parameters as information feedback in motor skill acquisition. *Journal of Human Movement Studies, 7,* 235–254.

Newsome, J. (1978). Dialogue and development. In A. Locke (Ed.), *Action, gesture, and symbol* (pp. 31–42). London: Academic Press.

Nickerson, R. S. (1975). Characteristics of the speech of deaf persons. *Volta Review, 77,* 342–362.

Ninio, A., & Bruner, J. S. (1978). The achievement and antecedents of labelling. *Journal of Child Language. 5,* 1–16.

Nittrouer, S., Munhall, K., Kelso, J. A. S., Tuller, B., & Harris, K. S. (1988). Patterns of interarticulator phasing and their relation to linguistic structure. *Journal of the Acoustical Society of America, 84,* 1653–1661.

Nittrouer, S., Studdert-Kennedy, M., & McGowan, R. S. (1989). The emergence of phonetic segments: Evidence from the spectral structure of fricative-vowel syllables spoken by children and adults. *Journal of Speech and Hearing Research, 32,* 120–132.

Norman, D. A., & Bobrow, D. G. (1976). On the role of active memory processes in perception and cognition. In C. N. Cofer (Ed.), *The structure of human memory* (pp. 114–132). San Francisco: Freeman.

Nottebohm, F. (1972). Neural lateralization of vocal control in a passerine bird. II. Subsong, calls and a theory of vocal learning. *Journal of Experimental Zoology, 179,* 35–49.

Oller, D. K., Eilers, R. E., Bull, D. H., & Carney, A. E. (1985). Prespeech vocalizations of a deaf infant: A comparison with normal metaphonological development. *Journal of Speech and Hearing Research, 28,* 47–63.

Ortega, J. D., DeRosier, E., Park, S., & Larson, C. R. (1988). Brainstem mechanisms of laryngeal control as revealed by microstimulation studies. In O. Fujimura (Ed.), *Vocal physiology: Voice production, mechanisms and functions* (pp. 19-28). New York: Raven.

Osberger, M. J., & Levitt, H. (1979). The effect of time errors on the intelligibility of deaf children's speech. *Journal of the Acoustical Society of America, 66,* 1316–1324.

Ostry, D. J., & Munhall, K. G. (1985). Control of rate and duration of speech movements. *Journal of the Acoustical Society of America, 77,* 640–648.

Ostwald, P. F. (1963). *Soundmaking: The acoustic communication of emotion.* Springfield, IL: Charles C. Thomas.

Oxendine, J. (1979). Emotional arousal and motor performance. *Quest, 13,* 23–30.

Oyama, S. (1979). The concept of the sensitive period in developmental studies. *Merrill-Palmer Quarterly, 25,* 83–102.

Paillard, J. (1988). Posture and locomotion: Old problems and new concepts. In B. Amblard, A. Berthoz, & F. Clarac (Eds.), *Posture and gait. Development, adaptation and modulation* (pp. v–xii). Amsterdam: Excerpta Medica.

Paivio, A. (1971). *Imagery and verbal processes.* Hillsdale, NJ: Lawrence Erlbaum.

Paivio, A. (1985). Cognitive and motivational functions of imagery in human performance. *Canadian Journal of Applied Sport Sciences, 10,* 225-285.

Palmer, J. M. (1973). Dynamic palatography. General implications of locus and sequencing patterns. *Phonetica, 28,* 76-85.

Panagos, J. M. (1974). Persistence of the open syllable reinterpreted as a symptom of language disorder. *Journal of Speech and Hearing Disorders, 39,* 23-31.

Parker, J. F., & Fleishman, E. A. (1961). Use of analytical information concerning task requirements to increase effectiveness of skill training. *Journal of Applied Psychology, 45,* 295-302.

Pavlicek, W., Geisinger, M., & Castle, L. (1983). The affects of nuclear magnetic resonance on patients with cardiac pacemakers. *Radiology, 147,* 149-153.

Pechmann, T. (1984). Accentuation and redundancy in children's and adults' referential communication. In H. Bouma & D. G. Bouwhuis (Eds.), *Attention and performance: X. Control of language processes* (pp. 417-431). London: Lawrence Erlbaum.

Perkell, J. S. (1969). *Physiology of speech production: Results and implications of a quantitative cineradiographic study.* Cambridge, MA: MIT Press.

Perkell, J. S. (1979). On the nature of distinctive features: Implications of a preliminary vowel production study. In B. Lindblom & S. Ohman (Eds.), *Frontiers of speech communication research* (pp. 365-380). London: Academic Press.

Perkell, J. S. (1981). On the use of feedback in speech production. In T. Meyers, J. Lavers, & J. Anderson (Eds.), *The cognitive representation of speech* (pp. 45-52). Amsterdam, The Netherlands: North-Holland.

Perkins, D. N. (1983). Why the human perceiver is a bad machine. In J. Beck, B. Hope, & A. Rosenfeld (Eds.), *Human and machine vision* (pp. 341-364). New York: Academic Press.

Perkins, D. N., & Deregowski, J. (1982). A cross-cultural comparison of the use of a Gestalt perceptual strategy. *Perception, 11,* 279-286.

Peterson, G. E., & Shoup, J. E. (1966). A physiological theory of phonetics. *Journal of Speech and Hearing Research, 9,* 5-67.

Pew, R. W. (1974). Human perceptual-motor performance. In B. A. Kantowitz (Ed.), *Human information processing: Tutorials in performance and cognition* (pp. 1-39). Hillsdale, NJ: Lawrence Erlbaum.

Piaget, J. (1952). *The origins of intelligence in children* (M. Cook, Trans.). New York: International Universities Press. (Original work published in 1936.)

Pierce, J. R. (1980). *An introduction to information theory: Symbols, signals & noise* (rev. ed.). New York: Dover.

Pinker, S. (1988). Visual cognition: An introduction. In S. Pinker (Ed.), *Visual cognition* (pp. 1-63). Cambridge, MA: MIT Press.

Pomeranz , J. R. (1978). Pattern and speed of encoding. *Memory and Cognition, 6,* 235-241.

Porter, R. J., Jr. (1987). What is the relation between speech production and speech perception? In A. Allport, D. G. Mackay, W. Prinz, & E. Scheerer (Eds.), *Language perception and production: Relationships between listening, speaking, reading and writing* (pp. 85-106). London: Academic Press.

Posner, M. I. (1978). *Chronometric explorations of mind.* Hillsdale, NJ: Lawrence Erlbaum.

Posner, M. I., Nissen, M. J., & Klein, R. (1976). Visual dominance: An information processing account of its origins and significance. *Proceedings of the 16th Congress of Applied Psychology.* Amsterdam, The Netherlands: Swets & Zeitlinger.

Preisser, D. A., Hodson, B. W., & Paden, E. P. (1988). Developmental phonology: 18–29 months. *Journal of Speech and Hearing Disorders, 53,* 125–130.

Pressley, M., Borkowski, J. G., & Schneider, W. (1987). Cognitive strategies: Good strategy users coordinate metacognition and knowledge. In R. Vasta & G. Whitehurst (Eds.), *Annals of child development* (Vol. 4). Greenwich, CT: JAI Press.

Pressley, M., & Levin, J. R. (1977). Task parameters affecting the efficacy of a visual imagery learning strategy in younger and older children. *Journal of Experimental Child Psychology, 24,* 359–372.

Pykett, I. L. (1982). NMR imaging in medicine. *Scientific American, 246,* 78–89.

Ready, B. G., & Bellezza, F. S. (1986). Encoding specificity in free recall. *Journal of Experimental Psychology, 24,* 169–171.

Reason, J. (1984). Lapses of attention in everyday life. In R. Parasuraman & D. R. Daview (Eds.), *Varieties of attention* (pp. 515–549). Orlando, FL: Academic Press.

Reitman, W. R. (1965). *Cognition and thought: An information processing approach.* New York: John Wiley.

Renfrew, C. A. (1966). Persistence of the open syllable in defective articulation. *Journal of Speech and Hearing Disorders, 31,* 370–373.

Requin, J. (1985). Looking forward to moving soon: Ante factum selective processes in motor control. In M. I. Posner & O. S. M. Marin (Eds.), *Attention and performance XI* (pp. 147–167). Hillsdale, NJ: Lawrence Erlbaum.

Requin, J., Lecas, J. C., & Bonnet, M. (1984). Some experimental evidence for a three-step model of motor preparation. In S. Kornblum & J. Requin (Eds.), *Preparatory states and processes* (pp. 139–174). Hillsdale, NJ: Lawrence Erlbaum.

Requin, J., Semjen, A., & Bonnet, M. (1984). Bernstein's purposeful brain. In H. T. A. Whiting (Ed.), *Human motor actions: Bernstein reassessed* (pp. 259–284). Amsterdam, The Netherlands: Lawrence Erlbaum.

Robb, M. P., & Saxman, J. H. (1990). Syllable durations of preword and early word vocalizations. *Journal of Speech and Hearing Research, 33,* 583–593.

Rondo, E. (1980). Intonation in discourse. In L.R. Waugh & C.H. van Schooneveld (Eds.), *The melody of language. Intonation and prosody* (pp. 243–278). Baltimore, MD: University Park Press.

Rothwell, J. C. (1987). *Control of human voluntary movement.* Rockville, MD: Aspen Publishers.

Rousselot, P. J. (1901). *Principes de phonétique expérimentale.* Paris: Welter.

Rozin, P., & Schull, J. (1988). The adaptive-evolutionary point of view in experimental psychology. In R. Atkinson, R. J. Hernstein, G. Lindsey, R. D., Luce, & J. Wiley (Eds.), *Steven's handbook of experimental psychology. Volume 1: Perception and motivation* (pp. 503–546). New York: John Wiley & Sons.

Rubin, E. R., House, A. S., & Stevens, K. N. (1955). Mechanical analog of fricative consonant articulation. *MIT Quarterly Progress Report,* pp. 10–12.

Rubow, R. (1984). Role of feedback, reinforcement, and compliance on training and transfer in biofeedback-based rehabilitation of motor speech disorders. In M. R. McNeil, J. C. Rosenbek, & A. Aaronson (Eds.), *The dysarthrias:*

Physiology-acoustics-perception-management (pp. 207–230). San Diego, CA: College-Hill Press.

Russell, G. O. (1928). *The vowel: Its physiological mechanism as shown by x-ray.* Columbus: Ohio State University.

Ryan, E. D., & Simons, J. (1981). Cognitive demands, imaging and frequency of mental rehearsal as factors influencing acquisition of motor skills. *Journal of Sport Psychology, 3,* 35–45.

Sage, G. H. (1984). *Motor learning and control: A neuropsychological approach.* Dubuque, IA: William C. Brown.

Salmoni, A. W., Schmidt, R. A., & Walter, C. B. (1984). Knowledge of results and motor learning: A review and critical appraisal. *Psychological Bulletin, 95,* 355–386.

Sapir, S., McClean, M. D., & Larson, C. R. (1983). Human laryngeal responses to auditory stimulation. *Journal of the Acoustical Society of America, 73,* 315–321.

Schach, R. T., & Sadowsky, P. L. (1988). Clinical experience with magnetic resonance imaging in internal derangements of the TMJ. *The Angle Orthodontist, 58,* 21–32.

Scheier, M. (1898). Über die bedeutung der Röntgenstrahlen für die Physiologie der Sprache und Stimme. *Neuere Sprachen, 5,* 40.

Schilling, R. (1930). Die elektro-palate und labiographie. *Bericht I. Tageszeitlich International Gesellschaft experimentall Phonetik, Bonn,* 44–48.

Schmidt, R. A. (1975). A schema theory of discrete motor skill learning. *Psychological Review, 82,* 225–260.

Schmidt, R. A. (1988). *Motor control and learning: A behavioral emphasis* (2nd ed.). Champaign, IL: Human Kinetics.

Schmidt, R. A., Young, D. E., Swinnen, S., & Shapiro, D. C. (1989). Summary knowledge of results for skill acquisition: Support for the guidance hypothesis. *Journal of Experimental Psychology: Learning, Memory, and Cognition, 15,* 352–359.

Schönpflug, W. (1985). Goal directed behavior as a source of stress: Psychological origins and consequences of inefficiency. In M. Frese & J. Sabini (Eds.), *Goal directed behavior: The concept of action in psychology* (pp. 172–188). Hillsdale, NJ: Lawrence Erlbaum.

Schunk, D. H. (1987). Peer models and children's behavioral change. *Review of Educational Research, 57,* 149–174.

Schwartz, R. G., & Leonard, L. B. (1982). Do children pick and choose? An examination of phonological selection and avoidance in early lexical acquisition. *Journal of Child Development, 9,* 319–336.

Scott, J. H., & Symons, N. B. B. (1974). *Introduction to dental anatomy,* (7th ed.). Edinburgh, Scotland: Churchill Livingston.

Sechenov, I. M. (1863–1975). *Biographical sketch and essays.* New York: Arno Press.

Secord, W. (1981). *Test of Minimal Articulatory Competency.* Columbus, OH: Charles E. Merrill.

Seligman, M. E. P., & Hager, J. L. (1972). *Biological boundaries of learning* (p. 464). New York: Appleton-Century-Crofts.

Seto, H. (1972). The sensory innervation of the oral cavity in the human fetus and juvenile mammals. In J. F. Bosma (Ed.), *Third symposium on oral sensation and perception* (pp. 35–75). Springfield, IL: Charles C. Thomas.

Seyforth, R. M., Cheney, D. L., & Marler, P. (1980). Monkey responses to three different alarm calls: Evidence of predator classification and semantic communication. *Science, 210,* 801–803.

Shadle, C. H. (1985). *The acoustics of fricative consonants* (Tech. Rep. No. 506). Cambridge, MA: MIT Research Laboratory for Electronics.

Shannon, C. E., & Weaver, W. (1949). *The mathematical theory of communication.* Urbana: University of Illinois Press.

Shapere, D. (1987). Method in the philosophy of science and epistemology. How to inquire about inquiry and knowledge. In N. J. Nersessian (Ed.), *The process of science. Contemporary philosophical approaches to understanding scientific practice* (pp. 1–39). Dordrecht, The Netherlands: Martinus Nijhoff.

Shapiro, D. C., & Schmidt, R. A. (1982). The schema theory: Recent evidence and developmental implications. In J. A. S. Kelso & J. E. Clark (Eds.), *The development of movement control and coordination* (pp. 113–150). New York: John Wiley.

Shapiro, D. C., Zernicke, R. F., Gregory, R. J., & Diestal, J. D. (1981). Evidence for generalized motor programs using gait pattern analysis. *Journal of Motor Behavior, 13,* 33–47.

Shawker, T., Sonies, B., & Stone, M. (1984). Soft tissue anatomy of the tongue and floor of the mouth. *Brain Language, 21,* 335–350.

Shea, C. H., & Kohl, R. M. (1990). Specificity and variability of practice. *Research Quarterly for Exercise and Sport, 61,* 169–177.

Shepard, R. (1981). Psychophysical complementarity. In M. Kubovy & J. R. Pomerantz (Eds.), *Perceptual organization* (pp. 279–341). Hillsdale, NJ: Lawrence Erlbaum.

Shibata, S. (1968). *A study of dynamic palatography. Annual Bulletin* (Research Institute of Logopedics and Phoniatrics, University of Tokyo), 2, 28–36.

Shick, J. (1970). Effects of mental practice on selected volleyball skills for college women. *Research Quarterly, 41,* 539–542.

Shiffrin, R. M., & Grantham, D. W. (1974). Can attention be allocated to sensory modalities? *Perception & Psychophysics, 15,* 460–474.

Shope, R. K. (1983). *The analysis of knowing.* Princeton, NJ: Princeton University Press.

Shriberg, L. D., & Kwiatkowski, J. (1980). *Natural process analysis (NPA): A procedure for phonological analysis of continuous speech samples.* New York: John Wiley.

Sidaway, B., Moore, B., & Schoenfelder-Zohdi, B. (1991). Summary and frequency of KR presentation effects on retention of a motor skill. *Research Quarterly for Exercise and Sport, 62,* 27–32.

Simms, R. E. (1963). The data underlying the concept of dyslalia. In S. E. Mason (Ed.), *Signs, signals, and symbols* (pp. 141–151). Springfield, IL: Charles C. Thomas.

Singer, R. N. (1986). Sports performance. A five-step mental approach. *Journal of Physical Education, Recreation, and Dance, 57,* 82–89.

Singer, R. N. (1988). Strategies and metastrategies in learning and performing self-paced athletic skills. *The Sport Psychologist, 2,* 49–68.

Smidt, G. L. (1990). Rudiments of gait. In G. L. Smidt (Ed.), *Gait in rehabilitation* (pp. 1–19). New York: Churchill Livingston.

Smit, A. B. (1986). Ages of speech sound acquisition: Comparisons of several normative studies. *Language, Speech, and Hearing Services in Schools, 17,* 175–186.

Smith, D. G., McCutcheon, M. J., Hasegawa, A., Christensen, J. M., & Fletcher, S. G. (1980). Computer based instrumentation for speech articulation research. In *13th International Conference on System Sciences, Volume III. Selected Papers in Medical Information Processing.* Honolulu, HA: Winston Periodicals.

Smith, G. F., Benson, P. G., & Curley, S. P. (1991). Belief, knowledge, and uncertainty: A cognitive perspective on subjective probability. *Organizational Behavior and Human Decision Processes, 48,* 291–321.

Smith, H. W., Fletcher, S. G., & McCutcheon, M. J. (1986). Optically transduced measurement and tracking of tongue height. In S. Saha (Ed.), *Proceedings of the 5th southern biomedical engineering conference* (pp. 66–72). New York: Pergamon.

Smith, N. (1973). *The acquisition of phonology.* London: Cambridge University Press.

Snow, C., & Ferguson, C. (1977). *Talking to children: Language input and acquisition.* Cambridge, England: Cambridge University Press.

Snow, C., & Hoefnagel-Höhle, M. (1978). The critical period for language acquisition: Evidence from second language learning. *Child Development, 49,* 1114–1128.

Solomon, R. L. (1982). The opponent process in acquired motivation. In D. W. Pfaff (Ed.), *The physiological mechanisms of motivation* (pp. 321–336). New York: Springer-Verlag.

Sparrow, W. A., & Irizarry-Lopez, V. M. (1987). Mechanical efficiency and metabolic cost as measures of learning a novel gross motor task. *Journal of Motor Behavior, 19,* 240–264.

Stark, R. E., Ansel, B. M., & Bond, J. (1988). Are prelinguistic abilities predictive of learning disability? A follow-up study. In R. L. Masland & M. W. Masland (Eds.), *Prevention of reading failure* (pp. 3–18). Parkton, MD: York.

Stetson, R. H. (1951). *Motor phonetics. A study of speech movements in action.* Amsterdam, The Netherlands: New Holland.

Stevens, K. A. (1987). Visual object perception from a computational perspective. In G. W. Humphreys & M. J. Riddoch, (Eds), *Visual object processing: A cognitive neuropsychological approach* (pp. 17–42). Hillsdale, NJ: Lawrence Erlbaum.

Stevens, K. N. (1971). Airflow and turbulence noise for fricative and stop consonants: Static considerations. *Journal of the Acoustical Society of America, 50,* 1180–1192.

Stevens, K. N. (1972). The quantal nature of speech: Evidence from articulatory-acoustic data. In E. E. David, Jr., & P. B. Denes (Eds.), *Human communication, A unified view* (pp. 51–66). New York: McGraw-Hill.

Stevens, K. N. (1975). The potential role of property detectors in the perception of consonants. In G. Fant & M. A. A. Tatham (Eds.), *Auditory analysis and perception of speech* (pp. 303–330). New York: Academic Press.

Stoel-Gammon, C. (1983). Constraints on consonant-vowel sequences in early words. *Journal of Child Language, 10,* 455–457.

Stoel-Gammon, C. (1985). Phonetic inventories, 15–24 months: A longitudinal study. *Journal of Speech and Hearing Research, 28,* 505–512.

Stone, M, Shawker, T. H., Talbot, T. L., & Rich, A. H. (1988). Cross-sectional shape during the production of vowels. *Journal of the Acoustical Society of America, 83,* 1586–1596.

Straight, H. S. (1980). Auditory versus articulatory phonological processes and their development in children. In G. H. Yeni-Komshian, J. F. Kavanagh, & C. A. Ferguson (Eds.), *Child phonology, Volume 1: Production,* (pp. 43–71). New York: Academic Press.

Straka, G. (1965). *L'album phonetique.* Quebec, Canada: PUL.

Strong, L. H. (1956). Muscle fibers of the tongue functional in consonant production. *Anatomical Record, 126,* 61–79.

Studdert-Kennedy, M. (1979). Speech perception. *Status report on speech research, SR-59/60* (pp. 1–22). New Haven, CT: Haskins Laboratory.

Studdert-Kennedy, M. (1984). Sources of variability in early speech development. In J. Perkell & D. Klatt (Eds.), *Invariance and variability in speech processes* (pp. 58–84). Hillsdale, NJ: Lawrence Erlbaum,

Subtelny, J. D., Pruzansky, S., & Subtelny, J. D. (1957). The application of roentgenography in the study of speech. In L. Kaiser (Ed.), *Manual of phonetics* (pp. 166–179). Amsterdam, The Netherlands: North Holland.

Suinn, R. M. (1980). *Psychology in sports methods and applications.* Minneapolis, MN: Burgess Publishing.

Summerfield, Q., & McGrath, M. (1984). Detection and resolution of audiovisual incompatibility in the perception of vowels. *Quarterly Journal of Experimental Psychology, 36,* 51–74.

Summers, J. J. (1981). Motor programs. In D. H. Holding (Ed.) *Human skills.* New York: John Wiley.

Suzuki, H. (1986). *Analysis of Japanese accent.* Unpublished study cited by Waibel (1988).

Tanaka, T. (1964). Development of the figure-cognition. *Psychologia, 7,* 207.

Templin, M. C. (1957). Certain language skills in children: Their development and interrelationships. *Institute of child welfare monographs, 26.* Minneapolis: University of Minnesota Press.

Thelan, E. (1979). Rhythmical stereotypies in normal human infants. *Animal Behavior, 27,* 699–715.

Thelan, E. (1981). Rhythmical behavior in infancy: An ethological perspective. *Developmental Psychology, 17,* 237–257.

Thelan, E., Ulrich, B. D., & Jensen, J. L. (1989). The developmental origins of locomotion. In M. H. Woollacott & A. Shumway-Cook, *Development of posture and gait across the life span* (pp. 25–47). Columbia: University of South Carolina Press.

Thelen, E. (1979). Rhythmical stereotypies in normal human infants. *Animal Behaviour, 27,* 699–715.

Thomas, J. R., Pierce, C., & Ridsdale, A. (1977). Age differences in children's ability to model motor behavior. *Research Quarterly, 48,* 592–597.

Thompson, R. F., & Bettinger, L. A. (1970). Neural substrates of attention. In D. I. Mostofsky (Ed.), *Attention: Contemporary theory and analysis* (pp. 367–401). New York: Appleton-Century-Crofts.

Tinbergen, N. (1951). *The study of instinct*. New York & Oxford, England: Oxford University Press.

Trabasso, T., Rollins, H., & Shaughnessy, E. (1971). Storage and verification stages in processing concepts. *Cognitive Psychology, 2,* 239–289.

Treisman, A., & Gelade, G. (1980). A feature integration theory of attention. *Cognitive Psychology, 12,* 97–136.

Trowbridge, M. H., & Cason, H. (1932). An experimental study of Thorndike's theory of learning. *Journal of General Psychology, 7,* 245–258.

Tuller, B., & Kelso, J. A. S. (1984). The timing of articulatory gestures. Evidence for relational invariants. *Journal of the Acoustical Society of America, 76,* 1030–1036.

Tulving, E. (1966). Subjective organization and effects of repetition in multi-trial free-recall learning. *Journal of Verbal Learning and Verbal Behavior, 5,* 193–197.

Turvey, M. T., Fitch, H. L., & Tuller, B. (1982). The Bernstein perspective: I. The problems of degrees of freedom and context-conditioned variability. In J. A. S. Kelso (Ed.), *Human motor behavior. An introduction* (pp. 239–252). Hillsdale, NJ: Lawrence Erlbaum.

Tyler, A. A., Edwards, M. L., & Saxman, J. H. (1990). Acoustic validation of phonological knowledge and its relationship to treatment. *Journal of Speech and Hearing Disorders, 55,* 251–261.

Udaka, J., Kanetake, H., Kihara, H., & Koike, Y. (1988). Human laryngeal responses induced by sensory nerve stimuli. In O. Fujimura (Ed.), *Voice production, mechanisms and functions* (pp. 67–74). New York: Raven.

Underwood, B. J., & Schulz, R. W. (1960). *Meaningfulness and verbal learning.* Philadelphia: Lippincott.

Van Gyn, G. H., Wenger, H. A., & Gaul, C. A. (1990). Imagery as a method of enhancing transfer from training to performance. *Journal of Sport & Exercise Psychology, 12,* 366–375.

Van Lawick-Goodall, J. (1968). Behavior of free-living chimpanzees of the Gombe Stream area. *Behavior, 13,* 165–311.

Van Riper, C. G., & Smith, D. E. (1954). *An introduction to general American phonetics.* New York: Harper.

Verbrugge, R. R., & Rakerd, B. (1986). Evidence of talker-independent information for vowels. *Language and Speech, 29,* 39–57.

Waibel, A. (1988). *Prosody and speech recognition.* San Mateo, CA: Morgan Kaufman Publishers.

Walker, B. E., & Fraser, F. C. (1956). Closure of the secondary palate in three strains of mice. *Journal of Embryology and Experimental Morphology, 4,* 176–189.

Walsh, T., & Diller, K. (1981). Neurolinguistic considerations on the optimal age for second language learning. In K. Diller (Ed.), *Individual differences and universals in language learning aptitude.* Rowley, MA: Newbury House.

Walter, W. G. (1966). The role of the frontal lobes in the regulation of active states. In A. R. Luria & E. D. Homskaya (Eds.), *The frontal lobes and the regulation of psychological processes* (pp. 156–176). Moscow, Russia: Moscow University Press.

Wassilieff, Von N. W. (1886). Ueber eine localisirte reflectorische Bewegung der Zunge. *Centrablatt für die Medincinischen Wissenschaften, 12,* 209–210.

Watkin, K. L., & Rubin, J. M. (1989). Pseudo-three-dimensional reconstruction of ultrasonic images of the tongue. *Journal of the Acoustical Society of America, 85,* 496–499.

Wehrli, F. W. (1990). Fast-scan magnetic resonance: Principles and applications. *Magnetic Resonance Quarterly, 6,* 165–236.

Weinberg, B. (1968). A cephalometric study of normal and defective /s/ articulation and variations in incisor dentition. *Journal of Speech and Hearing Research, 11,* 288–300.

Weinberg, R. S. (1981). The relationship between mental preparation strategies and motor performance: A review and critique. *Quest, 33,* 195–213.

Weinberg, R., Bruya, L., Garland, H., & Jackson, A. (1990). Effect of goal difficulty and positive reinforcement on endurance performance. *Journal of Sport & Exercise Psychology, 12,* 144–156.

Weir, R. (1962). *Language in the crib.* The Hague, The Netherlands: Mouton.

Weismer, G., & Ingrisano, D. (1979) Phrase-level timing patterns in English: Effects of emphatic stress location and speaking rate. *Journal of Speech and Hearing Research, 22,* 516–533.

Weiss, M. R., & Bredemeier, B. J. (1983). Developmental sport psychology: A theoretical perspective for studying children in sport. *Journal of Sport Psychology, 5,* 216–230.

Weiss, M. R., Bredemeier, B. J., & Shewchuk, R. M. (1985). An intrinsic/extrinsic motivation scale for the youth sport setting: A confirmatory factor analysis. *Journal of Sport Psychology, 7,* 75–91.

Welford, A. T., & Bourne, L. E., Jr. (1976). *Skilled performance: Perceptual and motor skills.* Glenview, IL: Scott, Foresman.

Wells, G. (1985). Language and learning: An international perspective. In G. Wells & J. Nicholls (Eds.), *Language and learning: An international perspective* (pp. 21–39). London: The Falmer Press.

Wells, R. S. (1947). Review of Kenneth L. Pike, The intonation of American English. *Language, 23,* 255–273.

Wentworth, N., & Witryol, S. L. (1990). Information theory and collative motivation: Incentive value of uncertainty, variety, and novelty for children. *Genetic, Social, and General Psychology Monographs, 116,* 301–322.

Wepman, J. M., & Hass, W. (1969). *A spoken word count (Children — ages 5, 6, and 7).* Los Angeles: Western Psychological Services.

Wever, E. G., & Lawrence, M. (1954). *Physiological acoustics.* Princeton, NJ: Princeton University Press.

Winitz, H. (1969). *Articulatory acquisition and behavior.* New York: Appleton-Century-Crofts.

Winitz, H. (1981). Input considerations in the comprehension of the first and second language. In H. Winitz (Ed.), *Native and foreign language acquisition* (pp. 296–308). New York: New York Academy of Sciences.

Wolf, M. B., Fletcher, S. G., McCutcheon, M. J., & Hasegawa, A. (1976). Medial groove width during /s/ sound production. *Biocommunication research report No. 1* (pp. 57–66). Birmingham: University of Alabama in Birmingham.

Wolfe, V. I., & Blocker, S. D. (1990). Consonant-vowel interaction in an unusual phonological system. *Journal of Speech and Hearing Disorders, 55,* 561–566.

Wood, S. (1979). A radiographic analysis of constriction location for vowels. *Journal of Phonetics, 7,* 25–43.

Wood, S. (1986). The acoustical significance of tongue, lip, and larynx maneuvers in rounded palatal vowels. *Journal of the Acoustical Society of America, 80,* 391–401.

Woodworth, R. S., & Schlosberg, H. (1954). *Experimental psychology.* New York: Henry Holt.

Wrisberg, D. R., & Ragsdale, M. R. (1979). Further tests of Schmidts's schema theory: Development of a schema rule for a coincident timing task. *Journal of Motor Behavior, 11,* 159–166.

Wurtz, R. H., Goldberg, M. E., & Robinson, D. L. (1980). Behavioral modulation of visual responses in the monkey: Stimulus selection for attention and movement. In J. M. Sprague & A. N. Epstein (Eds.), *Progress in psychobiology and physiological psychology* (Vol. 9, pp. 44–83). New York: Academic Press.

Wyke, B. (1974). Laryngeal myotactic reflexes and phonation. *Folia Phoniatrica, 26,* 249–264.

Wyrwicka, W. (1981). *The development of food preferences.* Springfield, IL: Charles C. Thomas.

Wyrwicka, W. (1988). Imitative behavior. A theoretical view. *Pavlovian Journal of Biological Science, 23,* 125–131.

Yando, R., Seitz, V., & Zigler, E. (1978). *Imitation: A developmental perspective.* Hillsdale, NJ: Lawrence Erlbaum.

Zelazo, P. R. (1976). From reflexive to instrumental behavior. In L. Lipsett (Ed.), *Developmental psychobiology: The significance of infancy* (p. 87). Hillsdale NJ: Lawrence Erlbaum.

Zelazo, P. R. (1983). The development of walking: New findings and old assumptions. *Journal of Motor Behavior, 15,* 99–137.

Zelená, J. (1957). The morphogenetic influence of innervation on the ontogenetic development of muscle spindles. *Journal of Embryological Experimental Morphology, 5,* 283–292.

Zemer, R. K. (1985). Foreword. *Radiology Clinic of North America, 23,* 379.

Zwislocki, J. (1975). The role of the external and middle ear in sound transmission. In D. Tower (Ed.), *The nervous system, Volume 3: Human communication and its disorders.* New York: Raven Press.

INDEX